Health Professional and Patient
INTERACTION

Health Professional and Patient

INTERACTION

SIXTH EDITION

Ruth Purtilo, Ph.D., P.T., F.A.P.T.A.
Center for Health Policy and Ethics
Creighton University
Omaha, Nebraska

Amy Haddad, Ph.D., R.N.
School of Pharmacy and Allied Health Professions
Creighton University
Omaha, Nebraska

Amy Haddad
May 10, 2006

W.B. SAUNDERS COMPANY
An Imprint of Elsevier Science
Philadelphia   London   New York   St. Louis   Sydney   Toronto

W.B. SAUNDERS COMPANY
An Imprint of Elsevier Science

The Curtis Center
Independence Square West
Philadelphia, Pennsylvania 19106

Publishing Director: Andrew Allen
Acquisitions Editor: Maureen Pfeifer
Associate Developmental Editor: Rebecca Swisher

Library of Congress Cataloging-in-Publication Data

Purtilo, Ruth B.
Health professional and patient interaction / Ruth Purtilo, Amy Haddad.—6th ed.

p. cm.

Includes bibliographical references and index.

ISBN 0–7216–9297–4

1. Medical personnel and patient. I. Haddad, Amy Marie. II. Title
   [DNLM: 1. Professional-Patient Relations. 2. Communication.]

R727.3.P87 2002

610.69'6—dc21   2001057638

HEALTH PROFESSIONAL AND PATIENT
INTERACTION, SIXTH EDITION   ISBN 0–7216–9297–4

Printed in the United States of America

Last digit is the print number: 9   8   7   6   5   4   3   2   1

With gratitude to the patients, professional colleagues, and students whose stories have enhanced the pages in this book—and enriched our lives.

RUTH and AMY

Preface

It is with anticipation that we present this sixth edition of *Health Professional and Patient Interaction* (HPPI). We believe that health care itself is in a period of profound transition. In the midst of change, basic foundations of the health professions become more important than ever. One such foundation is the health professional and patient relationship—the focus of this book.

We attempt in these pages to provide guidance in the complicated and challenging world of daily interactions that occur between health professionals and patients and to provide the tools to establish professional relationships built on respect.

This book should aid students by (1) enhancing their self-understanding; (2) helping them to clarify the dynamics of the health professional-patient relationship; and (3) developing their awareness of the larger societal and health care context in which the relationship takes place.

Respect is the thread that weaves together discussions regarding professional and patient encounters in the health care environment. Clarification of health professional and patient values sets the stage for exploring the context of interactions and the unique perspective that the health professional and patient bring to this relationship. HPPI includes the basic content from the foundational disciplines that support productive interactions in health care, such as sociology, psychology, anthropology, communications, ethics, and the most current clinical research. The purpose of this book, however, is not to discuss every topic in depth but rather to stimulate exploration of many topics.

In this new edition, we have attempted to continue to direct our focus to themes that cross many professions. A case originally directed to the nurse, technologist, physician, or therapist may be equally relevant to other health professionals as well. Part of the function of this book, therefore, is to show the extent to which different groups share common goals.

In some instances, it is necessary to assign meaning to key terms. We mention three here: (1) *Patient*—the person needing a health service, whether it be participation in a preventive program, diagnosis, evaluation, or treatment. (2) *On-site education*—the outside-the-classroom portion of the health professional's formal education, which takes place in a setting similar to that in which he or she will eventually seek employment. On-site education may begin early in professional preparation and progress from two or three hours a week to a full-time assignment. (3) *Clinical experience*—the composite of learning experiences to which the student is exposed during on-site education whether or not a given professional is involved in direct patient care.

The situations described and the names of patients, health professionals, and other persons in the case studies, appearing as examples or in the Questions for Thought and Discussion sections, are fictitious.

When the last word of a manuscript has been written, its life has just begun. In sharing our ideas with you, the reader, we hope that in turn you will be stimulated to share yours with others, thus making us all more knowledgeable in the exciting venture of human interaction based on respect.

RUTH PURTILO
AMY HADDAD

Acknowledgments

One of the great joys of preparing this sixth edition of *Health Professional and Patient Interaction* has been the opportunity for us to work together in its development—again.

In the years since the fifth edition appeared, we have received numerous letters in which readers have offered encouragement, suggestions, and critiques. Furthermore, both of us have discussed issues examined in the book with a large number of health professions students and faculty members around the country. We thank them for the growth we experienced during those encounters. Our colleagues will recognize portions of those discussions that have been incorporated into the sixth edition.

Several persons at W.B. Saunders Company have been outstanding in their guidance and support. We owe special gratitude to all the editors and their assistants who worked on previous editions and on this one. Many people have asked who provided the original drawings, which have appeared consistently since the first edition. It is with many thanks that we acknowledge Grant Lashbrook for his contribution.

The manuscript preparation of this edition was expedited by the able and efficient assistance of Oscar Punla, who coordinated permission requests; Helen Shew, who typed, proofread, and formatted the chapters; and Marybeth Goddard, who worked on parts of the final preparation with us. We extend our heartfelt thanks to them and to our husbands, Vard and Steve, who encouraged us and endured our long hours of preparation.

Contents

xii CONTENTS

PART ONE

Creating a Context of Respect

As you know from your own life, relationships never take place in a vacuum! They are always challenged by forces that may or may not be in your control. Therefore, as you enter into the pages of this book about the health professional and patient relationship, the first thing we bring to your attention are some features of your personal life, the health care environment, and the larger society that we believe have a profound impact on what you are able to do in that relationship.

Chapter 1 begins with a definition and discussion of respect. Respect is so central to a good working relationship between a health professional and a patient that you will meet the concept many times in your journey through this book. We describe how values—your own, those of the health professions, and society's—sometimes constitute a fertile oasis where respect can take root and grow and at other times create rough terrain through which you must pass gingerly. Overall, the chapter is optimistic, as are we, about your opportunity to develop, maintain, and help foster respect in the health professions.

In Chapter 2 we direct your attention to some key elements of the organization and institutions of health care: how certain physical environments, laws, regulations, and policies factor into your professional life. This is not a thorough treatment of the institutional dimensions of your practice; rather we pick areas that we judge to have the most influence on your relationships with patients, their families, and others. We show that respect is "institutionalized" through basic rights and responsibilities of health

1

professionals and patients, and we address the pivotal legal/ethical notion of informed consent, by which you establish your basic contract with a patient.

In Chapter 3, the final chapter of Part One, we give you an opportunity to think substantively about the rich diversity of social characteristics that individuals and groups bring to relationships. We ask you to consider ways you can learn to appreciate differences of culture and ethnicity, socioeconomic status, religion, age, gender, and sexual preferences and to show respect for people no matter what characteristics they have.

With these important considerations as background you will be prepared to proceed to the rest of the book.

CHAPTER 1

Respect: The Difference It Makes

CHAPTER OBJECTIVES

The student will be able to

- Give a brief definition of respect
- Describe why respect is so central to the success of the health professional and patient relationship
- Identify three spheres of values that constitute a "value system"
- List some "primary goods," both social and natural, and describe what Rawls means by "primary goods"
- Describe the value of character traits or "virtues" and their role in the realization of a good society
- Describe "autonomy" as a value in Western societies and how it affects decision-making within the health professions
- Discuss how professional values affect a professional who must treat patients whose values differ dramatically from his or her own
- Identify means by which health professionals can better understand a patient by exploring what that patient's values are

---

Having a dementing disease is a central fact in a person's life. But people are more than their disease, and as the person's own ability to express who he is through his words and actions fades, preserving his identity becomes more and more the job of those who love and care for him. Think of what you do to a person with Alzheimer's disease when you introduce him to someone by saying, "This is Henry. Henry was a lawyer." One man who was introduced this way gently interrupted: "I *am* a lawyer." This man was fighting to maintain his sense of self—an extremely precious thing—against the incursions of his disease. Those around him missed an opportunity to be his ally in this struggle.

J. and H.L. Nelson[1]

This excerpt about persons with Alzheimer's disease reminds us of how important it is to be respected and how tightly respect is woven into our sense of well-being. No matter how extreme our circumstances, we hope that others will show us respect and that we will be able to enjoy it ourselves. Whether you are preparing to enter a profession for the first time or are continuing to seek excellence in it, being able to show and receive respect is a key to the success of your identity as a professional. You might, in fact, think of respect as a linchpin that holds together your professional strategic plan. A strategic plan is the intentional process that individuals and groups periodically undertake to examine their strengths, weaknesses, opportunities, and challenges; the goal is to know which direction to take for success—or continued success—in a particular area. Without respect for (and from) others you will almost inevitably find the pattern you are weaving in your professional life to be off course.

Fortunately, in this book you will have a chance to reckon with the primacy of respect—for yourself, for patients and their families, and for your professional peers. You will be reminded that you should expect respect from others in their treatment of you. You will have a chance to identify where it can be found in your attitudes, communications, and conduct or where its absence is creating a barrier to effectiveness. You will receive ideas from us (and, we hope, through discussion of issues in this book, from each other) about how you can find, cultivate, and express respect in your everyday life as a professional.

WHAT IS RESPECT?

Respect comes from the Latin root *respicere*, which means to approach a person, group, idea, or object with regard or esteem. Other definitions emphasize the emotional component, that is, *feeling* esteem toward someone or something, which suggests that true respect requires more than learned behaviors devoid of deep attitudes. For instance, a polite act that appears to be respectful may be a mere shell of the real thing. When the discussion turns, as it will throughout this book, to respect between persons, there is an assumption that respect must be directed toward something in the person. That something is the person's dignity. The Latin word *dignitas* means worth. Therefore, the professional is encouraged to direct his or her respect to the very essence of the human being, to the person's basic worth.[2] This is usually referred to as the inherent dignity of persons. The respect you show to another person ultimately is a reflection of your willingness to look past positive or negative attributes to the very core of what makes the person human.

The notion of inherent dignity is so deeply ingrained into the idea of a profession that if you do not subscribe to such an assumption you may be in the wrong course of study. You may stop and ask, "But how can I know that at this stage of my preparation?" You may not, but we will help you learn how to make this assessment. Because respect and dignity are abstract concepts, we will help you look for them in various concrete shapes such as the tone of voice or title used to address a patient, the adaptation of your pace and language to meet the needs of a child or an elderly patient, your desire to be trustworthy, your presence during a crisis, and your willingness to work together with a patient's family and other professionals to reach his or her goal.

As you know, respectful concern or regard for one another is not confined to interactions within the health care system. In fact, respect for a person's dignity is a fundamental value in most religions and cultural traditions. In the health care setting this value is put into action as a response to the fact that patients are vulnerable in ways that do not exist outside of the health care context. Therefore, if you value respect, it is your responsibility to protect patients from any hint of exploitation or harm. To help you recognize and cultivate this type of respect, the first opportunity we give you is to examine your own values.

RESPECT AND YOUR VALUES

Values are deeply held attitudes and beliefs we have about the truth, beauty, or worth of a person, object, action, or idea. One criterion of a "true" value is that it has become part of a pattern of a person's life. In other words, values must not only be identified, but embraced and expressed. From what you have read so far you should be able to conclude that health professionals are expected to value attitudes and behaviors that allow respect for themselves, patients, and others to flourish. Suppose you say, "Well, I value my freedom to make my own decisions. I value self-confidence, honesty, and efficiency. Are those values consistent with respect?" They most likely are. For example, it is possible that you may honestly and with full self-confidence exercise your autonomy to disagree with a patient's decision to forego your professional advice, but still treat the patient with respect.

Taken together, your values constitute what can be called your *value system*. Some values in that system are highly specific to you. Some will be adopted through your cultural and/or professional subgroup. Still others are shared by virtually all humans. The unique value system for each person constitutes his or her idea of "the good life."

Values have their genesis in a variety of sources. We learn our early values from parents and other childhood friends, caregivers, teachers, religious leaders, and cultural influences such as TV. Values are imparted, taught, reinforced, and internalized. We incorporate many of them into our lives as a personal value system. We also exist in a complex world of bureaucracies and institutions. These influence us too, so that as we mature our values evolve with us. In his seminal work, Glaser presents a model that is very useful for us here.[3] One of his goals is to describe three spheres or realms in which values arise in the overall health care environment.

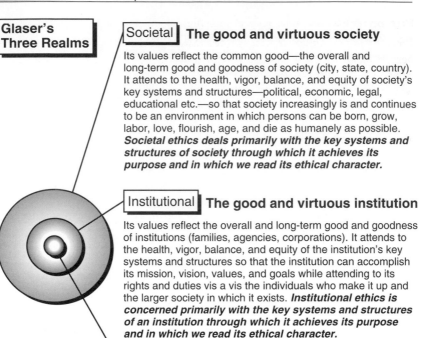

Glaser's Three Realms

Societal ▌ **The good and virtuous society**

Its values reflect the common good—the overall and long-term good and goodness of society (city, state, country). It attends to the health, vigor, balance, and equity of society's key systems and structures—political, economic, legal, educational etc.—so that society increasingly is and continues to be an environment in which persons can be born, grow, labor, love, flourish, age, and die as humanely as possible. *Societal ethics deals primarily with the key systems and structures of society through which it achieves its purpose and in which we read its ethical character.*

Institutional ▌ **The good and virtuous institution**

Its values reflect the overall and long-term good and goodness of institutions (families, agencies, corporations). It attends to the health, vigor, balance, and equity of the institution's key systems and structures so that the institution can accomplish its mission, vision, values, and goals while attending to its rights and duties vis a vis the individuals who make it up and the larger society in which it exists. *Institutional ethics is concerned primarily with the key systems and structures of an institution through which it achieves its purpose and in which we read its ethical character.*

Individual ▌ **The good and virtuous individual**

Its values reflect the good and goodness of individuals. It attends to the balance and the right relationships among various dimensions of a single individual (spiritual, mental, physical, emotional, etc.) as well as the values that support rights and duties that exist between individuals.

FIGURE 1–1

Note that Figure 1–1 highlights how our success as professionals depends not only on what we do in our person-to-person interactions but also on how we interact within institutions, which themselves have values, and the larger society in which we live. Both of these larger contexts place claims on us. His schema also helps us to better understand that each of three realms (i.e., the personal, the institutional, and the societal) have *legitimate* values that should be protected and furthered if the health care professions as a whole are to maintain their goals and integrity. The crunch comes when an individual professional like you faces a conflict in trying to honor legitimate but incompatible values in different spheres.

In the next pages we examine some issues that arise in each of the three realms.

Personal Values

Personal values are strictly one's own. Most people cherish more than one personal good, or value. Literature provides striking examples of the exception: Ahab braved the high seas relishing the thought of getting revenge on the great white whale, Moby Dick; Sir Lancelot suffered many grave adversities in his relentless quest for the Holy Grail; and, before his change of heart, Ebenezer Scrooge treasured money. The lifestyles of Ahabs, Sir Lancelots, and Scrooges are not the same as those of most individuals. Most people have many personal values, some more clearly defined than others, and go through life trying to realize several values simultaneously.

The process of developing values is the focus of values clarification. Values clarification provides the means for us to discover what values we live by. The following values rating exercise is helpful in identifying personal values and how these values play themselves out in real life. Consider the following statements and questions.

1. Values
    a. Individually, make a list of your 10 most important present values in order of importance.
    b. You can also compare your own personal values with your peers' values by following this procedure:
        (1) In groups of four or five, generate a composite list of the individual values.
        (2) Rank the items on the list (with each individual voting for three values).
        (3) Using the five most important values from the list, rate those values on the chart in Figure 1–2. To what degree do you agree with the ratings as they relate to your life?
        (4) Share information and any insights with the group.
    c. Now compare the list of your own highest ranking values with your own behavior.
2. Beliefs vs. Behavior: What Do You Really Believe?
    a. Using Figure 1–3, reflect on the following questions:
        (1) To what degree is your behavior consistent with your stated values?
        (2) If there is an inconsistency, why?
        (3) What values are different in the "outside world"?
        (4) What values are most difficult to live by in the outside world?
        (5) What are you going to do (if anything) to change your stated values and behaviors?[4]

As we suggested, sometimes your personal values will conflict with each other. An example is the case of a person who is excessively obese. Although there are many factors contributing to obesity, consider the obese person who finds security in consuming food. Unfortunately, his habitual eating eventually

	Strongly Agree	Agree	Neutral	Disagree	Strongly Disagree
Value 1					
Value 2					
Value 3					
Value 4					
Value 5					

FIGURE 1–2

causes his body to break down, and he is told by his physician that he can expect a shortened life span. At this point his basic value of *life itself* is endangered by the competing personal value of *feeling secure.* Because both of these values are essential to good health, treatment is often directed toward helping this person derive security from aspects of life other than eating. Similar examples can be made in regard to other life-endangering practices, such as smoking, alcohol and other substance abuse, or lack of good sleeping habits. As you will learn in Chapter 6, people who choose the health professions often are faced with stresses that lead to such value conflicts.

	Always	Most of the Time	Sometimes	Occasionally	Never
Value 1					
Value 2					
Value 3					
Value 4					
Value 5					

FIGURE 1–3

When patients seek your services it is almost always their own personal values that are driving them to do so. They believe rightfully that health professionals are there to help them be relieved of some forms of personal suffering. They value being or getting well. They seek comfort during chronic or life-threatening illness. They want you to help them maintain their value of health and optimize their functioning. Health care is, in fact, concerned primarily with personal values that are addressed through person-to-person relationships. Your professional preparation through the use of this book will include an opportunity to study and think about the challenges your own personal values pose and to identify many that do not create conflicts and will even facilitate your success. Can you think of some now?

Professional Values

Glaser's second sphere highlights values and conflicts that arise because our society is organized into institutions. Chapter 2 focuses on values and other characteristics of the institutional structures of health care—how they can assist in your desire to express respect and some places where they may hinder that goal. Many important and interesting values that govern health care institutions have come from the professionals who work within them. We introduce the idea of professional values here for two reasons: first, to assist you in understanding how professional values fit into all three spheres, and second, to allow you to identify some professional values that may already overlap your personal values.

Professions and professionalism have been the subject of much study and debate since the delineation of three traditional professions (law, medicine, and the clergy) during the Middle Ages. Today many still refer to a profession as a "calling" that requires total devotion, specialized knowledge, and extensive academic preparation. A calling implies a divine influence whereby the person is given special responsibility and privilege.[5] Therefore it is not surprising that the more recent term "profession" is a derivation of the verb "to profess," meaning affirmation or avowal (of something). From these root terms and interpretations the professions today are identified as groups whose members have responded to an opportunity to hold a special place in society, differentiated from those who simply hold a job or have an occupation.

Some health professions have articulated basic values that undergird their professional identity. For example, seven essential values for nursing are altruism, truth, esthetics, equality, freedom, justice, and human dignity.[6] Other professions have been less clear about the values that inform their practice, but they all share basic attitudes and behaviors that reflect values. For example, professions value having an organized body of specialized knowledge. This is slightly different from saying that a profession values a completely *unique* body of knowledge, because many developing health care disciplines draw from a variety of other knowledge bases.

Other values held by professions are as follows:

▪ Learning and use of the intellect
Preparation and practice should require a process largely intellectual in nature that demonstrates an exercise of judgment.
▪ Altruism, responsiveness to need
The profession's activity must serve the needs of society rather than the needs of a special interest group, usually for the benefit of that society, with an altruistic goal as opposed to a materialistic one.
▪ Identification as a group
The profession values a group identity and group consciousness that can be recognized by others.
▪ Public promises of ethical and competent behavior
The profession values being able to design and publicly articulate its own code of ethics and standards of practice.
▪ Lifelong devotion to the profession and its high standards
Attracting students with good intellectual and personal qualities who choose the profession as a lifelong pursuit is valued as opposed to attracting those using it as a stepping-stone to another career.[7]

Also, embedded in these values are others regarding the maintenance of expertise, commitment to social rather than personal goals, and willingness to exercise professional autonomy, compassion, and accountability for individual and collective behavior. Professions deeply value being in a position to gauge the quality of the performance of their peers. Society does grant professions a degree of autonomy in members policing each other. However, the lay public makes its own judgments about professional practice, as is the case exemplified in the cartoon of the woman and the balloon vendor.

Why is the balloon vendor being criticized? This purveyor of services has failed to live up to the expectations society has set for his "professional skills" and expertise, and therefore he should properly be ashamed. Of course, according to the values of a profession we have identified, the balloon vendor should not be considered a "professional." This cartoonist may also be poking fun at the fact that the term "profession" is applied widely today and, unfortunately, not always inappropriately.

The public is demanding more accountability from the professions, particularly in health care. As you will see in Chapter 10, there is a burgeoning use of the World Wide Web, TV commercials, and other means for the public to gain clinical information not previously available to them. There is also public skepticism that health professionals are not doing an adequate job of policing their members and bringing sanctions, such as enforcing restrictions on practice when professionals fail to comply with high standards of care.

As you enter your professional field you should be aware that the very make-up of health professions is evolving and with it some of their values. For example, the pharmacy profession is shifting from a male-dominated one to one

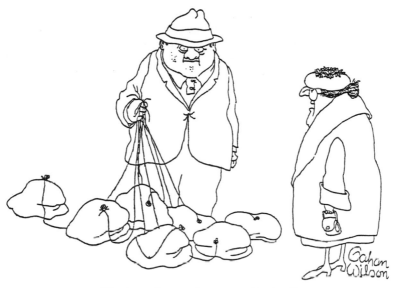

"You're a disgrace to your profession."

From Wilson, Gahan, *I Paint What I See*. 1971 Simon and Schuster, New York.

in which there is an equal distribution of men and women. Other professions today have a proportionately large number of older members than in previous decades, as is the case for nursing. How all of these factors will influence traditional professional values remains to be seen, but it certainly will be worth watching in the future.

Societal Values

One well-recognized characteristic of "the human condition" is that we, as human beings, organize ourselves into complex interactions among individuals and groups of individuals called societies. Glaser's third sphere highlights this dimension of influence too. Societies have values that come from our life together. With our ability to communicate and reflect, humans value being able to share their thoughts and ideas with each other. Humans are technological beings who value the use of tools to assist in the completion of daily tasks. We are historical beings who value building cultures based on the wisdom, mistakes, and knowledge of those who lived before us. We are political beings who value our laws that govern interaction, and aesthetic beings who create nonfunctional objects and value them for their beauty alone. Humans also perform rituals and are ethical beings, able to distinguish between right and wrong and to adjust behavior accordingly.[8] As a result, human beings rarely find satisfaction outside the contours of a society.

Because the individual identifies so strongly with his or her societal affiliation and in some places and times is identified entirely by it, it is not surprising that some values seem to be held in common by most or all members of the human community. However, it is more difficult to find full agreement beyond the most general values on which ones might be universally acclaimed. Literary and philosophical writings are replete with suggestions. Consider whether you agree that the following are generally accepted as universally held societal values.

Western societies seem to be organized on the principle that *human life* itself is a basic value and therefore ought to be sustained. Beyond that, certain other values are instrumental in ensuring a high quality of life.

Philosopher Rawls lists several "primary goods," reflecting his idea of the scope of basic societal values. *Social* primary goods include *rights, liberties, powers, opportunities, income, wealth,* and *self-respect.* (Self-respect, or what is commonly called dignity, is necessary for a person to have a sure conviction that his or her life plan is worth carrying out or capable of being fulfilled.) The realization of these goods is at least partially determined by the structure of society itself. *Natural* primary goods, also partly determined by societal structures but not directly under their control, include *health, vigor, intelligence,* and *imagination.*[9] Together, he says, these social and natural primary goods provide a sort of "index of welfare" for individuals in any society.

Other writers suggest certain character traits as the basic societal values that can produce a good life for the larger community; however, there is dispute over which character traits are the central ones. For instance, in ancient Greek thought, the virtues of temperance, prudence, justice, and fortitude were considered central. Early Christian thinkers argued that these alone were not sufficient and that faith in God, hope, and love were crucial. Other world religions and schools of philosophical thought also have contributed their lists.

A good example in modern Western societies of a value that has retained its hold and primacy is the value placed on individual autonomy. At no other time in history has there been such an emphasis on the importance of having control over one's own life, of independent functioning, and of radical self-reliance. Failure to succeed is often interpreted as not trying hard enough, and of subsequently becoming a burden.

As we discuss in Chapter 3, a changing ethnic and cultural milieu in Western societies may begin to change the primacy of autonomy. This may enhance aspects of our lives together in societies. For example, the social value placed on individual autonomy understandably places an immense burden on persons whose independence has been diminished by illness or injury. Somewhat paradoxically, this value of autonomous independence is juxtaposed with the value of conformity to societally established norms of behavior and dress. There is a "Catch 22" built into the idea that one must be an autonomous individual but must not be too different from others.

Of course, there are values other than those of autonomy and conformity that spring from the idiosyncrasies of a given society. Any time a person is placed

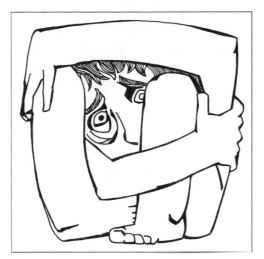

When a person is placed in a position in which it is impossible to live up to society's expectations, he or she may experience tremendous anxiety and discomfort.

in a position in which it is impossible to live up to society's expectations and the values it dictates, he or she may experience tremendous anxiety.

Whatever one's lot in life, the need to be accepted within the societal realm of values influences the well-being of almost everyone.

THE "GOOD LIFE" AND YOU

Examples of three sets of values have been presented—personal, professional, and societal. They have been discussed separately to emphasize their differences but in everyday life a person adopts a set of personal values that overlap in part and are harmonious with societal values. A schematic representation of such a person's value system is shown in the figure below.

Relationship between Societal
and Personal Values

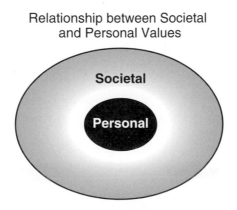

Societal

Personal

Here societal values are experienced by the person as a part of his or her personal values, but their source is distinct. We account for this perception by saying that persons have "internalized" social values so that they may become indistinguishable from their own personal preferences. Motivation for doing so usually arises from choosing to live harmoniously in society and experiencing personal benefit from it. One can live harmoniously by valuing mundane things such as obedience to traffic and other laws, adherence to practices of etiquette, and willingness to pay taxes. Personal benefits from internalizing societal values may include the opportunity for friendship and collegiality, economic independence, and help in cultivating certain virtues such as courage and compassion. In short, persons need personal values to individualize themselves. Most adhere to societal values to feel like an accepted part of their society and of humankind. Frankena says that everyone has some concept of what a good life involves so it is possible to say of anyone who lives according to his or her personal values, "That person has a good life." However, when a person's value system includes values that help to uphold and further society as well, we say that such a person *leads* a good life.[10] Moral approval and acceptance are afforded to the person who is concerned with societal well-being as well as his or her own and who tries to live in harmony with reasonable societal standards. Such an individual is perceived to be a sound citizen and a good person with a sense of personal identity.

Of course, not everyone adopts a set of personal values compatible with societal values or even with those of his or her own social or cultural subgroup. Such a person's value system is represented in the figure below.

In the extreme form, this person has not internalized any societal values. Such a person either desires not to live in harmony with society or, more likely, believes that there are no benefits to be derived from doing so. Some examples of people whose values clash with societal values are the hermit, the criminal, and

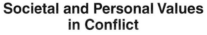

Societal and Personal Values in Conflict

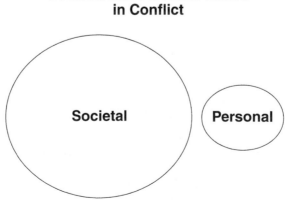

the saint or martyr. The hermit and criminal reject societal values and replace them with their own; the saint or martyr rejects societal values and replaces them with some "higher" set of values.

There are varying degrees to which such persons divorce themselves from societal values. On the one hand, the woman who drives through a red light to make it to her tennis match on time is replacing a societal value of obedience to traffic rules with the personal value of reaching her destination to play that game of tennis. On the other hand, the conscientious objector who performs alternative service is refusing to accept the societal value of engaging in war to protect one's country on the basis of following the antiwar dictates of a higher law. *Most* people experience some such conflict from time to time.

People who do not internalize societal values can be a source of discomfort to the majority of people in society, who accept the status quo no matter how unsatisfactory their existence may become. A good example is provided by the chorus of peasants in T. S. Eliot's *Murder in the Cathedral*. Here, Archbishop Thomas Becket comes to the city to indict those who have been oppressing the peasants through unjust laws and practices. One would expect the oppressed people to welcome him. But when the peasants hear that he is coming from France, they gather outside the cathedral, chanting:

> We do not wish anything to happen.
> Seven years we have lived quietly,
> Succeeded in avoiding notice,
> Living and partly living . . .
> O Thomas, return, Archbishop; return, return to France.
> Return, quickly, quietly. Leave us to perish in quiet . . .[11]

Rather than welcoming him, the peasants are afraid of this man with a vision.

It is not only peasants who are threatened by the person living outside the scope of societal values. The health professional, too, is sometimes wary of a person whose values are outside of a narrow, familiar norm. When faced with such a person, professional values become a major issue in the health professional's value system. These experiences challenge the widely accepted value in health care that respect for all persons is required even though a patient's specific values may differ dramatically from one's own. The professional value of respect for persons reminds us that the person deserves to be treated fairly and in a humane manner. Can you think of types of people whose personal values would be so far from your own or your society's (or both) that you would have great difficulty in treating them with respect? This is a good topic for discussion among you and your fellow students.

RESPECT FOR VALUES: YOURS AND OTHERS'

A first step toward respect in any circumstance is to learn more about the person. Not all patients will be reluctant to talk with you about what they consider to be important. On the contrary, most patients are eager to talk about their values.

Family and friends, when available, are also good sources. They are usually eager to assist, and an alert health professional will detect clues from casual conversation (e.g., "I'll tell you one thing; the fishing trip just wasn't the same this year without Joe"). Additionally, the patient's chart and other medical records offer information about the patient's social and medical history. All this information may help you understand the patient, even though you may not, in the end, like him or her any better.

Honoring That Values Change

In addition to being able to identify a patient's values, health professionals must work on the premise that everyone's values change from time to time. Unexpected opportunities, tragedy, and new insights all act as controls in a person's notion of what is considered valuable in life. However, the circumstances that force or enable most people to change their values usually evolve slowly, whereas those that force a patient to do so may appear in a matter of minutes or hours! We discuss this phenomenon in more detail in Chapter 8. A brief glimpse at the course of one patient's evolving values is illustrated in this story:

> Daniela Janowski was the star soccer player on her college team at Midtown State College. It came as a terrible surprise when in her mid-twenties she began to experience the debilitating symptoms of multiple sclerosis.
>
> It is 6 years later. She is almost totally unable to walk. Her weight has dropped to 90 pounds from her previous 125. She suffered one period of deep depression. She says now that she has "much to live for."

What types of values might Daniela have that would allow her to feel as if there is "much to live for" when so much has radically changed?

Reclaiming and Replacing Values

The process of reclaiming and replacing values may take weeks, months, or years for any of us. For one thing, the person who becomes a patient must learn what the illness or injury really means in terms of long-term impairment. Another woman who, like Daniela, had multiple sclerosis told one of the authors that it took her years to stop doing silly things that overstressed her. She said, "It was because I didn't *know* my disease; now I *know* it, like a friend, strange as that may sound. Not knowing was the hardest part. . . ."

As we reiterate in later chapters, the process of adjustment and acceptance is also based on the support of family, friends, and health professionals. The entire staff of health professionals can be instrumental in identifying possible new interests for a patient. The following are some general guidelines from Wright's classic work on physical disability for determining when a patient is faced with the need to change a value or alter a goal. Her suggestions apply to many kinds of change that must be endured:

1. Enlargement of the scope of values is indicated in the case of all-inclusive suffering, when the patient's problem is the inability to accept as valuable those aspects of life not closed to the person.
2. Subordination of values is indicated when the importance of the value has been overrated.
3. Containment of the negative effects of the change is needed.
4. When a value retains substantial importance, as in the case of physique, a person must not always compare what can be done now with what could be done before but rather concentrate on what can still be done.[12]

SUMMARY

Respect for others and enjoying it oneself are essential ingredients for a successful professional practice. Respect involves both attitudes and behavior that acknowledge your regard for another person's dignity, no matter what his or her attributes and circumstances are.

Our values are determinants of whether we will want and be able to express genuine respect for patients, their families, and other professionals. Some values arise from personal preferences while others become internalized over time through the influences of institutional affiliations and societal forces. Professional values are transmitted through the educational, clinical, and research institutions of health care. You can make good progress on your road to respectful interaction by identifying your own values, by developing a genuine interest in others' values, and by appreciating why both change over time.

REFERENCES

1. Nelson, J.L. and Nelson, H.L.: *Alzheimer's. Answers to Hard Questions for Families.* New York, The Hastings Center, 1996, pp. 22–23.
2. Johnson, P.R.S.: An analysis of "dignity." *Theor. Med. Bioethics.* 19:337–352, 1998.
3. Glaser, J.W.: *Three Realms of Ethics.* Kansas City, MO, Sheed and Ward, 1994, pp. 10–14.
4. Smith, M.: *A Practical Guide to Value Clarification.* La Jolla, CA, University Associates, Inc., 1977, pp. 160–161.
5. Sulmasy, D.P.: *The Healer's Calling. A Spirituality for Physicians and Other Health Professionals.* Nahwah, NJ, Paulist Press, 1997.
6. Essentials of College and University Education for Professional Nursing, Final Report. American Association of Colleges of Nursing, Washington, DC, 1986.
7. Rider, J.E. and Hartley, C.L.: *Nursing in Today's World: Challenges, Issues and Trends.* Philadelphia, Lippincott, 1995, p. 10.

8. Adler, M.J.: *The Difference of Man and the Difference It Makes.* 2nd ed. New York, Fordham University Press, 1993, p. 91.

9. Rawls, J.: *A Theory of Justice.* 2nd ed. Cambridge, Belknap Press of Harvard University, 1971.

10. Frankena, W.K.: *Ethics.* 2nd ed. Englewood Cliffs, NJ, Prentice-Hall, 1973, p. 62.

11. Eliot, T.S.: Murder in the Cathedral. In *T.S. Eliot: The Complete Poems and Plays 1909–1950.* New York, Harcourt, Brace, and World, 1952, p. 180.

12. Wright, B.: *Physical Disability: A Psychological Approach.* 2nd ed. New York, Harper & Row, 1983, pp. 143–144.

CHAPTER 2

Respect in the Institutional Settings of Health Care

CHAPTER OBJECTIVES

The student will be able to

- Compare the functions of health care institutions directed toward primary, secondary, and tertiary care
- List three major societal factors that have resulted in our present organizational structure of health care
- Compare public- and private-sector relationships and describe why health professional and patient interactions are public-sector relationships
- Compare the characteristics of total institutions and partial institutions of health care
- List at least three types of laws and policies that have a bearing on how you will practice your profession and what you should be able to expect from the institution in which you work
- Discuss the idea of patient's rights documents and the purposes they are designed to serve
- Describe the basis for and two major components of informed consent

I feel as though I have just come back from a foreign place worth reporting on . . .

This foreign place is, of course, the land of Hospital, a nation (a universe really) of its own, with which one quickly and progressively sinks into the role of patient, analogous in the way it transforms your personality and gnaws at both your assurance and sense of self to being a tourist in an unfathomable, dangerous land . . .

Meg Greenfield[1]

As you now have begun to realize, this book is about your work with people who need your service and how respect can be shown to them in your everyday interactions. In the process of learning what is required for respectful interaction, the organization and institutions of health care must be taken into account, but the individual patient's values and well-being should never be lost in the maze of these other considerations.

Some of you have seen paintings by the French impressionist painter Marc Chagall. His weightless figures hover in space, supported by clouds and celebrated by ethereal musicians. The heavenly environment Chagall creates suggests mystery, romance, bliss, and promise.

His work speaks to a deeper meaning: our environments always create certain expectations and evoke powerful feelings. They influence our attitudes and conduct in ways that sometimes we do not even understand. The quote at the beginning of this chapter—Meg Greenfield's observation about the land of Hospital—does not suggest bliss or promise. Her environment suggests unfamiliarity and even danger.

Today almost all health care is provided, administered, and managed through institutions. It follows that with rare exceptions every student reading this book will be employed within an institution. All individuals who are acting as a part of an organization (e.g., a health care institution) must take into account the well-being of the institution. Many times contracts for positions will include promises that one will abide by policies or specific behaviors for the good of the organization. Policies may include details about finances, ethical conduct toward other institutions, management issues, marketing, and loyalty to the institution. Your professional preparation will also include ways in which you will have to prepare yourself for specific policies, regulations, and other institutional dimensions of your work. Additionally, you will need to know how to respond when conflicts arise because of legitimate claims made on you by the patient and your employing institution. Throughout this book reference is made to how various types of institutions (e.g., nursing homes, industrial or school clinics, institutions for mentally ill persons, and health maintenance settings) impact what you as a health professional will face in your attempt to provide high-quality professional service.

The environment of health care is not easy to characterize because it is a complex web of ideas and beliefs woven into a modern fabric of health care facilities whose functions vary widely. At the same time, there are some silver threads of continuity that lend themselves to generalizations so that you can begin to understand what your work environment will be. You will need to know what it might look like to the patients who enter it, to health professionals who spend their days working in it, and to the larger community that supports it. As Glaser highlights in Chapter 1, the values of the institutions impact and are influenced by individuals' values and those of the larger society.

Glaser's scheme illustrates that the institutional organization of health care is not completely a "rational system" insofar as rational systems are oriented expressly to the pursuit of one specific goal and have a highly formalized social structure designed to meet that goal. Rather, in some regards it is more like an "open system" in which shifting and sometimes competing interest groups negotiate for their goals to be met.[2] Key values in addition to health often named as driving the changes in the institutional structures today in the United States are individual autonomy (free choice) and marketplace competition (free enterprise). As you consider the institutional environment, paying attention to these three realms should help you to identify key areas where individual, institutional, and societal values overlap and where they create conflicts that will require your best ethical reasoning, courage to resist inhumane institutional or societal policies, and commitment to implementing strategies of change in your workplace.

THE FUNCTIONAL ORGANIZATION OF HEALTH CARE

When you enter a program of professional preparation you may already have made a choice about your institutional setting insofar as the focus of your profession may be to maintain wellness or prevent illness or injury. Maintenance and prevention activities include careers in health spas, industry, free-standing "clinics" that provide prenatal or well-baby check-ups, and the like. You may want to engage in rehabilitation activities or respond to acute or chronic health care needs of persons who require primary, secondary, or tertiary care. These latter three designations are summarized in an article by Grumbach and Bodenheimer:

> Primary care involves care for common health problems and preventive needs (sore throats, sprained ankles, hypertension, and vaccinations) that account for 80% to 90% of visits to a physician or other caregiver. The secondary tier of care handles problems that require more specialized clinical expertise such as hospital care for a patient with acute renal failure. Tertiary care lies at the apex of the organizational pyramid, managing rare and complex cases such as pituitary tumors or congenital malformations.[3]

Facilities offering health care have continued to evolve too. Most health care facilities in the United States, Canada, and Great Britain are not restricted to one kind of service. There are tertiary care facilities such as burn hospitals or oncology centers and free-standing clinics for vaccinations, cardiac evaluations, diabetes and cholesterol tests, or other preventative measures, but the trend is toward comprehensive buildings housing "health plans" and away from institutions with one particular function. One large managed care organization (MCO) may have facilities and professionals to respond to the whole contin-uum of care. This approach represents a move toward more population-based models of care in which the goal is to define a target population of patients, define the health needs of this particular population, and then develop a community-based set of services to address that community. Not unusual today are complexes that involve many types of facilities and services. There may be a hospital, a nursing home, a clinic or several clinics housing various levels and types of care for ambulatory patients, home care services, supplier sources for durable medical equipment, and a pharmacy.

Why have we moved in one century from a system in which whoever could afford care was treated at home at the beginning of the 20th century to today's massive network of facilities?

Many have commented on this movement, identifying it with the efficiency sought through:

- Industrialization:
     the industrial revolution and its compartmentalization of public and private life functions;
- Urbanization:
     the movement of people to the cities and the resulting potential for increasing efficiency by offering a more centralized site for services; and
- Specialization:
     the emergence of specialized medicine necessitating a centralized site for coordination of care.

In other words, the institutional value of efficiency has dramatically influenced the style and design of health care services today.

There are many critics of the present approaches. For one thing, in spite of the movement toward larger health care networks such as the MCOs in the United States and elsewhere, critics maintain that our current organization results in fragmentation of services rather than continuity. Such critics suggest that these phenomena may be appropriate for the larger free market economy but compromise some important social values such as eligibility to receive service based on need. You will have an opportunity to help shape the new health care environment that will continue to develop as you enter your profession.

CHARACTERISTICS OF INSTITUTIONAL RELATIONSHIPS

Glaser nests the institutional dimensions of health care between the individual and the larger environment. It follows that the ability to show and receive respect in the work environment requires an understanding of several characteristics of relationships that take place in health care institutions compared to other settings. In this section we examine two aspects of health care institutions, namely their public rather than private nature and their role as partial rather than total institutions.

Public- and Private-Sector Relationships

"Public-sector" relationships are interactions reserved for public life. Therefore, individuals generally separate their lives into a private world of family and friends and a public world of other relationships designed to serve a useful purpose and then dissolve. Friendships are private-sector relationships, whereas student and professor or patient and health professional relationships belong to the world of institutional interactions (i.e., public-sector relationships). Understandably, both parties enter public-sector relationships with different expectations than would friends or two people preparing to become partners in marriage. The social boundaries that are maintained in a public-sector relationship permit rapid introduction and rapid separation when it is over, all the while promoting periodic cooperation. All public-sector relationships are characterized by abrupt changes from extreme remoteness to extreme nearness and the expectation that the relationship will be temporary. The opportunities for involvement in each other's life and well-being and the boundaries that must be honored in the goal of maintaining respect are addressed throughout this book, especially in Part Five.

The physical structure of an institution helps to enable an effective private- or public-sector relationship. Hospitals or schools, for instance, unmistakably are public buildings. What are some of the clues for this conclusion? Sometimes the environment where health care is administered mingles private- and public-sector environments. For instance, a home visit to a home-bound client may require that you go to his or her residence, knock on the door and be welcomed in as a guest would be, make your way across the living room among discarded pages of the morning paper, trip over the sleeping dog, and move a bathrobe from a comfortable overstuffed chair to sit down. However, the fact that your presence represents the type of public-sector relationship that takes place within the more obvious public-sector environment of health care institutions usually suffices to adequately set the tone for a public-sector interaction. Your conduct and attitudes, as is emphasized throughout this book, give the governing clues. At the same time, the type of institution can greatly enhance your effectiveness if it is designed to bring about the specific goals of health care as well as provide a humane and efficient environment overall.

Total and Partial Institutions

Another aspect of professional life is the ability to exert a certain kind of authority regarding your area of knowledge, respect the authority that other health professionals and administrators have because of their areas of expertise and roles, and, above all, recognize that the patient, client, and/or family brings the authority of knowing the person's values and life situation into the interaction. The design of institutions also can enhance the appropriate exercise of authority. To illustrate, recall your experience in a campus dormitory, airport, hospital, or other type of institution. Each has its physical design and function accompanied by certain rules, regulations, policies, and other constraints. We judge such constraints as legitimate if they seem to serve understandable goals of the institution, each other, or society. Almost 50 years ago sociologist Goffman advanced the understanding of institutions based on these observations, suggesting distinctions that are still useful today in dividing them into "total" and "partial" institutions.[4]

Total Institutions. On one side are *total institutions,* in which personal autonomy is totally or seriously compromised. They are places where, as Goffman describes it, "a large number of like-situated individuals, cut off from the wider society for an appreciable period of time, together lead an enclosed, formally administered round of life."[4] Usually professional and supportive personnel are the sole authority: they "run" the institution, and the assumption is that either the individual or society (and in some cases, both) benefit from the arrangement. Often a ritual act of donning the clothing of the institution (e.g., a nun's habit in a cloistered convent or a prison jumpsuit) further signifies the surrender of identity and autonomy and "the acquisition of a new identity oriented to the authority of the professional staff and to the aims and purposes and the smooth operation of the institution. . . ."[5] Although their functions vary, examples of total institutions are many: monasteries, nursing homes, long-term care facilities, hospitals for severely mentally ill or developmentally challenged persons, and prisons, for example.

Only a small percentage of health professional and patient interactions take place within the highly codified and rigid structure of a total institution. When they do, the patient's autonomy is compromised by illness, injury, or some social factor such as committing a felony. In this situation of uneven authority every precaution to respect the dignity of the person must be rigorously undertaken. Recognition of the vulnerability of such persons to abuse at the hands of even well-meaning individuals often necessitates writing special precautionary guidelines and policies for health care. For instance, there are especially stringent guidelines for protecting persons in such environments from abuses carried out in the name of important clinical research.

We believe that May summarizes the issue of total institutions in health care settings well, using the nursing home as an example:

> The nursing home occupies the same place in the psyche of the elderly today that the poorhouse and the orphanage played in the imagination of Victorian children. Even those who never set foot in such a facility fear it as fate.
>
> The deprivations that total institutions impose hardly argue for dismantling them. They have their place. But planners must give serious thought to their design, particularly to what might be called the moral significance of "turf."[6]

At several places in this book, particularly in Part Three, we revisit the idea of turf, those aspects of a personal living space and those dimensions of self-determination that can help to lend dignity in the midst of serious constraints as a result of health-related problems.

Partial Institutions. Along the continuum of institutional arrangements, most health care institutions can be classified as *partial institutions* because they constrain patients' or clients' autonomy in some important ways, but also allow for varying degrees of self-determination.

People entering such institutions are very concerned about the potential constraints they will face. Will they be able to go home from time to time during a long-term institutionalization and if so, under what conditions? Are children allowed to visit? May they see or be allowed to have pets? What will they be allowed to eat, and what kind of "time off" from a heavy schedule of treatments might they be able to negotiate? How much input will they have into changes in their diagnostic or therapeutic regimen? May they wear their own clothes? May they change doctors or other health care professionals without fear of retribution if there is reason to doubt the competence or disagree with other characteristics of the ones they have?

Your own autonomy in the institution where you work as a professional also will be constrained by policies for securing employment, regulations regarding employee conduct, expectations regarding the number of people in your care, and the other institutional peculiarities that will either enable or inhibit your ability to satisfy your professional and personal goals.

Health professionals are key vectors of change that can help create ways that respect can be expressed in humane and person-centered environments. As people talk about ways in which their autonomy and other values can be honored within the confines of partial institutions, you can think of ways to help realize those changes. In many areas of this book the authors assume that most interactions between health professionals and patients take place within an environment consistent with the characteristics of partial institutions.

THE INTERFACE OF INSTITUTIONS AND SOCIETY

In addition to the constraints and opportunities you, your colleagues, and your patients will experience from the design of the institution, your daily professional life in that institution will be affected by some laws and policies that govern all types of health care settings. The following pages illustrate some of the most widespread and important categories.

Laws and Policies Maintaining High Standards of Competence

In an effort to protect society from quacks and incompetent practitioners, all health care institutions that want to remain accredited by national and regional accrediting boards must take steps to assure that their professional staff are well qualified to do the work they say they can do. Laws of every state include professional licensing mechanisms whereby a person must pass a test and meet other qualifying characteristics to practice in that state. Some institutions go beyond the minimum requirements established by the state by adding continuing education requirements for their own professional employees. Today many health professionals are personally responsible for negligence and other types of conduct that lead to malpractice claims, so institutions increasingly are requiring individuals to maintain personal malpractice insurance. These requirements should not have a negative impact on your work and may even have a positive effect, since they have been developed over the years to help assure that the basic tenets of respect are maintained for all who need your services.

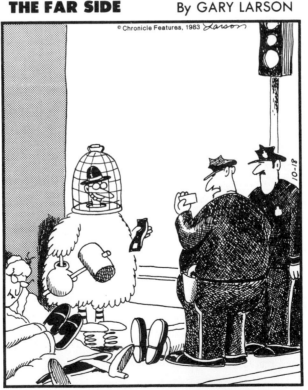

THE FAR SIDE   By GARY LARSON

"Well, I'll be darned . . . I guess he does have a
license to do that."

Laws and Policies Related to Discrimination

Several nondiscrimination laws have direct bearing on health care institutions in the United States. Some of these apply directly to health professionals as employees. Consider a few key examples:

- Title VII of the Civil Rights Act (1964) prohibits employers from refusing to hire an employee on the basis of race, color, sex, religion, or national origin.
- The Equal Opportunity Act buttressed and expanded Title VII in 1972.
- The Equal Pay Act of 1963 required that men and women are receive equal pay for performing similar work.
- The Age Discrimination and Employment Act prohibiting discrimination against persons 40 to 70 years old was passed in 1967.
- The Rehabilitation Act (Section 504) of 1973 required all employers to have an affirmative action plan that includes handicapped persons. Superseding this act was the Americans with Disabilities Act of 1990, which states that institutions with more than 25 employees cannot use a physical examination to deny employment.

Others laws have a direct bearing on your relationship with patients. For instance, prohibitions against some types of behavior such as touching a patient without his or her consent or sexual intercourse with patients often are written into state licensing laws as well as being reiterated in institutional policies and the ethical codes of professional organizations.

Other Laws and Policies

With the advent of the AIDS epidemic, numerous laws and policies have been implemented nationally and within institutions to try to decrease the accidental transmittal of infection through body substances to health professionals, among patients, or to others. The most notable of these is the Universal Precautions, a federal mandate requiring all health professionals to protect themselves and others by wearing certain types of gowns, gloves, goggles, and other equipment while treating any patient and by adhering to strict methods for handling body fluids. The requirements for the amount and type of protective clothing vary according to the likelihood of body fluids being transferred from patient to health professional or vice versa. For instance, an orthopedic surgeon may become splattered from head to toe with blood during surgery and may receive a puncture wound from the slip of a scalpel or from a splintered or protruding bone. A dietitian or an occupational therapist, in comparison, is not likely to be in a situation of direct and extensive contact with body fluids. Some health professionals have worried that the "space capsule" appearance of the protective garb is damaging to health professional and patient rapport, although everyone agrees with the necessity of minimizing transmittal of the AIDS virus and other pathogens that reside in body fluids.[7]

Depending on your area of service as a health professional you may be regulated by other laws and policies. Persons in the United States working in clinical or laboratory areas where blood and other body fluids are handled will be subject to an institution's standards as set out by the Occupational Safety and Health Administration (OSHA) for limiting their exposure to these potentially pathogenic substances and safe disposal of these materials.

If you work with patients or clients who have sexually transmitted or other infectious diseases, you may be required to report this information to your state's department of health. In some instances this may create an ethical conflict for you if you do not want to break the confidence of this matter entrusted to you by a patient.

Laws and regulations regarding the documentation of patient status, patient progress, and other patient information will affect you every day of your practice. The medical record is a legal document, as are many other types of reports and statements you prepare for billings, quality assurance reviews, and other activities requiring data about patients. Sometimes students treat documentation as a means of protecting their own interests legally. We prefer that you think of your documentation as a kind of travelogue of the journey you and the patient are taking during your professional encounter. Therefore, preparation of your documentation, like all other aspects of your interaction within the institution, should be undertaken first with respect for the patient's dignity and rights and then with respect for the type of professional you want the world to know you are.

Although this sampling of laws and policies is not intended to be exhaustive and focuses on laws of the United States, it illustrates the many types of constraints that come with the health professional's inevitable need to develop institutional affiliations with health care facilities.

Laws, Policies, and Change

We conclude this section with a short reminder that laws and policies are always in a state of flux. You should review all institutional policies and guidelines thoroughly before contracting to work in a particular institution. If upon review you judge that the laws and policies that you are asked to abide by in your place of employment will enhance your capacity to be respected and show respect in all areas of your professional interaction, they deserve to be followed. If they present major difficulties for you practically or ethically you should reflect seriously on your choice. At the same time, you have an opportunity throughout your career to help shape a better environment for health professions by working to change unworkable, unfair, or otherwise inadequate laws and policies.

Many health professionals feel impotent in the face of laws, regulations, and policies. To be sure, policy change is a complex process. Sociologist and American policy analyst Campbell suggests that policy change comes when a certain set of "policy windows of opportunity" open due to the coming together of ideas and people over time:

> Participants have different goals or preferences; the process is some sort of fight or bargaining; the result is determined by each participant's relative power, or by the amount of energy each is able and willing to expend on that issue, and how skillfully resources are deployed.[8]

The process of changing unacceptable laws and institutional policy requires willingness and courage. Some steps toward that end are documenting problems diligently, gaining an understanding of the formal and informal opinion leaders in the setting you wish to change, finding colleagues with whom you can link arms to develop effective strategies, and then persevering in the job of bringing about change.

RIGHTS, RESPONSIBILITIES, AND THE WORK ENVIRONMENT

All of the rights and responsibilities you will face in the institutional setting where you work will be spelled out in your contract and in the standing documents of the institution (e.g., bylaws and employee manuals). We have already mentioned some rights that are protected and responsibilities that are mandated by law. Like laws and policies, additional guidelines detailing your rights and responsibilities should be examined carefully for their potential to foster or hinder respect for you, your colleagues, and patients.

Patients' Rights Documents

In health care institutions patients, too, have rights and incur responsibilities. Some that are protected by law have been mentioned. However, other rights not addressed by legal guidelines have come to be accepted as important. Among the most helpful documents for understanding what they are is the American Hospital Association's list of patients' rights first published in 1975.[9] They have been updated several times but still are used as a prototype for many other institutions and groups today.

Among the rights listed are the rights to considerate and respectful care, accurate and complete information, participation (directly or through a legally appointed spokesperson) in health care decisions, privacy, and confidentiality (within constraints of the law). There are rights to information about the institution itself (e.g., who owns it and what its overall services are) and the right to have continuity of care. There are others, too, and as this book goes to press there is still debate in the United States about the necessity of a federally mandated Patients' Bill of Rights and how far the government should go to protect patients. What would you like to see included in such a nationally binding document?

Grievance Mechanisms

In recent years several professional organizations and institutions have created mechanisms to assist patients who believe their rights or other reasonable expectations are not being honored. Some institutions employ patient representatives, or "ombudsmen," whose job it is to listen to patients' problems and try to help solve them. Institutional ethics committees, highly encouraged by the Joint Commission on Accreditation of Health Care Organizations, are often useful for bringing together health professionals and patients and their families as they try to determine what to do next in complex life-and-death decisions or to help resolve conflicts among various members of the group. There have been recommendations that health care institutions hire mediation specialists to try to reach consensus about areas of conflict or dissension.

INFORMED CONSENT: THE BASIC CONTRACT GUIDING INTERACTION

We conclude this chapter on the institutional settings of health care with a close look at informed consent in the health professional and patient relationship. An institutional mechanism for gaining informed consent (or refusal) from patients or their surrogates will be found in virtually every health care institution. It is *sine qua non* the most basic contract guiding institutions and professionals in their interaction with patients.

The need for mechanisms ensuring informed consent rests on the assumption that both health professionals and the institutions of health care themselves place patients in a potentially vulnerable position. The patient's say-so or "agency" is threatened by this imbalance of power and the goal of informed consent is to help level the playing field between health professional and patient.

Informed consent involves informing a patient of what is to be done to him or her, including the potential risks and desired outcomes, and obtaining the patient's consent to (or refusal of) the procedure.

Disclosure of Relevant Information

Currently, there is debate over how much information must be provided to enable a person to make an intelligent decision regarding treatment. One school of thought in health care maintains that it is impossible to provide the information in all of its detail. Members of this group base their argument on the complexity of treatments, which, they say, patients cannot understand. A second school maintains that it is inadvisable to provide information; that to do so can only harm the patient. This is a particularly delicate issue in the matter of treatments for mental illnesses for which the therapist believes a favorable outcome can be attained only by keeping certain information from the patient. Providing information is problematic, too, for health professionals who wish to give a placebo to a patient who is finding no relief from pain killers. As soon as the patient knows a sugar pill or other inert substance is being substituted for a prior "real" medication, the placebo becomes ineffective.

Proponents of a third view argue that information does not harm, but rather that knowledge sets a person free by allowing the patient to retain control over the events of his or her life. In a context of a total or partial institution, the goal should be to maximize the patient's autonomy as much as possible. The language a health professional or other employee of the institution uses to describe the details should be personalized to maximize each person's comprehension. In other words, the standard used for determining the type and amount of disclosure should be one derived from the knowledge of each individual patient, although there lingers a dispute about the depth of information that health professionals must give to patients. There is agreement about the type of information that must be shared. Patients should be told the proposed treatment in terms they can understand. This includes information about the diagnosis and prognosis, a general notion of the treatment involved, and the desired outcome. The patient should also be given information about alternatives to the proposed treatment, which may include doing nothing, and the risks involved for each.

Giving or Refusing Consent

The patient's consent or refusal is the sign that she or he is not being coerced into any course of action. Obtaining consent is also a means of enforcing the implicit rules of the relationship, which say that the health professional will neither harm the patient nor be unfaithful to the task of helping the patient.

Although informed consent is a potent mechanism for honoring patient's preferences, it is not a fail-safe protection from difficult decisions or even outright conflict among health professionals themselves or between them and patients or families. One form of difficulty is that sometimes what the patient considers best for himself or herself is not consistent with what the health professional considers best. Consider, for example, the story of Mrs. Mathilda Martin:

> The patient, Mrs. Martin, was a 54-year-old woman who was transferred to this tertiary care hospital's critical care unit from an outlying community hospital with a principal diagnosis of acute anterior wall myocardial infarction (i.e., a heart attack). Secondary diagnoses were acute pancreatitis, disseminated intravascular coagulation, acute respiratory failure, acute renal failure, and lactic acidosis. The patient was given ventilator support. Because of her medication and increasing medical problems, she was alert only periodically, but was responsive when directly addressed. There were no written advance directives.
>
> Mrs. Martin had been hospitalized in 1990 for acute pancreatitis. She also had a psychiatric history of anxiety and depression and had been

consistently treated with Haldol and Prozac for several years. Mrs. Martin had attempted suicide about 10 years ago.

Her family consisted of a supportive husband (Gene Martin), an adult daughter (Martha), the daughter's husband, and a 15-year-old grand-daughter (Rachel). The Martins also had a son (Jake) who lived in the Midwest. He was not present at the hospital. Jake also had a history of depression and suicide attempts. The family informed him of his mother's serious condition but purposely kept him out of the decision-making loop, fearing his acting out if he saw his mother fulfilling his possible latent wish. Mr. Martin and Martha consistently voiced agreement that Mrs. Martin should make her own decision regarding terminal weaning (removing ventilator support and keeping her comfortable with no plan to reinstate use of the ventilator, even if she stopped breathing). Mr. Martin said that his wife and he had talked about potential end-of-life situations. She clearly stated that she did not want to be kept alive if it meant living in a more debilitated state or if the quality of her life would be compromised more than it already had been.

During the first three days of hospitalization Mrs. Martin was consistently aware and responsive. She was presented with the possibility of pancreatic surgery or drug treatments to relieve the excruciating pain of her pancreatitis. She was told that surgery had a high risk of mortality and her chance of coming out of the operating room alive was less than 50%. Recovery would require extensive respiratory care with possible placement for a period of time in an extended care facility where she would be in a program for redevelopment of skills for activities of daily living. Within these first three days it also become clear that she would have to undergo dialysis. Mrs. Martin declined more medical intervention and expressed a desire to discontinue ventilator support.

With Mrs. Martin's decision and the support of her husband and daughter, the attending physician agreed to terminal weaning. In a further phone conversation with the daughter on the day before the scheduled wean (the fourth day of hospitalization), the attending physician hesitated about the matter and told her he had requested a consultation from the ethics committee.

At this point, Mr. Martin and Martha became angry and distraught about the seeming reversal and the calling of "more people"—i.e., the ethics committee. . . .[10]

If you were the attending physician, what might have caused you to change your mind, if anything? The concern of this physician was that he should discontinue treatment only when it no longer was doing any good, and he began to doubt that treatment was futile. Where did the breakdown in communication occur, and what could have been done to prevent this unhappy state of affairs? Sometimes health care institutions feel trapped by patients who refuse treatments that health professionals believe are important or insist on treatments that health professionals believe are inappropriate, when these same patients are too ill or incapacitated to be discharged. At other times patients insist on going home before the health professionals believe they are ready. They are said to have left "AMA"—against medical advice. They may be asked to sign a document confirming that they have been informed of the physician's judgment but are choosing to act contrary to his or her advice.

Much more refinement of the concept and limits of informed consent and related mechanisms still is needed. Great strides have been made toward recognizing and honoring patients' preferences as an integral aspect of decision making in health care institutions.[11] At the same time, problems do remain. The process of gaining informed consent is designed to ensure that the health professional's and institution's promises to help and to not inflict harm are kept. However, daily interaction with the patient cannot depend on acquiring the patient's (or family's) written consent every step of the way. Trust must underlie the consent process and whatever else goes on in the setting; it promotes feelings of relatedness and allows the procedures to flow smoothly. In short, if informed consent mechanisms are substituted for other aspects of a humane environment, institutions will not succeed in respecting the patient's dignity.

SUMMARY

This chapter highlights that a respect-filled health care environment requires the cooperation and responsible participation of individuals, institutional leaders, and society as a whole. Your own efforts will be fruitless without institutional support. At the same time, respect is so fundamental that you have an opportunity and duty to exercise it at all levels: as an individual professional, as an employee of the institution, and as a citizen. We ended this chapter with a focus on informed consent—a basic legal and ethical process whereby respect is brought down to the most personal level of your interactions with the people you are preparing to serve in your professional role.

REFERENCES

1. Greenfield, M.: The land of Hospital. *Newsweek,* June 30, 1986, p. 74.
2. Scott, W.R.: *Organizations: Rational, Natural and Open Systems.* Englewood Cliffs, NJ, Prentice Hall, 1981.
3. Grumbach, K. and Bodenheimer, T.: The organization of health care. *JAMA* 273(2):160–167, 1995.
4. Goffman, E.: *Asylums.* Garden City, NY, Anchor Books, 1961, p. xiii.
5. May, W.: *The Patient's Ordeal.* Bloomington, Indiana University Press, 1991, p. 146.
6. May, W.: *The Patient's Ordeal.* Bloomington, Indiana University Press, 1991, p. 127.

7. U.S. Department of Health and Human Services, Public Health Service, Centers for Disease Control, Atlanta, *Morbidity and Mortality Weekly Report,* 36(suppl 25): 55–65, 1987.

8. Campbell, J.C.: *How Policies Change: The Japanese Government and the Aging Society.* Princeton, NJ, Princeton University Press, 1992.

9. American Hospital Association: *A Patient's Bill of Rights.* Chicago, American Hospital Association, 1992 [1975].

10. Kuczewski, M.K. and Pinkus, R.B. *An Ethics Casebook for Hospitals: Practical Approaches to Everyday Cases.* Washington, DC, Georgetown University Press, 1999, pp. 21–22.

11. Purtilo, R.: *Ethical Dimensions in the Health Professions,* 3rd ed. Philadelphia, Saunders, 1999, pp. 126–133.

CHAPTER 3

Respect in a Diverse Society

CHAPTER OBJECTIVES

The student will be able to

- Define cultural bias and personal bias
- Identify three sources of personal bias that interfere with respect toward persons or groups
- Distinguish factors that may cause negative perceptions of another person from factors leading to a positive "halo effect"
- Define prejudice and how it is related to discrimination
- List primary and secondary characteristics of culture
- Describe ways that the label of "race" is problematic even though it continues to be used
- Describe how gender discrimination, ageism, and discrimination based on ethnicity affect the health professions and some ways you can counter their disrespectful dimensions
- Define cultural sensitivity and cultural competence and describe the steps to achieving each

---

Why, a cabdriver would go the wrong way down a one-way street to pick up a white woman. White women are the best fares. Don't cause you no trouble. Don't hassle you. Worst fares are young black men. I call 'em 'yo' boys. Nothing but trouble. I won't pick them up, and *I'm* black, in case you hadn't noticed.

Washington, DC, cabdriver, July 2000

The first two chapters discussed the value context of individuals, as persons and professionals, and the institutional environment. Respect also involves sensitivity to individual and group differences. Thus, you may discover that, even with deep understanding of your personal values and clarity about the goals and values of the place where you work, respectful interaction still does not result. Yet to be considered is the fact that each person interprets actions, facial expressions, choice of words, and other forms of communication according to his or her cultural conditioning and past experience. All of these interactions take place within a society that, at least within the United States, has been described as a "melting pot" in which all of the various cultures and beliefs blend together. Some hold that the melting pot description of the United States is no longer accurate and that it is more like "chunky stew," a stew savored both for the character of the individual ingredients (ethnically-derived differences) and for the delicious melding of flavors (social integration).[1]

In this chapter, we examine some of the differences you will encounter in clinical practice and the barriers (e.g., personal and cultural biases, prejudices, and discrimination) that get in the way of appreciating differences and inhibit respectful interaction.

BIAS, PREJUDICE, AND DISCRIMINATION

A *cultural bias* is a tendency to interpret a word or action according to some culturally derived meaning assigned to it. Cultural bias derives from cultural variation, discussed later in this chapter. For example, some cultures view smiles as a deeply personal sign of happiness that is only shared with intimates. Others view smiles as an indication of general friendliness to be shared with any and all. It is quite possible that another can interpret a friendly smile on the part of one person as disingenuous or inappropriate. Regarding health care, attitudes toward pain, methods of conveyance of bad news, management of chronic illness and disability, beliefs about the seriousness of illness, and death-related issues vary among different cultures. These different kinds of beliefs about disease and illness have an impact on health care-seeking behavior and acceptance of the advice and intervention of health professionals. Understanding a patient's concept of health is critical to the development of interaction strategies that are acceptable to the patient.

A *personal bias* is a tendency to interpret a word or action in terms of some personal significance assigned to it. It is found largely in what is commonly called prejudice. Personal bias can derive from culturally defined interpretations but can also originate from a number of other sources grounded in personal experience. The individual internalizes the cultural attitudes until he or she believes them to be entirely personal. Put another way, a personal bias is an individual's feeling about a particular person or thing that colors his or her interpretation of it. The bias can lead to more favorable or less favorable judgments than are merited. This process is similar to that of internalizing societal values described in Chapter 1.

Understanding the way personal biases influence us and their effect on our attitudes and conduct is important to the health professional. Whenever bias is present, it affects the type of communication possible between the persons involved and therefore must be recognized as one determining factor in respectful interaction. None of the documents outlining patients' rights support an ethical or legal right permitting professionals to refuse care or show any kind of disrespect on the basis of their personal biases. The Washington, DC, cabdriver quoted at the beginning of this chapter expresses a negative personal bias based on his experience with certain passengers. How does it show up in his comments?

The cabdriver's comments also show another side to his judgments: in some cases, personal bias may produce a positive personal bias or "halo effect" on certain individuals; that is, two people may have common interests or characteristics, and their camaraderie is immediately apparent. How is the halo effect at work in the comments of this Washington, DC, cabdriver? While showing favoritism on this basis alone is not permissible in the patient and health professional relationship, common interests can, of course, have legitimate positive effects on the relationship between two persons working together.

Consider, again, the *negative* personal biases of the cabdriver. He is discriminating against young, black, male passengers. Discrimination is negative, different treatment of a person or group. Usually it is derived from prejudice. Prejudice is "an aversive or hostile attitude toward a person who *belongs to a group,* simply because he belongs to that group, and is therefore assumed to have objectionable qualities ascribed to that group."[2] In this way we see how prejudicial attitudes manifest themselves in discriminatory behavior.

In short, every exchange between a patient and health professional undoubtedly will be influenced by cultural differences and other sources of personal bias. Sometimes these feelings will create an attitude of prejudice and a desire to discriminate. In Chapter 2, you were introduced to some of the laws that help define the legal limits to which discrimination can be pushed within the health care environment. However, despite legal guidelines, discrimination occurs craftily and evasively. You must watch for it in yourself and others because both parties involved are inevitably injured by the interaction. Consider your initial reaction to the cabdriver's statement. Were you offended? Were you perhaps a little sympathetic to the driver's situation? Whatever your reaction, it should give you a glimpse into your own prejudices.

Gordon Allport, in his definitive work, *The Nature of Prejudice* (which, although written over 45 years ago, is still widely considered an authoritative study), warns, "It is a serious error to ascribe prejudice and discrimination to any single taproot, reaching into economic exploitation, social structure, the mores, fear, aggression, sex conflict or any other favored soil. Prejudice and discrimination . . . may draw nourishment from all these conditions and many others."[3] It should be emphasized that treating people differently because of race, religion, ethnicity, or gender does not necessarily imply prejudice and discrimination. Respect for differences includes understanding when those differences should count, how they inform the responses of people, and the process of caring for them.

What can you learn from the previous pages? One thing you can discern is that developing effective interaction skills with others must begin with self-examination and consideration of what cultural differences mean to you. This is not as easy as it may seem at first glance. It requires that you enter into a

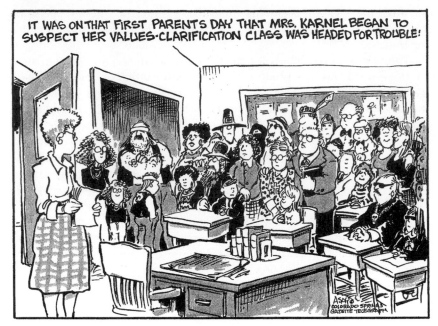

By permission of Chuck Asay and Creators Syndicate.

"difficult dialogue"; that is, you are asked to reconsider long-held assumptions about individuals and groups that raise questions about your values and beliefs. Engagement in this type of activity may lead to feelings of discomfort and uneasiness.[4] These uncomfortable feelings result from the limited experience most of us have in interacting and talking with individuals different from ourselves.

We explore here a variety of differences, both obvious and subtle, that exist between people, such as differences in language, one of the most basic reasons for miscommunication—why, for example, even when we speak the same language, we may hear what a patient says but not understand its true meaning. Once you become aware of your often-unconscious biases you can more easily avoid being controlled by them in your interactions with others. Furthermore, by becoming aware of your hidden biases, you will be less likely to form inappropriate judgments about patients, colleagues, and others and more likely to remain sensitive and open to differences that influence your interactions with them.

RESPECTING DIFFERENCES

We live in a multicultural society. Sensitivity to cultural differences today has increased owing to the various minority rights movements over the last several decades and the fact that there is an ever-growing percentage of ethnic minorities in the United States. As the new millennium begins, ethnic minorities comprise 27% of the U.S. population. Reliable estimates indicate that their numbers will increase to 37% in the year 2025.[5]

In California, Texas, and Florida today's ethnic minorities should reach numerical majority early in the 21st century.[6] This growing diversity has strong implications for the provision of health care. There is a significant underrepresentation of minorities in the health professions, which contributes to the disparity in the health status of whites and other minority groups—blacks, Hispanics, Asian Americans, American Indians, Alaskan natives, and Pacific Islanders.

Depending on where you live, you may be more or less aware of the percentage of persons from cultural and racial backgrounds that are different than your own who are living in your community. One way to identify the various cultural groups in your area is to use data from the U.S. Census Bureau, which is organized by state. You can access the most recent information by going to the home page of the U.S. Census Bureau (http://www.census.gov). There are tables for each state and you can find the cultures represented, the languages spoken, and other information about where you live and work.

In almost every health care setting, you will interact with patients of backgrounds different from your own. Certain differences are obvious; others are hidden. The iceberg model illustrates how much remains below the surface in our interactions with others.

Health professionals are generally aware of a patient's race, gender, and language. They might be able to make educated guesses about age and ethnicity. With this limited information about potential differences a professional can

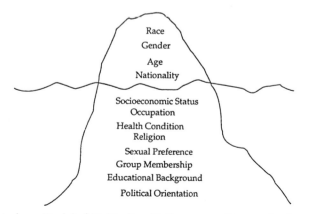

Iceberg Model of Multicultural Influences on Communication.

From Krepp, G.L.: Effective Communication in Multicultural Health Care Settings. New York, Sage Publications, Inc., © 1994. Reprinted by permission of Sage Publications, Inc.

adjust communication patterns and approaches accordingly. However, it is more difficult to assess a patient's socioeconomic status or place of residence, two differences that can have as profound an effect on a patient's health beliefs or behavior as do visible attributes such as race and gender. The differences that are hidden may create more stress than those that can more readily be identified.

Even with experience, you may sometimes fail to appreciate significant differences in others with whom you interact. It is a continual challenge to look below the surface at the differences that affect interactions with patients and devise strategies to overcome barriers and facilitate communication. Many such differences have come to be viewed collectively as being characteristics of a person's "culture." Using a broad definition, we describe *culture* as the beliefs, customs, technological achievements, language, and history of a group of similar people.[7] So you can think of culture in terms of primary characteristics such as race, gender, age, and ethnicity and secondary characteristics such as place of residence, sexual orientation, and socioeconomic status.[8] We turn your attention to a difference that is the root of numerous conflicts between social groups—race.

Race

Race is one characteristic of culture almost always mentioned in discussions about cultural differences. However, even the distinctions used by the U.S. Census Bureau constitute a system that some claim is based on outmoded concepts and dubious assumptions about genetic difference. "In fact, race is poorly correlated with any biologic or cultural phenomenon other than skin color, which makes it a useless classification for biomedical or social research."[9] One of the authors was visiting South Africa during the apartheid years, where laws were based on "racial" distinctions. A geneticist and anthropologist with whom she worked noted that the most accurate way to talk about races was to say that so-and-so was "classified as" white, or black, or another race. They wanted to emphasize the social construction of this potent label. At present the idea of race has social meaning, assigns status, limits opportunities, and influences interactions between health professionals and patients.[10] Take a moment and reflect on which racial category presently being used to classify people in the United States (e.g., white, black, Hispanic, Asian American, American Indian, Alaskan native, or Pacific Islander) you most closely claim as your own. Is it a perfect fit, or is there room for additional categories to describe who you really are? The same difficulty with racial identification can occur with your patients as well.

Although it is generally true that patient treatment and counseling are more effective when obtained from members of one's own race, it does not mean that patients *must* be treated by members of the same race. First of all, this would not be possible because there are so few minority health professionals. Second, it is possible to learn how to appropriately handle the health care of minority groups different from our own racial and ethnic backgrounds through sensitivity, knowledge, and skills in cross-cultural communication.

There are other barriers to be overcome between patients and health professionals that are, unfortunately, deeply tied to race. "Many minorities don't have access to medical care in general, due primarily to issues of both race and economic class. Underlying these issues is the cultural history of African Americans in the United States and their mistrust of the medical establishment."[11] There are ample historical reasons for minorities to mistrust the health care system. For example, in the not-too-distant past, black patients were refused treatment at "white only" hospitals. Some were undertreated and deceived in the infamous Tuskegee syphilis study. Gaining the trust of patients whose race is different from one's own is a challenge, but not an insurmountable one if a health professional can show that her or his aim is to provide optimum care personally and minimize and eventually eliminate disparities in care.

One of the first steps in reducing disparities in the health care setting is to be aware that they exist. For example, not long ago one of the authors participated in an ethics consultation regarding an extremely ill newborn. The black parents of the baby looked around the table of health professionals gathered for the meeting. The father quietly commented, "I'd feel a whole lot better about this if there was one black face other than ours at this table." Although everyone present was there for the good of the baby and his family, the lack of representation of someone of the parents' skin color was a significant barrier to the discussion and, ultimately, to the decisions made. If the father had not made the comment, the health professionals involved probably would never have noticed the circle of white faces surrounding the black couple.

The preceding example indicates that there may be justifiable reasons to consider race when making clinical decisions. Another situation in which race (and ethnicity) may be a reason for differential treatment is when certain medications are prescribed because both can affect disease pathophysiology and drug metabolism.[12] Race and ethnic background can also influence dietary habits and other activities of daily living that have a direct impact on health care outcomes. Although different treatment based on race or ethnicity may be justified in special cases such as those mentioned, it is the exception, not the rule. You must remain alert for unjustified differences in care based on race or ethnicity.

Gender

Gender issues interact with other primary and secondary characteristics of culture to shape a person's identity. There are many implications for assessment and treatment of patients based on differences in gender. Gender inequities exist in health care just as they do in society at large. Women in the United States have a history of unequal access to sources of economic and political power.[13] This is especially true for black women or older women who experience the combined impact of race, gender, and age discrimination. Although it is important that gender inequities in health care be remedied, it is also important to simultaneously acknowledge those differences that should be taken into consideration and accommodated in planning and delivering care.

Let us take as an example the preferences of patients regarding the gender of their physician. Numerous studies have documented the fact that 20% to 56% of women explicitly prefer a female physician for women's health problems.[14, 15] Because most women feel uncomfortable and perhaps embarrassed during a gynecological examination, they may prefer female physicians because they are familiar with the female body and have firsthand experience with the examination. If women are more comfortable with the examination, then they will be more likely to follow through with checkups and follow the recommendations of the physician. All things considered, women's health care provided by women should result in better health care outcomes. Once again, it is not always possible, or desirable, for women health professionals to provide health care to women patients. The challenge is for male health professionals to adopt behaviors and communication styles to compensate for the difference in gender from their patients. Of course, the same is also true for female health professionals working with male patients.

The preference for a health professional who is of the same sex may not only be personal but may also be a cultural or religious one. Many cultural groups are very concerned about modesty and may require that only a female health professional examine a female patient's genitalia or be present when the patient is undressed. Gender differences regarding modesty can have direct implications for diagnosis and treatment, as is evident in the following case:

> A 50-year-old female peasant from Mexico is seen in the clinic. The patient's 35-year-old son accompanies her. The woman has been coming to the clinic for some time. Her son usually interprets because she does not speak English. An interpreter who is employed by the clinic is called because the son has to leave for work and cannot stay and translate for his mother. Before they enter the room, the physician discloses to the female interpreter that he is concerned about whether the health problems claimed by this woman are real or imagined. She has been in the clinic three times before, each time with different vague and diffuse complaints, none of which make medical sense. The physician learns through the translator that the woman has a fistula in her rectum. In her previous visits, she could not bring herself to reveal her true symptoms in the presence of, and therefore to, her son as he interpreted for her. She was so embarrassed that she invented other symptoms to justify visits to the physician. She wanted someone else to interpret, but did not know how she could ask since she would have to speak through her son.[16]

Although some of the problems in this example occurred because of differences in gender, these problems were compounded by differences in language. The case offers insight into the problems that can arise when language is a primary barrier. In a sense, the clinic was fortunate to have an interpreter on-site. This is not always the case and you might have to rely on family members for translation. If a family member is the translator, you should pay attention to the gender of the translator as well as to the translator's relationship to the patient, because this can impact what the patient is willing to share. Language barriers are a critical stumbling block to the delivery of health care. There are several web sites such as http://www.omhrc.gov/CLAS and http://www.hhs.gov/ocr/lep that provide information on the newly issued national standards for culturally and linguistically appropriate services.

Age

The particular form of stigma associated with being old is related to the prejudices of an ageist society. The word ageism was coined to designate the discriminatory treatment of old people (as sexism was coined to describe the systematic devaluation of one sex on both an individual and a societal basis).

Older adults are constantly confronted with ageist conduct. Unfortunately, ageist conduct occurs in the health care environment as well. Older patients often receive less attention or are denied services based on their age alone. Physical and psychological problems may not be addressed because health professionals assume that they are normal for an older person. Older patients are often overmedicated and experience the effects of poorly coordinated care. Regardless of their state of health or physical ability, an elderly patient is commonly met with a patronizing attitude. Ways in which you can overcome the tendencies to engage in ageist behavior are discussed in more detail in Chapter 17.

Ethnicity

Ethnicity refers to a person's sense of belonging to a group of people sharing a common origin, history, and set of social beliefs. Recall from the broad definition of "culture" earlier in this chapter that ethnicity counts as one of the primary characteristics of culture along with race, age, and gender. Ethnicity may also refer to an individual's place of geographical or national origin, one of the secondary characteristics of culture.

It used to be very easy to identify an ethnicity-based cultural variation because one could readily distinguish between the various ways of doing things in various parts of the world. Frequently, early explorers were stunned by the practices they encountered as norms in cultures, and all too often they used the occasion to minimize the importance of the cultural practices of other societies. Even 100 years ago, the "American way" differed significantly from the "European way," and these two were easily distinguished from the "African way" or the "Far Eastern way." Today, in most parts of the world, a large variety of influences such as telecommunications and the presence of foreign visitors impact what used to be traditional, homogeneous cultures. Although the United States has a history of immigration from various parts of the world, "Never before has the United States received immigrants from so many countries, from such different social and economic backgrounds, and for so many reasons."[17] A result is that it is often more difficult to sort out and identify specific cultural differences that modify behavior in various ethnic groups.

Sometimes as a health professional you may have a difficult time remembering that members of an ethnic group cannot be expected to be homogeneous. Their ethnicity is only one characteristic of the culture or cultures they bring to their present experience. For example, an outstanding physician and friend of the authors grew up in rural Nigeria, studied as an undergraduate in Scotland, took her medical training at Johns Hopkins University in Baltimore, Maryland, and now practices in the heart of Midwest America. When asked if she had difficulty "adjusting" to the Midwest, she said that she simply brought along to "this new culture" the best of what she had the opportunity to accumulate along the way! At times, each of us becomes aware of cultural beliefs held by an individual that, on the surface, seem to be incongruent. For example, a Chinese American may be highly assimilated into the majority culture and seek mainstream health care for a gastrointestinal disorder yet also seek care from a traditional Chinese healer who might prescribe herbs or other forms of alternative therapies. Because we can identify with individual variations in our own cultural beliefs and the blending of seemingly opposite beliefs that can occur within us as individuals, we must appreciate the profound variability that can exist within cultural groups.

One of the widest cultural gaps you will encounter in your role as a health professional is that created by the "ethnocentrism" of health professionals. (Although separate professions often are not thought of as cultures in themselves, they are.) Ethnocentrism is the belief that one's own cultural ways are superior. Health professionals often believe that their way is best and so are guilty of *medical* ethnocentrism. In fact, while you are a student you are learning and adopting the culture of your chosen health profession. The culture of a health professional encompasses the interrelationships of professional values, beliefs, customs, habits, and symbols. You are learning the cultural meaning that your profession gives to concepts such as pain, disability, disease, and illness. You will find that even within the culture of the health professions, there are different meanings and understandings of identical phenomena. Thus, as an individual you may share the same ethnic origin, race, and gender as the patient you are working with and yet not hold the same beliefs and perspectives about some important things related to what his or her care should involve.

The following poem, used here with the author's permission, demonstrates how difficult it can be to reach across the ethnic (and other cultural) gap between health professional and patient:

4/2

She came into the room smiling.
"This is the real thing," said the interpreter.
"*Sientese*," I said, gesturing to the chair, grateful for my limited Spanish.
I asked her questions about cancer and illness.
"Only Americans talk of dying of cancer," she said.
I asked her questions about cancer and illness.
"Look in the eyes, you can tell by the eyes," she said.
I looked in her eyes.
I asked her questions about cancer and illness.
"The *curanderas* use objects and herbs for healing.
They have their own way of speaking.
No one else understands them."
She looked at me.
"That's all," she said. She stood.
that's all that's all that's all
whispered ancestor spirits
holders of ancient wisdom
written in Aztec
kept in jars and pots
herbs animals
stones
goat's milk
"That's all," she said.
she smiled
she left the room.

—*Jolene Siemsen*

Socioeconomic Status

The vast majority of U.S. and Canadian health professionals are white, with average incomes that are in the middle to high economic range when considered globally. The income level and accompanying higher social status of health professionals tend to create barriers to interacting with patients. "Ethnic minority groups and economically disadvantaged individuals may have particular difficulty feeling in control within a setting dominated by well-educated professionals."[18] The difference in socioeconomic status may hinder patients from asking you important questions, hinder you from empathizing with patients, and limit your knowledge of the practical everyday obstacles that prevent or facilitate the ability of patients to pursue medication or treatment regimens.[19] The following case highlights the challenges patients face just getting to a medical appointment.

A young mother and her two small children, a toddler and a 3-month-old, leave their apartment at 7:00 A.M. for a 9:00 A.M. clinic visit. With the baby in a stroller and her son at her side, they head for the bus stop that is four blocks from their home. The first bus is late because of icy conditions. She will have to transfer three times to get to the clinic and walk a block or two at each stop. She gets to the clinic 45 minutes late for her 9:00 A.M. appointment. The medical assistant at the intake desk looks at the clock as the mother signs in and says, "Couldn't you have called if you were going to be late?"

We will address different interpretations of time in Chapter 10, but in this case there is no disagreement about what is "on time." The medical assistant does not understand the meaning of having to be dependent on public transportation or the hassle of using a pay phone while juggling two small children in the cold. The fact that this patient actually made it to the clinic is testament to her desire to receive care. Yet, this fact becomes lost in complaints about the patient's tardiness and lack of consideration for the clinic staff. Health professionals may take for granted owning a car or a mobile phone, items that would be completely beyond the financial means of many patients.

The difference in social class and economic status also affects the type and frequency of interaction between patient and health professional outside the health care setting. The informal networks that exist in neighborhoods and communities provide opportunities to establish cooperation, exchange information, and determine appropriate behavior. "For instance, minority patients might be described as 'noncompliant' by clinicians (who, mainly, have been socialized in a white urban middle-class milieu) when, in fact, the patients are 'following the rule,' but rules that are based on a different set of principles."[20]

Outsiders can make unintentional errors in judgment because they under-estimate the effects of ethnicity, age, or class on insiders' responses or actions; that is, individuals born or socialized into membership of the group. Outsiders must work to "get in," to gain, build, and maintain trust with a group.[21]

Level of education is another difference between health professionals and patients related to socioeconomic status. Although patients may respect education in the abstract, they may also be suspicious that you will use your education to take advantage of them rather than to assist them. Patients may also be too intimidated to admit when they do not understand something. For fear that they will be seen as ignorant or superstitious, patients may neglect to mention that they are also seeking alternative methods of care or providers. Even when patients are well educated, they may not speak the dominant language well enough to adequately express themselves. For example, a French tourist in the United States was in a minor accident that required an emergency room visit. The patient, an attorney, spoke some English, but told the nurse in the triage unit that she would feel better if she could talk to someone in French because, "I lack eloquence in English." You may understand what the French patient means if you have struggled to make yourself understood across a language barrier. It is important to remember that the "language" of health care is often foreign to patients as well. In Chapter 10 we discuss in more detail how language and vocabulary, which are partially a result of education, can facilitate or block what patients perceive as respect from you.

Occupation and Place of Residence

One of the first questions we often ask a new acquaintance in a social setting is, "What do you do?" We deeply identify with our occupations in mainstream American culture. Some would go so far as to say that their occupation defines who they are more than their ethnicity or other primary characteristics. Occupations shape how people see the world and what they value. The importance of a person's occupation is sometimes seen more clearly when injury, illness, or retirement forces a change in occupation. How patients occupy themselves, whether they spend their time in the formal workforce or not, can give important cultural clues that have an impact on health care beliefs and decisions.

We do not often think of place of residence as a cultural variable in our interactions with patients, yet there is increasing evidence that place of residence has an impact on how patients think about health. For example, certain health beliefs and practices sometimes are different between urban and rural patients. Rural patients, because of their environment, must often travel a considerable distance to see a health professional. Thus, rural patients are more independent than their urban counterparts. Another significant difference between rural and urban dwellers is the way health needs are viewed. Rural dwellers, both male and female, from a variety of locations, tend to determine health needs primarily in relation to work activities.[22]

A striking example of the impact the values held by rural dwellers can have on health decisions is evident in the following case:

> Michael T. is a 61-year-old wheat farmer. He maintains his large and profitable family farm with the help of his wife, three sons, and occasional hired help. He has managed and actively worked on the same farm for almost 40 years. Mr. T. attended the state university for 2 years, studying agribusiness. By his state's standards he is well educated; he is in the middle-income bracket. During the harvesting season, he often works parts of the fields alone with the help of rented heavy farm equipment. Two years ago while working in this way, he caught the middle finger of his right hand in a moving part of his equipment while he was adjusting a machine component. He could not pull his finger free, and the injury was quite painful. Mr. T. realized that it might be some time before anyone would come to his aid. The weather was changing, and he needed to

complete the harvesting work in the field to avoid damage to the wheat crop and prevent additional equipment rental costs. He decided to pull his hand free, severing his finger at its base. He was able to control the bleeding with a tightly bound handkerchief, and he completed harvesting the field.

When he returned home, his son drove him to the nearest town, 57 miles away, where he sought care in the hospital emergency room.

Before continuing with the rest of the case, consider what your reaction might be if you were the first health professional to interact with Mr. T. when he arrived at the emergency room. Do you think Mr. T. is brave, stupid, shortsighted, practical, hard-working, frugal, or a combination of these characteristics? If you had been in his position, what would you have done? How might these personal values and cultural beliefs affect your ability to interact with Mr. T.? Let us return to the case and see how the health professionals involved responded to the situation.

The physician who saw Mr. T. was very distressed that he had not retrieved the digit and sought care immediately. While dressing Mr. T.'s wound, the physician explained that, with prompt action and air ambulance transport to the state's major medical center, it might have been possible for the finger to be reattached. Fortunately Mr. T. did not develop an infection or other serious complication after his injury. He was able to manage his farm as usual once he healed. When he tells neighbors about the story of this event, he often comments, "It simply goes to show you that, if you go to those doctors too soon, you end up with lots of unnecessary treatment and bills."[23]

Whether a patient lives on a farm, in the inner city, or in the suburbs, you must be mindful of the impact place of residence can have on interactions with patients. This is especially true when the patient does not have a permanent place of residence or is homeless. The challenges of working with patients whose only home is the streets include major issues such as ensuring the safety and basic well-being of the patient, but also practical considerations unique to this environment such as the need for access to a bathroom or to a source of drinking water. Persons who live on the street either by choice or necessity are part of a subculture that is often hidden from view and require openness and understanding from health professionals.

Health Status

Another fundamental difference between patients and health professionals is that patients are experiencing the effects of illness or injury in some way and health professionals generally are not. What is unique about this difference is that all of us will experience the loss of ability to function normally at some point in our lives, whether temporarily or permanently. All of us will be in the role of patient at some point in our lives. Susan Wendell comments,

> Most of us will live part of our lives with bodies that hurt, that move with difficulty or not at all, that deprive us of activities we once took for granted or that others take for granted, bodies that make daily life a struggle.[24]

Patients occupy a role that has certain expectations. "Good" patients are cooperative, pleasant, honest, and quiet. Patients are in need of care or service and this automatically places them in a position of lessened power and control. Because it is almost a certainty that you will be a patient sometime in your life, it is possible to maintain a connection with this reality as you care for others. The possibility that you could just as easily be the patient, an idea sometimes referred to as reciprocity, should not be forgotten.

Religion

Another feature of culture that influences interaction with patients is religious beliefs. Religion gives meaning to illness, pain, and suffering. Religious beliefs are often most apparent when a patient is seriously injured, critically ill, or dying. For example, the Christian faith, with its valuing of human life and belief in eternal life, states that whereas a struggle for health can be meaningful, a struggle against death at all costs to the point that the effort becomes a torment is nonsense.[25] The Christian cultural view of the dying process and death itself influences treatment decisions and may promote requests for symbolically meaningful activities such as receiving the sacraments.

A different view of illness is evident with believers in Islam. "The word Islam means to submit; that is, to submit their lives to the will of God (Allah). A fatalistic worldview is common whereby the person attributes the incidence and outcome of a health condition to 'inshallah.' This belief can make preventive health behaviors or self-care programs difficult to institute. Because God is perceived to be in control of the outcome, what can humans do?"[26] Christian and Muslim beliefs are widespread and relatively well known; therefore, health professionals may not find much difficulty in recognizing them. Religious beliefs that are far removed from mainstream religious traditions may challenge health care professionals' understanding, tolerance, and willingness to make accommodations.

Sexual Orientation

In modern society, sexual orientation is yet another characteristic of culture that may elicit biased responses to a person. A homosexual is one example of a person who causes anxiety for some. His or her sexual orientation, rather than country of origin or skin color, becomes the basis for another's personal bias against him or her. The homosexual community is extremely diverse, but one commonality among gay men and lesbians is that they often hide their lifestyle for fear of prejudicial attitudes and discrimination. Thus, the homosexuality of patients may be somewhat invisible. However, given the number of men and women who report being homosexual (and that number is probably an underestimate of the actual total), it is highly likely that most health professionals provide care to gay, lesbian, or bisexual patients whether they know it or not.

In an interesting study, undergraduate health professions students focused on their discomfort with a variety of persons from differing cultural groups. The students reported the most consistently negative attitudes toward lesbian, gay, and bisexual people.[27] Because of unexamined homophobia, many health professionals react with shock or thinly veiled unease when patients reveal that they are homosexual or bisexual.

In addition to the negative attitudes expressed by health professionals toward patients with a sexual orientation different from their own, gay, lesbian, and bisexual patients find themselves in a health care system that is built on heterosexual assumptions to the extent that women who seek gynecological or obstetrical care may not even be asked about their sexual history. Lesbian and gay patients' partners may not be formally acknowledged in a health care system. These are only a few of the barriers that gay, lesbian, and bisexual patients may face as they seek health care. Providing sensitive, culturally appropriate care requires taking the patient's sexual orientation fully into account and assuring that the information is used to optimize the patient's quality of care. For some readers this will involve preparation before they have an opportunity to interact with homosexual patients. The first step is being aware of feelings of homophobia. These feelings should be consciously addressed and myths regarding gays, lesbians, and bisexual individuals should be dispelled.

CULTURAL SENSITIVITY AND COMPETENCE

The overall lesson to be gleaned from the preceding description of various cultural characteristics is that the atmosphere in health care must rest on fully appreciating what each culture brings to the richness of our society and on acceptance, not on fear and misunderstanding.

What is needed is an approach to each patient, client, and colleague that takes into account cultural differences. Culture-sensitive care includes knowledge, mutual respect, and negotiation.[18] Knowledge begins with a desire to understand the other person, but one of the first steps in becoming culturally aware is to examine your own cultural background. "Examine how each of the following areas affects your view of health and health care: health beliefs, communication styles, health-care system in the country of origin, and social structures."[29] It is often difficult to grasp our own views, so one method of obtaining this information is to interview family members, parents, or grandparents to understand where your attitudes toward health care came from. Here are some sample questions to get you started:

1. When faced with an injury or illness, did your family member first seek out the help of a health professional or someone else?

2. If someone else, who and why? How does your family view pain? Are you supposed to be "good" and keep quiet about pain or are you supposed to complain so that pain will be relieved?

3. What home remedies are used for everyday health problems such as headaches, minor burns, or stomach upset?

To reach a point of mutual respect, it is helpful to analyze your experiences and comfort level with people from cultures other than your own. Table 3-1 provides you with an opportunity to do so. Although the authors of the table use some different names for categories of people than those we have been using, the exercise will help you reflect on your own posture toward people who may be

TABLE 3–1. Experience and Comfort with Diverse Groups of Patients

Group	Level of Experience (1 = none, 2 = a little, 3 = some, 4 = a lot)	Level of Comfort (1 = not at all comfortable, 2 = somewhat uncomfortable, 3 = somewhat comfortable, 4 = very comfortable)
African Americans		
Jewish		
Hispanics		
Asian Americans		
Native Americans		
Gay men		
Lesbians		
Bisexuals		
Terminally ill		
HIV-positive		
Women on welfare		
Homeless		
Mentally handicapped		
Blind people		

From Eliason, M.J., and Raheim, S.: Experiences and comfort with culturally diverse groups in undergraduate pre-nursing students. *J. Nurs. Educ.* 39(4):162, 2000.

different from yourself.[30] First consider your experience working or socializing with each group (none, a little, some, or a lot), then consider how comfortable you would be working with patients from each group (not at all, somewhat uncomfortable, somewhat comfortable, or very comfortable). When you have completed the table, look at the patterns within your answers. What does this tell you about how you might react to certain groups of patients? Where does your greatest discomfort lie?

In Chapter 1, you were reminded to approach each interaction with mutual respect. This means, among other things, consciously avoiding unfair judgments about other people's traditions, values, and beliefs. We are much more likely to respect a patient's decision or action if we understand its rationale. Misunderstandings can result in harm to the patient in that he or she may hesitate to seek medical attention or follow the advice of someone so out of touch with his or her beliefs.

One barrier to mutual respect is the tendency for health professionals to adopt stereotypes and expect certain behaviors from patients from a particular culture simply because they are from that culture. Avoid scripted remarks such as "Jewish patients believe . . ." or "All Chinese patients practice . . ." because it is impossible to generalize from one patient to an entire culture. "Although some behaviors may appear similar within an identified cultural group, the astute health provider must assess for differences both within and between groups to plan appropriate care."[31]

Finally, you must learn the basic skills of negotiation. This means finding a place where you can feel confident in the exercise of your professional judgment yet incorporate the beliefs and values of patients into their treatment plan to achieve mutually desirable outcomes.

Culturally competent care is knowledge about, and sensitivity to, the different experiences and responses individuals may have because of a variety of characteristics of their lives.[32] Appendix 3-1 (The Berg Cultural/Spiritual Assessment Tool), included after the references in this chapter, is a concise guide to help you assess a patient's cultural background. This tool works best as a scripted interview guide. Not only can this and other tools be used as a starting point in your interactions with patients, but this tool also presents an opportunity for patients to think about how their cultural backgrounds influence the health care they receive. The goal of culturally competent care is to provide care characterized by respect. Such care is meaningful and fits with cultural beliefs and ways of life for those involved.

SUMMARY

The issues relevant to showing respect in the midst of diversity must continually be examined and reflected upon. Any time cultural variations and personal biases become a basis for prejudice or discrimination, these destructive tendencies and conduct will be increased by other distinguishing differences among individuals as well. The only constructive approach to evaluating human differences with the goal of showing respect is to take each experience as an opportunity to learn more about the rich diversity of the human condition and to take what one learns as a gift that will enrich one's own life.

REFERENCES

1. Spencer, M. and Markstrom-Adams, C.: Identity processes among racial and ethnic minority children in America. *Child Dev.* 61:290–310, 1990.
2. Allport, G.: *The Nature of Prejudice.* Reading, MA, Addison-Wesley, 1954, p. 8.
3. Ibid, p. xii.
4. Baldwin, D. and Nelms, T.: Difficult dialogues: impact on nursing education curricula. *J. Prof. Nurs.* 9(6):343–346, 1993.
5. United States Department of Commerce, U.S. Census Bureau, Population Division, Population Projections Branch. Washington, D.C., 2000.
6. Bessent, H. Closing the gap: generating opportunities for minority nurses in American health care. In *Strategies for Recruitment, Retention, and Graduation of Minority Nurses in Colleges of Nursing.* Washington, DC: American Nursing Publishing, 1997.
7. Johnson, F.A: Contributions of anthropology to psychiatry. In Goldman, H. (ed.): *Review of Psychiatry.* 2nd ed. Norwalk, CT, Appleton & Lange, 1988, pp. 167–181.
8. Purnell, L.: A description of the Purnell model for cultural competence. *J. Transcult. Nurs.* 11(1):40–46, 2000.
9. Hahn, R.A.: The state of federal health statistics on racial and ethnic groups. *JAMA* 267:268–271, 1992.
10. Pinderhughes, E.: *Understanding Race, Ethnicity, and Power.* New York, Free Press, 1989.
11. Schmidt, L.: Addressing ethnic and cultural diversity in end-of-life care. Posted May 25, 2000. Available at http://www.lastacts.org.
12. Hines, S.E.: Caring for diverse populations. Intelligent prescribing in diverse populations. *Patient Care* 34(9):135–136, 139–140, 142, 2000.
13. Conway-Turner, K.: Older women of color: a feminist exploration of the intersections of personal, familial and community life. *J. Women Aging* 11(2/3):115–130, 1999.
14. Kerssens, J.J., Bensing, J.M., and Andela, M.G.: Patient preferences for genders of health professionals. *Soc. Sci. Med.* 44:1531–1540.
15. Delgado, A., Lopez-Fernandez, L.A., and Luna, J.D.: Influence of the doctor's gender in the satisfaction of users. *Med. Care* 31, 795–800.
16. Haffner, L.: Translation is not enough: interpreting in a medical setting. *West. J. Med.* 157(3):256.
17. Portes, A. and Rumbaut, R.: *Immigrant America: A Portrait.* 2nd ed. Berkeley, University of California Press, quote on p. 7.
18. Ramer, L., Richardson, J.L., Cohen, M.Z., Bedney, C., Danley, K.L., and Judge, E.A.: Multimeasure pain assessment in an ethnically diverse group of patients with cancer. *J. Transcult. Nurs.* 10(2):94–101, 1999.
19. Waitzkin, H.: *The Politics of Medical Encounters: How Patients and Doctors Deal with Social Problems.* New Haven, CT, Yale University Press, 1991.

20. Fineman, N.: The social construction of non-compliance: implications for cross-cultural geriatric practice. *J. Cross-cult. Gerontol.* 6:219–228, 1991.
21. Kauffman, K.S.: The insider/outsider dilemma: field experience of a white researcher "getting in" a poor black community. *Nurs. Res.* 43(3):179–183, 1994.
22. Bushy, A.: Rural determinants in family health: considerations for community nurses. In Bushy, A. (ed.): *Rural Nursing,* Vol. 23. Newbury Park, NY, Sage, 1991, p. 133.
23. Long, K.A.: The concept of health: rural perspectives. *Nurs. Clin. North Am.* 28(1):123–130, 1993; quote on p. 126.
24. Wendell, S.: Toward a feminist theory of disability. In Holmes, H.B. and Purdy, L.M. (eds.): *Feminist Perspectives in Medical Ethics.* Bloomington, Indiana University Press, 1992, pp. 63–81; quote from p. 66.
25. *Care of the Dying: A Catholic Perspective,* St. Louis, The Catholic Health Association of the United States, 1993, p. vii.
26. Haddad, L.G., and Hoeman, S.P.: Home healthcare and the Arab-American client. *Home Healthc. Nurse* 18(3):189–197, quote on p. 192.
27. Eliason, M.J., and Raheim, S.: Experiences and comfort with culturally diverse groups in undergraduate pre-nursing students. *J. Nurs. Educ.* 39(4):161–165.
28. Chrisman, N.J.: Transcultural care. In Zschoke, D. (ed.): *Mosby's Comprehensive Review of Critical Care.* St. Louis, Mosby, 1986, pp. 58–69.
29. McDonagh, M.S.: Cross-cultural communication and pharmaceutical care. *Drug Topics* Sept. 18, 2000, pp. 97–98.
30. Eliason, M.J., and Raheim, S.: Experiences and comfort with culturally diverse groups in undergraduate pre-nursing students. *J. Nurs. Educ.* 39(4):162, 2000.
31. Bechtel, G.A., and Davidhizar, R.E.: Integrating cultural diversity in patient education. *Semin. Nurse Manag.* 7(4):193–197, 1999, quote from p. 194.
32. Meleis, A.I.: Culturally competent care. *J. Transcult. Nurs.* 10(1):12, 1999.

APPENDIX 3–1: Introduction to the Berg Cultural/Spiritual Assessment Tool

by David Berg

The Berg Cultural/Spiritual Assessment Tool is a guide to a patient-focused, scripted dialogue between a provider and patient. It is different from other assessment tools in that it looks at both culture and spirituality simultaneously. These two threads are so delicately woven together in the tapestry of our sacred story and inner journey that we seldom separate them. Only in the Western industrialized world has a sacred-secular split developed. This assessment process allows providers to place a patient within a cultural/spiritual context while recognizing a patient's individual uniqueness at the same time. It assists providers in establishing a trusting therapeutic alliance with their patients, empowers the patient to become a more active participant in their healing journey and helps patients to give voice to their own sacred story. Go through the tool first completing it as a patient would. This allows the provider to become familiar with the process and also to begin to recognize his or her own cultural/spiritual story.

This tool works best when the provider approaches the patient and invites him or her into a one-to-one dialogue using the assessment tool as a scripted interview guide. Whenever possible invite patients to write their own answers to the questions. Sit with them as they go through the process, responding to questions, assisting them when necessary and reframing questions when appropriate. If patients are resistant to a particular question, simply move on to the next question. After they have completed the assessment go back over it with them briefly, summarizing the highlights of the personal story they have shared. Clarify where that is necessary. Have the patient complete question #7 on the summary sheet. This will place them on a cultural continuum and help the provider to better understand their responses to questions on the assessment tool. Summarize the information from the interview on the summary sheet and place the tool on the patient's chart. This process will require an investment of time, but the results make it worthwhile. The tool needs to be adapted for different populations and settings.

There is also a Youth edition of this tool. For further information the author can be reached at: David Berg, 2412 27th Avenue South, Minneapolis, Minnesota 55406; E-mail: davidfberg1990@msn.com.

Berg Cultural/Spiritual Assessment Tool (Adult Edition)

Culture is the total way of life of any group of people. It is the way they learn to think, feel, believe and act. Everyone has a culture. Spirituality is whoever or whatever gives ultimate meaning and purpose in life. This assessment has value only as you are honest. We are interested in getting to know and help you to be respectful of you. We are not intrested in labeling or judging you.

Fill in the best answer(s) in the space provided or circle the best response(s). Leave blank those questions which do not apply.

1) Name _____

2) Date of Birth _____

3) Community where you were born _____

4) Important places you have lived _____

_____

5) What is your cultural/ethnic identity? **(Circle all answers that apply and fill in the blanks when needed. This does not refer to your citizenship.)**

    Native:

        Tribe(s)

Ojibway	Menominee	Pueblo	Cree
Dakota	Mohawk	Navajo	Cherokee
Lakota	Ho-Chunk	Innuit	Other _____

        Band _____

        Clan/Society _____

        Are you an enrolled member?   YES   NO   DO NOT KNOW

    African-American _____   West Indian (country of origin)_____

    African (country of origin) _____   Tribe _____

    Arab (country of origin) _____   Palestinian   Israeli

    Asian

Indian	Hmong	Cambodian	Chinese
Korean	Lao	Vietnamese	Japanese	Other _____

    European American (country of origin) _____

    Hispanic/Latino/Chicano (country of origin)_____   Puerto Rican

    Bi-cultural _____   (e.g., Afro-European, Afro-Asian)

    Tri-cultural _____

    Do you identify with one of these particular groups? Which one?_____

    Other_____

    Do not know cultural identity _____

6) Who raised you?_____

7) Do you have family members or friends who you visit regularly?   YES   NO
  If yes, how often do you spend time with them?_____

8) What language did you learn first? _____

9) Is English the only language spoken in your home?   YES   NO
  If no, what other language(s) is spoken? _____

10) What language(s) do you speak most easily? _____

11) Were you adopted?   YES   NO
  If yes, please indicate your thoughts/feelings about your adoption. _____

_____

12) Within your community, is there a specific group or organization that is important in your life? If so, what is it? _____

_____

13) Have you or your parents immigrated to the U.S. or Canada?   YES   NO
   a) If yes, did you spend any time in a refugee camp?   YES   NO
   b) If yes, did you experience abuse in a refugee camp?   YES   NO
   c) Did someone else in your family spend time in a refugee camp?   YES   NO

14) In your community where you live are most of the people who you do things with members of your cultural/ethnic group?   YES   NO

15) Have you ever been in a place where most of the people were of another cultural identity than yours? YES   NO   If so, what are you feelings? _____

16) Have you ever visited a traditional healer (medicine men/women, shaman, curandero, etc.) for healing?   YES   NO

17) Are there spiritual rituals you participate in for healing purposes?
YES   NO   If so, describe them ____   _____

_____

18) Circle the word which best describes your own sexual identity.
   Straight   Gay/Lesbian   Bisexual   Transgender

19) Name some of your special traditional cultural/ethnic customs (activities) that you regularly participate in (e.g., music, food, dances, holidays, feasts, festivals). _____

_____

20) What are you proud of in your culture? In your culture what means the most to you?

_____

21) What are the words or names you have heard about your cultural identity that have hurt you?

_____

22) Are there experiences you have had which have made you feel uncomfortable with your cultural identity? If yes, please describe _____

_____

23) What religion/spirituality do you practice? (Circle the most accurate answer(s).

Judaism	Muslim	Confucianism	Ancestor Worship
Native	Hindu	Taoism	Satanism
Wicca	Buddhism	Shintoism	Animism
None	Other_____		Christian: Protestant Catholic
			(What church?) _____

24) What are the traditional religious/spiritual practices, customs, and holidays in which you participate?

_____

_____

25) If you are Christian, have you been baptized?   YES   NO   DO NOT KNOW

Figure continued on following page

26) If you are Native, have you participated in a traditional naming ceremony and received an Indian name?
 YES   NO   What is it? _____

27) If you are Jewish,   a) have you been bar/bat mitzvahed or confirmed? YES   NO
                         b) do you live in a kosher home?   YES   NO

28) If you are Muslim,   a) have you taken the shahadah?   YES   NO
                         b) do you have a Muslim name?   YES   NO

29) Do your children have the same religious/spiritual beliefs?   YES   NO   DO NOT KNOW
 If no, please explain _____
 _____

30) List at least two caring people who you trust. a) _____
 b) _____

31) How do they show their care for you? _____
 _____

32) What is something you have done which gives you a sense of healthy pride? _____
 _____
 _____

33) Give an example of when you acted independently in a healthy way _____
 _____
 _____

34) What's one thing you have done to help someone else without pay? _____
 _____
 _____

35) How did you feel after the above experience? _____
 _____

36) What gives you hope? _____
 _____

37) I pray (circle all the answers that apply)
 a) often   b) when I'm in trouble   c) at bedtime
 d) when I feel thankful   e) in the morning   f) when I eat
 g) five times a day   h) never   i) sometimes

38) During the past year I felt close to my Higher Power/God/Universe (circle all the answers that apply)
 a) in the church/synagogue/mosque b) in a sweat lodge   c) never
 d) listening to music   e) alone in quiet   f) in nature
 g) with special friends   h) during troubled times   i) with family
 j) on the streets   k) other _____

39) Who or what has the most influence in your life today? _____

40) What gives meaning and purpose to your life? _____
 _____

41) Is there a spiritual/religious group that nurtures and supports you?   YES   NO
 If yes, what is the group? _____

42) Describe personal practices you follow to stay in good health.
 _____
 _____
 _____

43) Is there anything else that your health care provider should know?
 _____
 _____
 _____

44) If someone helped you complete this assessment, were you satisfied with their help?   YES   NO

Cultural /Spiritual Assessment Summary

Name_____ Date_____

This Cultural/Spiritual Assessment was completed by_____

Please update as indicated.

1) Cultural Identity

2) Spiritual Identity

3) Sexual Identity

4) Cultural / Spiritual Mentors

5) Client Cultural / Spiritual Strengths

6) Cultural/Spiritual Loss / Separation / Struggles

7) Client position on cultural continuum; check all the following that apply.

      _____ follows only traditional culture

      _____ is isolated and/or alienated from dominant culture

      _____ rejects traditional culture as evidenced by adopting external features of dominant culture; for example, style of clothes, behavior patterns and habits, changes in values, etc.

      _____ lives in two worlds (is accepting of dominant culture while maintaining important attachments to traditional culture)

      _____ lives without particular cultural awareness

      _____ is primarily influenced by the dominant US culture

8) Recommendations for Treatment

9) Considerations for Post-Treatment

10) Recommendations for Spiritual Care

PART ONE

Questions for Thought and Discussion

1. In what important ways is professional education similar to and different from other types of formal education?

2. Review the characteristics of a profession. Apply these characteristics to your particular profession. Which do you meet? Which do not seem to apply? Why?

3. You are the supervisor of an ambulatory clinic. You recognize an increase in the number of recent immigrants from Kosovo in your patient population. What should you do to prepare your staff to care for these patients?

4. Some native American Indians and native Hawaiians see illness as part of a harmony-disharmony pattern for which actions of family members are responsible. How might this view of illness affect your work with these patients?

5. Your first encounter with a health care institution is in your professional education program. It has policies and regulations regarding your interactions with faculty and peers. Obtain copies of these documents and discuss how they facilitate or hinder respectful interaction.

6. You are treating a 24-year-old woman whose diagnosis is cervical cancer. You do not know if she is aware of her diagnosis. One day she asks you to get her medical chart for her from the nursing desk. "The 'Bill of Rights for Patients' in this hospital says that I have a right to accurate information and I figure that is where I will get it." What will you say to her? What will you do? Why?

PART TWO

Respect for Yourself

Part Two focuses on you, the health professional, as an individual, because a key to all respectful human interaction lies in respecting yourself through better understanding. When you and your colleagues enter the health professions you bring with you your own unique combination of abilities, needs, values, and fantasies. As we discussed in Chapter 1, you expect to incorporate these into the positions you will assume as health professionals.

Chapter 4 addresses your student experiences. The questions asked in this chapter are fundamental to promoting respect for yourself in the health professions: "What is professional education?" "What is expected of me during this period of professional preparation?" "How does it affect me as a person?"

Chapter 5 focuses on respect for yourself as you assume a professional role. Although not all health professions place people in the role of direct patient or client contact, some of the most challenging aspects of professional life are in the clinical setting when one is acting as a professional "helper." A health professional's attitudes toward and understanding of the clinical setting influence the effectiveness of interaction with patients. The role of the health professional as one of a whole matrix of persons caring for a patient is examined, with attention devoted to the importance of being a good player on the health care "team." Newer dimensions of interaction (e.g., through computer technologies) also are examined.

Chapter 6 discusses the joys and challenges of maintaining healthful attitudes and behaviors during your lifetime, emphasizing ways to help you retain your satisfaction with your choice of profession. Included are sections on how to make time for yourself, how to develop good work habits, and how to utilize the strengths of the community of persons with whom you will work.

By the end of Part Two, you should be better able to view yourself as respectfully as others will in your several possible roles as a health professional.

CHAPTER 4

Respect for Yourself as a Student

CHAPTER OBJECTIVES

The student will be able to

- Identify three kinds of learning that take place during professional preparation
- Identify the environment in which each kind of learning takes place
- Explain similarities and differences between the classroom and on-site settings of professional preparation
- Identify four types of skills associated with professional practice
- Name eight steps in acquiring skills needed for professional practice
- List five procedures that should assist the student in adjusting to the on-site education phase of professional preparation
- Describe the characteristics of critical thinking and their role in professional problem-solving
- Evaluate several sources of student anxiety and some methods of addressing it effectively

"I'm a student nurse," I began by way of introduction. "Could we sit down somewhere and talk?"

Ann led the way with shaky steps to a small table and two chairs. Ruth followed us and stood behind her mother and played with her necklaces.

I asked Ann, "How long have you had this shakiness?"

"Started two days ago," Ann replied.

"Has this happened before?"

"Sometimes, but not this bad."

I had seen a few patients react to antipsychotic drugs this way, but not this severely. At least I thought it was a reaction to the medication. Maybe Ann drank as well, I didn't know how to ask her if she did . . .

A. Haddad

HOW THE DESIRE TO HELP WILL HELP YOU

Most students know that they would like to be able to help people when they apply for a place in an education program for a health profession. They also know that they may have moments when they will feel very uncertain of how to proceed to accomplish that end, like the student nurse above who is in her first semester of working in a home setting. Often, although not always, this desire arises because students have had the experience of their own illness or injury and have been helped by a professional whom they have come to admire or a friend or loved one was ill and dying, and health professionals showed able assistance and compassion in caring for the person.

Sometimes the desire to help is nurtured by a student's recognition that he or she has a talent for being a good listener or for helping friends when they are in trouble. Other students have actually had an opportunity to save another person's life or in other ways have intervened constructively, and that experience has been instrumental in their desire to be of service.

The desire to help is not always the primary or only factor that leads people to choose a career as a health professional. Love of science, the desire to be in a "people-oriented" line of work, the desire for status, and a career that promises to provide a good salary and high satisfaction are other important and understandable motivators. However, the desire to help is probably the factor that will most assist a student in staying true to his or her course of study when the going gets rough. One of the best "survival tactics" during professional education is to identify early on a teacher or other professional role model who manifests the spirit of generosity that is so central to being a helpful person, and be in touch with that person frequently.

HOW DO I BECOME AN EXPERT?

Preparation for work in the health fields is different from that for other fields. While students in other programs of study are partying on Friday afternoon, the health professions student may be at the clinic or laboratory carrying out an education internship or field work requirement; while roommates are still trying to get out of bed in the morning, it is not unusual for the health professions student to be on the way out the door; and, while most careers do not require students to adopt a set of "professional" attitudes, behaviors, and ethical guidelines, the health professions do.

Education in the health professions is preparation for carrying out a lifelong commitment and for realizing a certain type of lifestyle. Identity as a health professional carries with it expectations on the part of society, as well as privileges and responsibilities. You will be considered an "expert" in your field, but more than that, as a professional you will be looked on as a person whose knowledge, skills, and attitudes can make the world a better place and improve individuals' lives. In choosing to be a health professional, you are in essence deciding on the types of activities that will take up the best energy of the best days of your life. The preparation, then, is central not only to what you will do but also who you will become in your own eyes and in the eyes of others.

What can a health professions student expect during the years of formal education? Three types of learning experiences will predominate: the acquisition of basic concepts and theories, the mastery of professional skills, and the attainment of attitudes appropriate to one's role as a health professional. Each will have its place in the preparation for effective and respectful interaction with patients, colleagues, and society.

The following pages discuss these three areas of learning (knowledge as theoretical concepts, skills, and attitudes) to help you understand more fully why you are asked to pursue particular learning activities in the classroom or other professional setting.

Knowledge (Theoretical Concepts)

Traditionally, education in the health professions required knowledge of the classics and, as the scientific age developed, basic sciences. Today, the foundation of required knowledge is much broader.

What knowledge does a person need to become a competent health professional? Knowledge in the sciences still provides a foundation for understanding the body and the natural forces acting on it, and knowledge in the behavioral sciences of psychology, sociology, and anthropology provides understanding of people's needs and behaviors and of how these needs and behaviors affect interaction. Knowledge in the liberal arts exposes one to the great political, religious, and philosophical ideas and establishes one's own link with history. An awareness of pertinent economic and legal concepts allows one to practice more competently in the complex world of health care institutions today. Knowledge of statistics and computers furnishes a baseline for research design and other data analysis and communication functions. Theoretical knowledge underlying the techniques relevant to one's profession lays the foundation for applying specific professional skills.

Knowledge can be acquired effectively and efficiently in a classroom setting or through independent study. In the classroom, large numbers of people can listen to one lecturer impart information and answer questions; discussions may readily follow. Each individual can then supplement the lecture and discussion material with as much outside study as he or she deems necessary. The student's grasp of the material can be determined by written or oral examination. If the only type of learning needed for professional competence were acquisition and integration of knowledge, there would be no need to include extensive laboratory experience or clinical education in the preparation of health care providers. Already one begins to see that education for professional health care practice is different from the formal preparation for most other careers.

Skills

At the time they enter their professional curriculum, students are usually more accustomed to classroom learning than to laboratory and clinical learning. In the years of professional preparation, more time in the laboratory and clinic is required for the acquisition of skills. The student's acquisition of all the skills needed for professional practice creates the milieu in which he or she will be able to exercise independent professional judgment. This type of independent functioning is one mark of a true professional. Only with experience will full mastery of a skill be realized, but all components for enabling that mastery must be presented in the professional preparation period.

The acquisition of skill often requires long, tedious hours of practice. The frustration that sometimes accompanies mastering a skill was illustrated in a story related by a friend who was trying to teach her 7-year-old daughter how to use cross-country skis. They came to a hill, and the mother gave the child explicit instructions about how to position her body, hold the poles, and maneuver the skis to succeed in this new challenge. Next, the mother demonstrated the process. The child, who had been watching intently, pushed off down the slope and immediately fell. Reflecting on the experience, the mother said, "I forgot to tell her, 'If you do everything exactly as I do it, and then fall the first few times you try it, you'll be able to do it.' " Likewise, a student who observes an apparently simple skill may find that it takes weeks of repetition to master that skill and avoid regrettable mistakes.

Consider the following four basic skills needed for competence in a health profession.

Technical Skill. This is the ability to safely and effectively apply a given technique to secure a diagnosis, conduct an evaluation, or provide a treatment. The medical technologist analyzes the contents of a sample of blood or other body fluids. The physical therapist conducts a gait analysis to determine what is needed to restore optimal functioning. The respiratory therapist identifies and regulates the output of the proper balance of gases. In each case, mastery includes an intricate coordination of mind and body, as well as the exercise of sound judgment. The application of techniques requires skillful management of oneself, and of the technical equipment of one's profession.

Skill in Interpersonal Relationships and Communication. A health professional interacts with a wide variety of people during the course of a day: other health professionals, support personnel, patients or clients and their families, students, visitors, administrators, and business contacts such as professional equipment salespersons. This activity demands that the health professional understand appropriate conduct in different types of relationships. It means being able to accept responsibility as a supervisor and constructive criticism as one who is supervised. It involves learning what caring means in the professional role and demands tact, diplomacy, consistency, and forthrightness. It also requires listening as if your patient's or client's life depended on your hearing—and it may! Much of this book focuses on the means whereby you can gain and exhibit skills in communication. We will especially focus on this in Chapter 10.

Teaching and Administrative Skill. There are numerous teaching and administrative opportunities for health professionals. Education of individual patients or clients and the larger public is essential in virtually every health field today. Whatever your choice of profession, you will probably be required to engage in educational activities geared to patients or clients, families, students, other health professionals, and support personnel. Administrative skills also are essential. Among the tasks requiring such skills are the following: (1) organization and implementation of workable solutions to potential problems; (2) setting reasonable short- and long-term goals for the department or other workplace setting; (3) fair, objective evaluation of oneself and others; (4) wise allocation of equipment and supplies; and (5) maintenance of a cost-effective operation.

Research Skill. Skill in research is required to develop a good research question, design a project, formulate a hypothesis, and collect and analyze data to determine whether the hypothesis is correct. In the past, the health professions have relied on findings from this *quantitative* type of research. In addition, *qualitative* research is conducted today and may require the conduction and interpretation of in-depth interviews or other narratives designed to highlight important areas of understanding about the type of problem or phenomenon at hand. Highly specialized or simple equipment available within a health facility may be utilized. Honest, accurate reporting of findings is imperative to ensure high standards of practice. As today's students enter practice, their reimbursement will be based on scientific evidence; thus, the term "evidence-based practice." Research will confirm that an intervention effectively fulfills the intended goal.

To understand better how students usually acquire the skills for professional practice, consider the following steps. The student

1. Acquires knowledge related to the skill
2. Experiences the skill applied to himself or herself
3. Applies the skill to a classmate
4. Observes a professional person using the skill
5. Assists the professional person in using the skill
6. Is closely supervised in the first attempts to use the skill alone
7. Satisfactorily uses the skill in a variety of situations, with decreasing amounts of direct supervision
8. Is tested for safe application and beginning mastery of the skill

Note the progression from classroom to professional setting in this process. Number 1 can easily take place in a classroom, on a computer, or with the help of a programmed text; numbers 2 and 3 must take place in the skills laboratory. Numbers 4 through 8 take place in the workplace setting where a variety of situations are available, perhaps initially with simulated patients/clients and then with "real patients" and decreasing amounts of direct supervision. Thus, the basics needed to assume eventual mastery of professional skills require that only a part of the training be in the classroom.

As a student, you should expect to encounter appropriate teaching styles and type and amount of supervision during the various steps of your professional preparation. The greatest challenge to educators is to shape their approaches to guarantee that you acquire the skills you will need. It is their moral obligation to provide you with this guidance at each step of your professional preparation.[2]

Attitudes and Character

During your student years, efforts are made to teach and reinforce attitudes that will prepare you well for professional service. Many of them are related to the necessity of cultivating approaches that are devoid of the negative biases discussed in Chapter 3. Consider the following questions related to attitudes.

1. Do you consider yourself a helper? Under what conditions might you resent having to help? How do you expect people to respond to you after you have done your best to help them?

2. How do you react to a person who is mentally or physically impaired? Do you feel pity? Embarrassment? Discomfort? Compassion? All of these?

3. What qualities of life make it worth living? Are most older people more ready to die than younger people? Would some people be better off dead? If you were to become seriously ill or have a serious accident, what changes in your present status would be the most difficult to accept? Why? How will this affect your response to people who are facing adjustment to such changes?

Your attitudes toward helping, the qualities that you believe make life worth living, and your own personal integrity, discussed in later chapters, are among the most central to your success as a professional.

One important attitude to acquire or cultivate during your student years is a love of learning itself; it is best planted during this period if it is to flourish in later years. This attitude can actually have a strong bearing on your success as a professional. May described ten characteristics required for success in the health professions, identified through a study at the University of Wisconsin–Madison. Among them was a *commitment to learning;* described as the ability to self-assess, self-correct, and self-direct as well as the willingness to continually seek new knowledge and understanding.[3] Unfortunately, the competitive nature of some academic programs and the "drive" instilled in many young people today to succeed may take the joy out of learning and replace it with attitudes of anger or resentment for having to study all the time. Faculty and students should work together to avoid this catastrophe. The sense of adventure in approaching an unknown horizon of professionalism should govern your experience. Taylor Caldwell, in *The Sound of Thunder,* said of learning, "It is life's greatest adventure; it is an illustrated excursion into the minds of noble and learned men, not a conducted tour through a jail. So its surroundings should be as gracious as possible, to complement it."[4] The physical environment should be an encouragement too. Institutions in which professional education takes place must take responsibility to make the student work and leisure environment conducive to learning through design of the building inside and out. Students have a responsibility to help maintain it too, by treating it as a resource to be respected.

ON-SITE EDUCATION: NEW CHALLENGES

You should now be familiar with three kinds of learning that take place during professional preparation: knowledge, skills, and attitude/character formation. In addition, you know the environments in which each kind of learning most efficiently and effectively takes place. With this baseline, you are ready to explore the nature of the relationship between classroom and on-site professional education.

On-site education is called by different names in different professions. It may be called clinical education, clinical fieldwork, clinical clerkships, rotations, or internships. On-site education introduces the student to the peculiarities of the work environment. The quality and quantity of teaching that take place are determined by such wide-ranging and unpredictable variables as the availability of patients or clients and the availability of other professionals who can monitor and guide the students. This learning environment is much less controlled than that in the classroom. New smells, sounds, and sights combine with new tasks to present a weighty challenge to the best of classroom students. Almost all students find it the most exciting part of their educational experience, and faculty who work on-site as teachers and supervisors benefit from the opportunity, too. Refinement is one of the most important functions of on-site education. Refinement implies that the student has the basic materials with which to work, but new materials will be introduced to improve on the "basics" by introducing subtleties, gracefulness, and efficiency. The basic materials consist of the person's own individual qualities and previous learning. The new materials include (1) large numbers of patients or clients with different problems, (2) several manifestations of a single pathological condition, (3) time limitations, (4) multiple professional responsibilities related to the work environment (e.g., documentation and participating in staff meetings), and (5) assimilation of particular techniques into workable evaluation or treatment programs. The desired outcome is the competent professional person.

There is inherent wisdom in getting off to a good start in any new venture, and a few practical guidelines apply to a student who is beginning the new venture into on-site education. A general rule is to acknowledge that one is entering an environment that has its own players, peculiarities, and habits. Respect for the fact that the student is in someone else's territory is key. Fortunately, most educators in the on-site setting extend themselves to try to help students feel accepted, but the student may find the situation awkward anyway, at least initially. It is rather like going into someone else's home and being told to "make yourself at home." It takes time to be able to feel at home, no matter what the host or hostess says. When awkwardness is present, neither timidity nor arrogant self-assurance will serve the student or the educational process well. We remember a medical student telling us about her awkwardness at the nurse's station on her first clinical rotation. She had received a thorough orientation from her physician supervisor, who then left.

> I just stood at the nurse's station waiting for someone to ask me what I wanted or tell me what to do. Nobody paid any attention to me. I felt like I was at the grocery store, wanting to check out, but nobody noticed that I was there. It was awful.

At the other extreme, one of us observed a nursing student at a large university hospital treating the staff nurses and office personnel with sheer rudeness. Later, he said that he could not understand why he had felt like an intruder at the nurse's station when he was almost "one of them." It was quite obvious to observe that it was because he was acting like an intruder. Both of these students could have been helped by following a few simple suggestions. The amount of discomfort can be greatly, perhaps completely, diminished by the following procedures:

1. Always introduce yourself to the key players, even those who do not seem to be "important."
2. Try to assess in advance the usual protocols and ways of doing things in this setting.
3. Ask explicit questions about the expectations of the supervisor.
4. Assume that some people will be suspicious or perplexed by a newcomer, and prepare to respond to their questions or comments in a nondefensive and instructive manner.
5. Assume that everyone basically wants you there, in your role. They would not have you there if they were not invested in your learning. If you have any reason to believe otherwise, you should discuss it with your faculty advisor.

In on-site education, a good general rule is to follow some of the same etiquette expected of a good houseguest. Busy staff do notice when someone comes in and participates politely in the work that has to be done. Taking part in the ongoing life of the work environment is viewed as a positive contribution: the student is seen as an effective team member. Therefore, act as if you are a member of the staff's team by showing genuine interest in their work, their professional challenges, and especially in the patients' or clients' well-being. The awkwardness of the setting almost always gives way to a sense of belonging when a student takes this type of initiative.

During the on-site educational experience, the moments of awkwardness decrease as independence and responsibility mount. In this phase of your education, you are learning the maneuvers that enable you to proceed deftly toward the goal of full professional competence.

CRITICAL THINKING: AN ESSENTIAL TOOL

The primary purpose of any health professional education is to prepare students adequately for their responsibilities in their chosen profession. As we have noted, one important part of this preparation is to ensure that the student has factual knowledge, adequate skills, and appropriate attitudes to perform activities, at first with supervision and then alone. But, even with the most comprehensive preparation, there will be details that will not be included. Furthermore, as advances in the health sciences continue, some things imparted in your basic education will not be correct. Therefore, health professionals must be able to review and update knowledge and skills not presented in their basic education.

The Art of Critical Thinking

To successfully meet challenges that are novel or unexpected requires the ability to think critically. Obviously this text cannot provide complete training in critical thinking. It is even questionable if it would be possible to develop a "how-to" manual in critical thinking. It is worth the effort, however, to take some time to present guidelines to the art of critical thinking and to specifically focus on one aspect, that of detecting emotional and psychological factors people sometimes use to win arguments or prove a point.

Critical thinking requires time and silence. Just as we exercise our bodies, we need time to exercise our minds. Initially, you might find that your mind is quite undisciplined and jumps from one idea to the next with little pattern or coherence. After a while, it is possible to see familiar themes in our thoughts. We must also guard against the common misconception that merely thinking is wasting time.

Critical thinkers are neutral toward the environments in which they find themselves. This does not mean that they are uninterested. It means that they are able to view the place and people in a situation objectively and to take in the whole of the experience.

Critical thinkers can size up a situation, get to the point of what is happening, and observe general principles behind the specifics of circumstances. As will be noted many times in this text, listening carefully to what people are trying to tell you is an invaluable skill in the interaction between health professional and patient.

Listening is also essential to critical thinking to move from personal perspectives to the perspectives of others involved in a clinical situation.

Psychological Factors in Critical Thinking

The practice of health care also involves the ability to discern credible, logical reasons that people use to justify their views or recommendations from those that are illogical and emotional. This is not to say that emotions are trivial or should be suppressed. However, without thought, feelings can cause one to lose perspective. A common device used to avoid rational arguments and to persuade others emotionally is a logical fallacy. A fallacy is an incorrect way of reasoning. People use illogical thinking and wild leaps from one thought to another because they do not pay attention. It is easier than the demands of concentrated thought, and emotional arguments are generally more compelling initially than logical ones.

Although the list of the types of fallacies is long, two are the most common. Because sustained attention to clarity and the flow of an argument are difficult, many people commit the dual fallacies of being ambiguous and jumping to hasty conclusions. One commits the fallacy of ambiguity by not defining key terms. Complex problems require complex terms that are open to a variety of interpretations and that need definition for the parties involved to understand each other. Individuals who do not listen well in the first place may hear only the last thing that has been said and thus steer the argument in a totally different and unconnected direction, resulting in a hasty, and perhaps harmful, conclusion.

These components of critical thinking—sensitivity to illogical arguments, good listening skills, and the ability to transcend the present and see general principles—can be learned and practiced in all facets of life, not just professional life.

FINDING MEANING IN THE STUDENT ROLE

The stresses that students face often are directly related to the transitional nature of their position: they are not fully professional but are beyond being a lay person. The process of going from being a classroom student to an "intern" on-site to a full professional means you are constantly changing roles. In trying to find your exact function on the health care team, you may find that students are sometimes "put in their place" by patients and professionals alike. A case in point involves a nursing student who mustered the courage to call a physician to clarify a medication order. Although the student had identified herself at the outset of the call, when she finished sharing her concerns the physician responded, "Okay, you may have a point. Now put a real nurse on the line and let me talk with her." That kind of response hurts, no matter how confident you might have felt when you made the call. This grey zone of being "betwixt and between" gives rise to some of the types of anxiety we explore next.

Why Do I Feel Anxious?

The bad news is that most anxiety directly arising from the pressures of student life is difficult to avoid completely since much is due to the transitory role of students. The good news is that most of it will pass for the same reason! However, for many students, at least three serious questions may be the focus of anxiety, and each is worth attending to. The first is "Am I/can I get prepared well enough to pass the courses and complete the degree requirements?" This type of insecurity is most evident just before an exam, and when you can attach your anxiety to something as concrete as an exam, it is possible to deal with it. (Usually we test whether we are indeed competent enough by actually taking the exam!) The second question, "Do I have what it takes?" is rather like the first but is more fundamental. It may arise from the troublesome suspicion that other students and your professional models have qualities that you seem to lack or from the fact that you have responsibilities that compete for your attention.

Both questions may be related to your assessment of your intellectual or moral capacities as well as to your physical or emotional limits. They are questions often asked by students who fail an exam or experience the rather common reaction of feeling faint the first time they see a badly injured patient, observe surgery, or are unexpectedly overwhelmed by a noxious odor.

The third question is "Can I afford to stay in school?" Many students feel burdened by the financial demands that an education places on them and their families. Anxiety about having to take another loan or find a job or the possibility of having to drop out of school altogether is more common than is sometimes supposed.

Anxieties related directly to student life affect many students' performance. However, anxieties arising from nonstudent issues also can impinge on student success when one fails an exam or cannot concentrate on course work or must miss important sessions. An impending divorce, either one's own or that of one's parents or child, an unwanted pregnancy, the news that a loved one is seriously ill—these and many other problems can influence a person's performance dramatically.

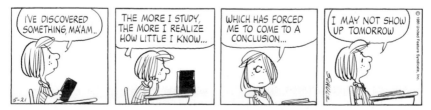

PEANUTS © NEA. Reprinted by permission.

Some students worry about their choice of profession. This is understandable: it is a big decision. Pressures on young people to decide what they are going to be lead many to choose a career early in life, sometimes as early as junior high school. At the same time, a growing number of students who have raised children or spent many years in another line of work also are choosing formal education in the health professions. Their anxiety often springs from the belief that they are acting on their last chance to realize a dream, may be too old to compete in a job market apparently geared to the young, or are not giving enough time to family.

Much is at stake in making the correct judgment about a field of study. In short, both younger and older students are confronted by a dilemma faced by able, highly qualified students in every field. You may not only ask, "Is this what I want?" but also ponder the far more difficult question, "Is this what I want more than the other good opportunities open to me?"

How Can I Respond Constructively to Anxiety?

Most students do go through a skeptical, questioning phase. You can do several things to respond well and go on to enjoy your choice of life's work:

Identify the Source. One of the most important steps in dissipating the destructive tension associated with anxiety is to identify the source of the anxiety. However, this is not always easy and may require help from someone else.

Share Feelings with a Friend or Trustworthy Classmate. The sting of anxiety is that it can alienate you from others who know that you are acting strangely but do not know why. If you discuss the anxiety and try to get at the root of it, you have overcome the powerful feeling of isolation of the experience. An amazing side effect of this process is that you may find out how common these feelings are. By knowing that others, too, are feeling the same anxiety, you feel less "crazy" or "out of joint" with the world.

Seek Professional Help. Sometimes talking with a friend is not adequate, and you may benefit from the help of a professional. In such cases, usually a few minutes with an instructor or counselor will help you discover why you feel anxious and depressed. In other instances, the treatment for anxiety may require an extended course of intervention over weeks or months. Sometimes counseling with a professional provides insights into the breadth of possibility available in the field. For instance, the student who does not enjoy the treatment or evaluation activities of his or her chosen profession may enjoy research, teaching, design, administration, writing, or consulting in the same general field. The family member concerned about the hours required at the workplace may find that another profession allows for more regularity and control over schedules. Because of the many opportunities open to the health professional, it is highly likely that the choice of a vocation in the health professions was a wise one.

In all of these methods, the key to decreasing anxiety, once its source is identified, is to attend to it so that it does not ruin what would otherwise be an exciting adventure.

REAPING THE REWARDS OF PERSEVERANCE

This chapter, focusing on student life of health professionals, would be incomplete without a short postscript on the rewards of persevering.

The health professions continue to be among the most rewarding and challenging careers available today. Most educational programs select from a large pool of applicants, ensuring the high quality of the peers with whom you will spend your professional career. The opportunity for personal growth and professional advancement is high in almost all health profession fields. The daily work is varied and engaging. When you complete your formal study, there will be an awareness of how you can help to make the life of another person, indeed the lives of many other persons, better. Fortunately, students usually do learn how to celebrate the successful completion of various aspects of their journey by end-of-term parties, post-exam indulgences, and other markers. The educational programs themselves contribute through milestone events such as events after the board exam, pinning or capping ceremonies, and, of course, commencement. The more reminders you can give yourself along the way, the better! Because the rewards of persevering to the end are many, the following chapters are designed to assist you in maximizing the wealth of experiences open to persons in the health professions. Read on, and plan for a fine future.

SUMMARY

This chapter highlights some fundamental challenges, anxieties, and anticipations faced during the student years, each of which contributes to the complex and demanding journey traveled in pursuit of your goal to become a health professional. It also provides guidelines for helping to get past the barriers when the going gets rough. The emphasis on preparedness through the acquisition of knowledge, skills, and ennobling attitudes should help you remain focused on why you are here reading this book in the first place. Your goals should be to enjoy the student role, be prepared for its challenges when they come, understand it, and then leave it respectfully behind for your new life as a professional.

REFERENCES

1. Haddad, A.: Spring semester. In Haddad, A. M. and Brown, K. H. (eds.): *The Arduous Touch: Women's Voices in Health Care*. West Lafayette, IN, NotaBell Books/Purdue University Press, 1999, p. 116.
2. Purtilo, R., Shaw, B., and Arnold, R.: Obligations of surgeons to team members. In McCullough, L., Jones, J. and Brody, B. (eds.): *Surgical Ethics*. New York, Oxford University Press, 1998, pp. 302–321.
3. May, W., Morgan, B., Lemke, J., et al. Model for ability-based assessment in physical therapy education. *J. Phys. Ther. Educ.* 9:1–2, 1995.
4. Caldwell, T.: *The Sound of Thunder*. New York, Doubleday, 1957, p. 19.

CHAPTER 5

Respect for Yourself in Your Professional Capacity

CHAPTER OBJECTIVES

The student will be able to

- Distinguish between the characteristics of being an intimate and a personal helper
- Compare important aspects of social and therapeutic helping relationships, describing why maintaining this distinction in everyday practice affects your self-respect as a professional
- Identify some mechanisms for assuring optimal care when your own areas of competence do not allow you to fully meet a person's health care needs
- List four criteria for referral of patients
- List some strengths and potential problems inherent in the team approach
- Identify and discuss two respect-enhancing goals that the interdisciplinary health care team approach is designed to meet
- Compare the values realized through team decisions that are hierarchy derived and those that are community-derived
- Describe conditions that enable you to realize self-respect through lifelong learning habits

---

The goal of health professional education is to assist students in becoming a professional. What does it mean to "be professional"? Much has been written elsewhere about that question. Suffice it to say here that any description of a professional would contain the integration of a body of knowledge and skills and the proficient and effective delivery of the same. The authors believe that in the profession of health care, proficient and effective delivery requires a "therapeutic use of one's self" while interacting with clients.

If health care consisted of "working on bodies" alone, perhaps a consideration of the self would not be necessary. But the fact remains that health care involves people interacting with people....

C.M. Davis[1]

As this quote suggests, the result of years of professional preparation as a student is that you will become prepared to take action by enabling people to remain in or regain good health and be relieved of suffering when they have not been able to avoid the ravages of illness or injury or the deleterious effects of aging or their environment.

Although health professionals work in many environments, the term "clinician" usually is used to specify aspects of their work that involve care of patients or clients. Thus, this chapter continues on the course of following you from your role as a student in the classroom and in on-site training to that of a person with full professional capacity.

In this chapter we briefly introduce you to several professional capacities that, if nurtured, will serve you well. These include being in a position to help, being able to engage in certain activities that distinguish your everyday relationships from professional ones, and having the opportunity to use some mechanisms for increasing your effectiveness through shared responsibility with team members. We conclude with a final section on the valuable resource of lifelong learning. Together these capacities will also help assure that you will experience deep satisfaction and self-respect in your professional roles.

DEVELOPING YOUR CAPACITY TO HELP

In the traditional use of the term, the "helping professions" referred only to those that provided prolonged, one-to-one contact with patients. Today, the usage has been expanded to include all health professionals, whether their skills are used in direct person-to-person contact or in working through others, because the overall goal is to benefit individuals in society. Therefore, the way you use your capacities to help others will affect the self-respect you will enjoy over the course of your professional life. One important dimension of such development is to learn to distinguish between intimate and personal modes of helping.

Intimate versus Personal Help

Helping ranges from performing highly intimate acts to performing simple, personal ones, depending on the depth of involvement in which you engage another person. Intimate help is what you offer to someone whom you love deeply or for whom you are willing to do a big favor. The offer of intimate help in its most extreme form means that you would be willing to risk danger to yourself for this person. In contrast, personal help is what you are willing to offer acquaintances or strangers when giving directions, assisting a person physically, or donating money to a good cause. Personal help demands an investment in the well-being of others but should be distinguished from intimate involvement, the latter of which is reserved for families and close friends. Professional helping falls within the category of personal rather than intimate helping.

Social Helping Relationships

A related way to view helping relationships concentrates on the tools and activities used rather than on the degree of involvement with the other person. Any help in which your resources for providing help are not specific, well-defined, professional skills can be called social helping. Social helping takes many forms because the number of tools for helping are as infinite as one's own resources. One helps a child cross the street, one helps lessen an old man's loneliness by paying him a visit, or one helps a neighbor in need by lending her five dollars. This type of helping stems from an unselfish or "altruistic" motive of wanting to benefit someone else. There is an interesting and growing body of literature in the field of evolutionary psychology that debates whether we have an *inherent* inclination to express caring or compassion.[2]

Others' offers of help seem to grow out of a desire to fulfill their own needs.[3] Persons with functional impairments often are victims of those whose desire to fulfill their own needs reaches neurotic proportions.

A sobering example of this was related by a health professions student. On weekends, the student cared for a 13-year-old boy with paraplegia who ambulated with the help of a wheelchair. One Saturday, the student and boy

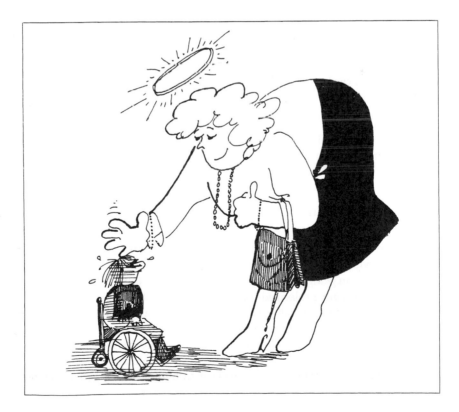

way the help is perceived by others. Recall Chapter 3: negative personal and cultural bias and the danger of prejudicial attitudes or discriminatory behavior create barriers to genuine caring. The patient's personality, motives, and other characteristics have power to influence how health professionals respond, as is evident in the following case:

> When Eddy Underhill was admitted to the Veterans Affairs Medical Center again, no one was surprised. He was well known to the staff in the emergency room and to most of the personnel who had been there for any length of time, and none of them were glad to see him. Eddy lived in a furnished room in the poorest section of town, where his veteran's pension was enough to cover his rent plus enough alcohol to keep him drunk almost all the time. Occasionally, he would spend money on food, but never if it meant going without booze.
>
> This time he was admitted with impending delirium tremens, a life-threatening condition resulting from alcohol withdrawal. Often such admissions would occur toward the end of the month when his money ran out, and scavenging could not net him enough money to keep him drinking. Other times he was admitted for pneumonia, contracted after spending a winter night unconscious in the gutter, or bleeding from esophageal varices, or trauma from falling on the street or being beaten up by thugs.
>
> Jesse Sampson, a young chaplain who had recently begun working at the hospital, started to visit Eddy after his acute withdrawal symptoms had subsided. Eddy had some degree of brain damage from chronic alcohol abuse but was garrulous and enjoyed "shooting the breeze" with this young man who came to see him every day. Chaplain Sampson was very different from the doctors and nurses at the hospital, who spent as little time as possible with Eddy. The chaplain would sit down in a chair next to the bed as if he was not in a hurry to be somewhere else. He would ask Eddy questions about himself and his life as if he really cared about the answers. Eddy told Jesse that booze was his only friend and that his life was lonely, but seemed warmer and more convivial when he was drunk. He had no family. His friends were the other people on skid row. He had no ambitions. Life was hard and pretty senseless, and he just wanted to get through it as easily as he could. He appreciated being brought to the hospital when he was in really bad shape. There it was warm, and he got decent food, but most of the people treated him with thinly veiled disgust. This often made him angry. "I'm a gomer [get out of my emergency room], you know. They hate my kind, but they can't come right out and say so, so they try to ignore me. They wish I would die, and sometime I will. Would serve 'em right. But they won't care—they'll just keep on goin' about their prissy and proud ways. They think they are so good hearted, but they don't know what it's like to live on the street. To be alone with

your only friend, the bottle. It's my life and I got a right to do what I want. I served my time in the war, and I got a right to be in this hospital, to come in here and get dried out and get a little food. I'm an old man. I got a right."[5]

How many sources of potential negative bias can you identify in this story? Mr. Underhill is the type of patient who can cause much consternation for health professionals. The example set by the chaplain is not always easy to follow, although most would applaud the chaplain's caring approach. What would *you* do to try to help this patient? What things about him would you find difficult to accept?

This dramatic instance is not the only type of challenge you will encounter. For example, some patients who initially seek your services seem to resist any kind of help, even though you judge that the services offered should benefit them. For these patients, receiving help may be seen as a sign of weakness, even though their suffering has driven them to your door. Other types of patients might surprise you. Sometimes people who are lonely do not comply with your efforts to help because if they do they will lose the benefit of your company. (For some major challenges patients face, see Chapter 7.) These and other examples highlight the fact that the wish to help is not always easily accomplished.

Carl Rogers, a psychologist who studied relationships in depth, defined a positive helping relationship (whether intimate or personal, social or therapeutic) in the following manner:

> By this term I mean a relationship in which at least one of the parties has the intent of promoting the growth, development, maturity, improved functioning, improved coping with life of the other. The other, in this sense, may be one individual or a group. To put it another way, a helping relationship might be defined as one in which one of the participants intends that there should come about, in one or both parties, more appreciation of, more expression of, more functional use of the latent inner resources of the individual.[6]

BEING AN EXPERT HELPER

In Chapter 4 you were introduced to steps that are required to become an expert. Everyone who enters the health professions has had the opportunity to provide help to someone who needs it. This chapter so far describes how such help in the role of a health professional is personal and therapeutic rather than intimate and social. Expert help always involves a high level of competence in some area. For example, some students have had experience teaching a sport or hobby or some other type of skilled activity to someone. Some health professions students today are entering second careers, and so they have been expert in some area of the workforce. Doing a job well is closely tied to feelings of self-respect, so making sure you are in a situation where your best self can be expressed is extremely important.

Being an expert helper in the health professions usually necessitates working closely with people. Occasionally a student gets as far as the clinical setting before discovering how much time must be spent in actual patient or client contact and/or with professional colleagues. For some, this is not what they anticipated, and they conclude that, while being an expert is great, being an expert helper entails demands that do not suit their personality.

It is difficult for someone who has already entered a program in the health professions to concede that he or she does not like working closely with people. Fortunately, some institutions offer preadmission testing through personality inventories and aptitude and interest tests that can help applicants gain insight into the type of work site that is an apt fit. The good news is that this person is usually not in the wrong profession, but, rather, may become one of those professionals who pursue the relatively scarce but rewarding careers in areas where little ongoing contact with other people is required. Such careers include some types of laboratory work, research, design (of equipment or departments), and some areas of management and writing. What better way is there to demonstrate a concern for others than to contribute to the high standards and productivity of the health professions by working in these less socially demanding areas? A different problem faces students who want to work with people and find that this is not going to figure significantly in their role within a chosen profession. If you are one of them you may want to consider entering a health profession where more interpersonal contact is the norm.

SHARED RESPONSIBILITY FOR OPTIMAL CARE

A clinician's role traditionally was geared to helping a patient over a period of time. This role can now be expanded to include limited contact with individual patients or, in some instances, indirect contact through supervision of assistants and referrals to other professionals. In the next few pages we examine two mechanisms available to you to help you succeed in providing optimal care.

What about Working with Assistants?

In many health professions a dramatic change in professional functions is occurring with the introduction of an "assistant" level into the field. The term itself sometimes adds confusion because some assistants, such as physician's assistants, are health professionals themselves and may enjoy the benefit of assistants who aid them. Other assistants are trained to become a part of the support staff for therapists, technologists, or other more highly educated professionals. What difference do assistants make? One negative consequence is that some individuals who entered a health profession with the understanding that they would provide help through direct interventions with patients or clients are finding that activities they thought were a part of their professional responsibility are now being carried out by assistants. When this is the case these individuals may experience less respect for what they themselves are doing than they had hoped for. As one professional said, "Why did I spend all those years learning my profession when my job turns out to be supervising assistants and aides who get to have all the fun of direct care?" A positive consequence is that professional assistant programs were introduced to help provide lower-cost optimal care, to create employment opportunities for those who did not want to or could not pursue a longer and more arduous professional preparation, and to alleviate serious personnel shortages in many health fields. Some health professionals needlessly feared that assistants would take over treatment procedures entirely, leaving the professional with evaluation and administrative tasks only. This has not proven to be the case. Even in fields in which assistants are used widely there are key areas of direct evaluation and treatment that you as the health professional must continue to provide; other means of assuring optimal care can often be more efficiently be administered by a supervised assistant.

Assistants are in the health care system to stay. The task of more highly prepared professionals is to focus on the responsibility of providing the best care possible at the lowest cost, a responsibility that is shared with assistants. In some cases, this means the professional will become a competent, respectful supervisor to the person directly performing procedures previously performed by a health professional. For the assistant it will involve respectfully accepting such supervision.

When Should I Refer Patients to Other Professionals?

"Referral" has been a time-honored method of ensuring that a person who seeks professional services will receive optimal care by not having to depend completely on one professional's capabilities and resources. It acknowledges that you cannot always be expected to single-handedly manage that person's health care needs. Sometimes health professionals are reticent to refer a patient to someone else, even though she or he can do the job more effectively and even though it is in the patient's best interest. Reasons are that health professionals do not take their jobs lightly, become attached to patients with whom they have been working, or find it painful to admit "failure."

You should take steps to implement referral when progress is hindered (1) because you are not experienced in appropriate techniques or do not have adequate equipment for providing proper services to that particular person, (2) because you and the patient have a serious personality conflict, (3) because you experience a negative bias toward the person (or group to which the person belongs), or (4) because of a detrimental amount of dependency between the patient and you (for details see Chapter 11).

Optimal care, then, entails using the time-honored referral system to extend your professional resources. It requires self-knowledge: knowing when and where to refer the patient for further evaluation or treatment. In this manner, your integrity as a professional helper can be maintained, and your self-respect will be enhanced because of your good judgment.

TEAMS AND TEAMWORK

Work with assistants and the practice of patient referral are two examples of how teamwork can enhance your self-respect. We end this chapter with a section that more fully addresses the challenge of working as part of an interdisciplinary health care team because almost all health care today is provided through the team approach.

Teams were developed to try to effect several important goals in patient care. First, because of specialization, it became obvious that professionals must band together to provide coordinated and comprehensive care. One goal of teamwork was to provide protection against the complete fragmentation of services that could result from more specialization.

The second goal grew from the belief that team-coordinated care is more likely to ensure that the patient's many needs are met in a manner that shows respect for that person as a *unique individual.* In other words, despite the importance of coordinated and comprehensive care, no one today judges this as the sole criterion of good health care. Health professionals must also fulfill the stringent requirement of tailoring care to suit the individual who receives it. The hope is that the deeply held moral ideal of respect for persons (including yourself!) is best realized by the team approach because it allows the patient to be viewed from many different perspectives and by also drawing on others' resources when appropriate. As one of us reflected in an article on teamwork:

> A good intervention must fit within the context of the patient's needs, hopes, and fears. For example, following a shoulder disarticulation for cancer a person who is well qualified medically to be fitted with an upper extremity prosthesis may be opposed to it on esthetic, financially burdensome, or religious grounds. Assuming that the person understands the ramifications of each of the options, withholding the prosthesis would be judged the morally good course of action despite the technical advantages of the prosthesis. Thus, the patient or candidate's well-being becomes the reference point for judging whether the person is being treated with respect and for ultimately determining the moral worth of the treatment program.[7]

In addition to these two goals, teams have been welcomed by institutions because they are an efficient mode of health care delivery and create a sense of mutuality among team members themselves. Health care institutions are made up of two broad categories of actions: actions flowing from hierarchy-derived decisions and those flowing from community-derived decisions.

Within the hierarchy, the power to make decisions flows from very few persons to affect very many. Power differentials are necessary and accepted. The power and responsibility weigh heaviest at the top. A value realized by this mode of functioning is efficiency.

In contrast, within the community framework the power to make decisions is more equally diffused throughout the institution or at least among the members of a health care "team." Power differentials are less obvious. Professionals with different skills function together with mutual support and as task-sharers. Values realized by this mode of functioning are equality and mutuality.

Therefore, two important values are realized in the two forms of activity—efficiency and mutuality. The idea of the health care team is that all team members are working together cooperatively and efficiently toward the professional *and* institutional goal of optimal care.[8]

In summary, the team itself can become a means of support, growth, and increased effectiveness for the health professional who wants to maximize his or her personal strengths while performing necessary professional tasks.

SELF-RESPECT AND LIFELONG LEARNING HABITS

It has been said that the era in which you are entering the professions is "the era of information." An article by sociologist Peter Drucker entitled *Age of Social Transformation* looked at the latter years of the 20th century as the time when we "moved into an economic order in which knowledge, not labor or raw material or capital, is the key resource; a social order in which inequality based on knowledge is a major challenge. . . ."[9]

In an era of intense research, information highways, and the lightning swift electronic transfer of knowledge, it is understandable that you cannot be expected to learn everything during the years of initial professional preparation. Fortunately the usual face-to-face continuing education mechanisms are being augmented by many computer-generated online opportunities.

Just as evidence is mounting that you can remain physically fit over a lifetime, you can also think of lifelong learning as "professional development."

Once you "get in the habit," you will look forward to the many opportunities for learning that confront you almost every day. Virtue is knowing your limits. The posture that you are always in a position to learn more will help you continue to feel deep respect for yourself as someone who is "up on the latest" and able to use the cumulative knowledge and skills available to you.

SUMMARY

When you become a health professional you will assume many roles in the course of your chosen career. Self-respect is an essential component of satisfaction over the course of that career. Understanding the appropriate nature of the help you proffer is one key resource. Maintaining your competence, meeting challenges, and remaining compassionate are other important conditions for the self-respect you will attain in your lifelong efforts. This chapter has provided some pathways for that task. Surely you will find others.

REFERENCES

1. Davis, C.M.: *Patient-Practitioner Interaction.* 3rd ed. Thorofare, NJ, Slack, Inc., 1998, p. 5.
2. Wright, R.: *The Moral Animal: Why We Are the Way We Are: The New Science of Evolutionary Psychology.* New York, Pantheon Books, 1994, pp. 12–13.
3. Cassell, E.: Recognizing suffering. *Hastings Cent. Rep.* 21(3):24–31, 1991.
4. Wright, B.: *Physical Disability: A Psychological Approach.* New York, Harper & Row, 1960, p. 224.
5. Purtilo, R.: *Ethical Dimensions in the Health Professions.* 3rd ed. Philadelphia, W.B. Saunders, 1999, pp. 235–236.
6. Rogers, C.R.: *On Becoming a Person.* Boston, Houghton Mifflin and Co., 1961, pp. 39–40.
7. Purtilo, R.: Ethical issues in team work. *Arch. Phys. Med. Rehab.* 68:318–326, 1988.
8. Purtilo, R.: Interdisciplinary health care teams and health care reform. *J. Law Med. Ethics* 22(2):121–126, 1994.
9. Drucker, P.F.: The age of social transformation. *Atlantic Monthly* November 1994, pp. 53–92.

CHAPTER 6

Enhancing Self-Respect through Good Personal Habits

CHAPTER OBJECTIVES

The student will be able to

- List some positive goals health professionals can realize by attending to their own needs and sources of satisfaction
- Assess some reasons why health professionals may fail to take precautions to safeguard their own health
- Identify two approaches for constructively adopting good work habits
- Distinguish the strengths of a Sisyphus-type approach to professional tasks from those of a Pandora-type
- Identify some characteristics of solitude and why it is important
- List four ways to help ensure that you will make time for leisure, play, and solitude
- Identify bonds among health professionals fostered by several forms of common language

Often, the transition from student to professional nurse can be a traumatic experience. Many of us find ourselves enveloped in a highly technologic, automated, bureaucratic system for which we may not be prepared. We may become increasingly aware that the individual can become more and more powerless with respect to the system, and we may find ourselves resisting submergence and loss of personal identity. What becomes of essence, then, is how we as nurses, as persons, choose to respond to this environment; how we choose to define ourselves and name our own meanings in a system where things are already named, where tradition, routines and habitual practices prevail. Our authenticity lies in keeping in touch with ourselves as persons, in adhering to a personal value system and having the courage to resist peer pressure for mediocre practice should such pressure exist. This does not mean that we will not aspire to a certain "group belongingness" or participate in team effort—these are essential to personal and professional survival. What it does mean is that we do not succumb to loss of personal identity or abdicate personal responsibility and accountability for our actions. . . .

M.J. Nelson[1]

In Chapter 1 you were introduced to the idea that persons' well-being depends in part on their ability to identify and shape their lives in a manner consistent with their own values and those that help to build a stronger community. In this final chapter of Part Two we return to some of the general themes found in Chapter 1 and focus them specifically on you, to give you an opportunity to think about your own personal health and well-being. The basic question we ask for your reflection is, "What kinds of attitudes and activities can you cultivate to stay authentically *you*—healthy, satisfied with your job, and able to integrate your professional and personal goals?" As the nurse in the above excerpt observes, the very essence of ourselves depends on successfully meeting this challenge. It may be the ultimate indicator of self-respect. The chapter progresses along two major lines of thought: (1) nurturing yourself and (2) building strong personal and professional support networks.

SELF-RESPECT THROUGH NURTURING YOURSELF

Today there is a general belief that individuals are ultimately responsible for their own health. Do you agree? It certainly is the case that people feel better, look better, and are able to function more fully when nurturing their own sense of well-being, seeking balance in their lives, and mapping a life course that has opportunity for changing priorities. None of these goals ever comes easy! Some readers of this book have just completed study for their preprofessional degree, giving up other pleasures and competing responsibilities to qualify for professional preparation. Some have come from a period devoted to work in another field, to parenting, or to recovery from trauma. Whatever their history, it is likely that all persons have familiarity with the challenge of creating a life that has balance between work and play and between home and workplace and that presents them with many options.

The challenge of keeping these life-affirming goals in the forefront is a not new one: the ancient Greek philosopher Aristotle built his entire approach to ethics on the idea that one must take charge and build a life of excellence based on similar goals. Central to his approach was the idea that persons must always seek the mean between extremes of character. Today, hints for striking a "healthy balance" in life are the topic of books on literally rows of book shelves in the psychology, self-help, and health sections of your local bookstore. The next time you are there, take a look! Clearly, acknowledging the benefits of nurturing yourself to stay healthy physically, mentally, and spiritually and actually being successful in doing so are not the same! In this chapter insights

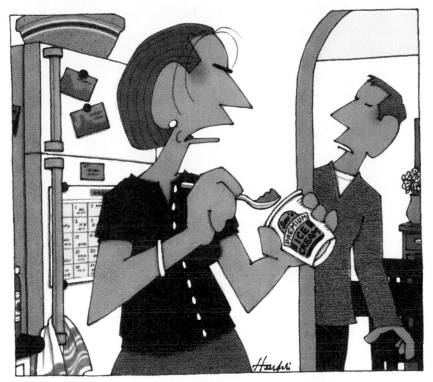

"I'm not eating. I'm self-medicating."

and suggestions are offered to help you succeed to the extent that healthfulness is within your control.

Overcoming Illusions of Invulnerability

Many health professionals are so used to being helpers that they perceive themselves as "the strong ones," immune to illness or debilitation. Goethe, in his *Elective Affinities*, illustrates that everyone has a potential for organizing a world that fits his or her illusions:

> And so they all, each in his own way, reflectingly or unreflectingly, go on with their daily lives; everything seems to have its accustomed course, for indeed, even in desperate situations where everything hangs in the balance, one goes on living as though nothing were wrong.[2]

To make matters worse for health professionals, ethical codes and oaths in the health professions do not provide encouragement to health professionals to take good care of themselves. It is as if they, too, deny the health professional's vulnerability. Throughout history, all of the major codes have been duty oriented and have emphasized the health professional's responsibility to *others*, with a striking degree of negligence in talking about responsibility to one's own self. This is not surprising, since, as you also learned in Chapter 1, a professional by definition is one who provides an important service to others. In fact, there was so much emphasis on serving others that some early documents in nursing and medicine suggested that one's dedication might lead to death in times of plague or other danger. Medical historians tell us that the physician Galen suffered nightmares for the rest of his life owing to his feelings of guilt after he fled the plague of Rome to save his own life and that of his family. The good news is that today martyrdom is out! However, ethical codes of the health professions have been slow to incorporate the importance of taking good care of yourself as a value, even though you are obviously in a better position to serve others when you are acting from a position of strength yourself. The need to respect your own limits and survival instincts seems to be a blind spot in most writings about professionalism. Review the ethical code of your chosen field to see if your leaders have incorporated this important aspect of professional life.

In the presence of psychological reasons for adopting a feeling of invulnerability and in the absence of clear ethical guidelines to foster self-care, the challenge to the person entering the health professions is to forge a path that will serve him or her well over the years. We offer two general suggestions: the first is to adopt generative approaches to your tasks; the second is to take time for yourself. Although they may be obvious, the particulars of how to go about each of these deserve attention.

Adopting Generative Approaches to Professional Tasks

As we said, bookshelves are filled with prescriptions for more effectively managing your time, stresses, and responsibilities in the workplace. Some authors suggest personal strengths and habits as reasonable starting points for developing health-supporting work habits. Two characters from Greek mythology, Sisyphus and Pandora, offer contrasting models that many professionals seem to imitate in trying to cope with the many projects and responsibilities related to professional life. Whereas neither, taken alone, is adequate, some aspects of the two models taken together can create a balanced approach to stresses and problems in the workplace. They also illustrate some behaviors to avoid when one organizes priorities and approaches tasks.

One model is Sisyphus.[3] He is portrayed as possessing competence, single-mindedness, and perseverance. As a king, being "held responsible" required that Sisyphus willingly place himself in a position of decision-making and accept as an integral aspect the consequences (sanctions) that would follow if he did not complete his job well. In the Sisyphus approach, the major challenge is to pursue the completion of a task with undying diligence.

Although he is portrayed as a male figure, his approach is by no means limited to male health professionals today! The Sisyphus type of health professional is decisive, acts autonomously, competes with vigor, but generally sees little need for input from others. Things are going well when he is "in control." When colleagues offer assistance, noting that his shoulders seem weighed down by his work, he responds, "It's not heavy, it's my duty!"

The person who adopts this approach fosters and values efficient decision-making within our highly bureaucratized and fragmented structures of health care. The Sisyphus-type health professional also places a high value on competence. One can see that Sisyphus-type traits support specialization in the professions, in which each contributor has a highly competent but narrowly defined role to play—an important quality because specialization is so pervasive in health care today.

The emphasis of the Sisyphus model on holding oneself fully accountable for one's activities makes this type of health professional supportive of accountability-oriented procedures such as informed consent, institutional review mechanisms for clinical research, outcomes management, and quality assurance policies.

With so many positive values fostered by the Sisyphus approach, one may not be surprised that an entire social workers' code of ethics is organized around the concept and language of "responsibility"[4] and that the codes of numerous associations of the health professions place it centrally in their ethical guidelines. In fact, one might ask, has this approach any shortcomings at all?

As in so many of the Greek tragedies, the major shortcoming is revealed in the plight of the focus of our attention, the main character. Sisyphus was not a well-liked fellow, although that did not create the major problem for him. His activities were such that during his tenure as king of Corinth he had betrayed a secret of Zeus, incurring the wrath of the gods, who doomed him to Hades. As the administrators of *this* efficiently-run institution tended to do, they drew on his strengths in deciding what his eternal task would be. Sisyphus has to forever roll a heavy stone uphill, which forever rolls down again. He keeps pushing, never reflecting, never getting help, never trying an alternative route, and never attempting to renegotiate the terms—always pushing up the same path again and again and again . . . ad infinitum.

His accountability is awesome; the fastidious persistence with which he exercises his task is exhausting. He is rigorously responsible, *but he never quite succeeds.*

What would happen if only once, just once, Sisyphus would break away to try the alternative route up the back side of the mountain, or better yet, around it? Suppose if only once he'd say, "Phooey, this isn't going to work. I'm going to bed!" Although his dogged persistence generates much activity, the tragedy of

Sisyphus is his inability to recognize that his goal may be attainable by some other route.

There is another problem with the Sisyphus model. Modern-day Sisyphus-type health professionals are becoming immortalized, too—in the literature of "burnout." Burnout is the term applied to a person's state of emotional and physical exhaustion due to extreme stress. The demands of professional life can be exhausting, and most leaders today are not placed in immortal bodies with immortal minds and spirits. The dogged persistence of the Sisyphus approach can squelch an extremely able person's ability to exhibit competence, produce a closet substance abuser, or cause chronic rage and depression. This burnout phenomenon destroys some of the most committed leaders in the professions.[5–7] There is mounting evidence that these destructive habits all too often have their start during the years of preparation for a profession.[8] The strains are so exhausting that eventually the morning sun is robbed of anticipation, joy is bleached into boredom, meaninglessness—like the morning fog in Carl Sandburg's poem—comes "on little cat feet," obscuring the promise of the horizon.

Because there is such a high price to pay for many who adopt a Sisyphus approach only, it is worthwhile to consider alternative or additional modes of functioning as a professional. It seems that some of the serious difficulties accompanying a strictly Sisyphus approach can be mitigated by weaving them skillfully with Pandoran traits. Therefore, let us consider this model.

Pandora was a leader in her own right, being the first mortal woman. She was playful, imaginative, and mischievous. Her inquisitiveness was unbridled. Her optimism and ingenuity were a delight to behold.[9]

Virtues required for operating within this model include the acknowledgment of surprise, ability to embrace rather than to oversimplify ambiguities, willingness to accommodate uncertainty, courage to act in the face of the unknown, optimism, risk-taking, love of the lyrical, a propensity for dancing rather than for marching, and a comfort level with improvisation.

One can readily see the contrast with the model of Sisyphus and begin to assess this model's strengths (which, again, may be expressed by members of both genders). Imaginative exploration is required to overcome the uselessness, in some situations, of trying old—even time-tested—routes for today's changing health care system demands. The weakest link in the chain of the Sisyphus approach is the inability to cope with what is new and uncertain.

Preparation for addressing problems created by uncertainty seldom is addressed adequately in formal professional programs of study. Still, uncertainty faces the health professional almost every day. One physician observes:

> In my own practice, I came to dread the simple complaints such as colds, viruses, and headaches, not so much because I was worried that I was missing something serious, but because people seemed so disappointed with the indefinite results of my examination and treatment. I am sure that if the time were all accumulated

and tallied, I have literally spent days trying to explain the uncertainty of medicine to often understandably unwilling patients. . . .[10]

This physician's anxiety is understandable! The health professions are very knowledge-intensive: in other words, you are rewarded by society for what you know. Accurate knowledge is important because if you do not know key information you may cause harm to a patient, client, or institution. At the same time, no one knows everything about how to reach the ends worth achieving through professional interventions. Even for the most knowledgeable health professional, the problem of uncertainty lays in the variability of the human condition—including the variability of different patients' responses to a given intervention.[11] Part of what professionals faced with uncertainty must deal with in today's environment of technological possibility is the urge to intervene as new complications arise. Sometimes an intervention will help to solve one problem, but the patient does not seem to have benefited overall, so that in the end the treatments are "spot-welded" onto the patient without consideration of the overall context of his or her life situation.[12]

The uncertainty combined with the urge to intervene leads to anxiety about whether one really is doing what is best. This set of circumstances can be extremely dissipating to one's self-respect because it is so closely identified with not causing harm to the patient. Because everyone errs at some time, Blustein and others have urged health professionals to cultivate the (neglected) virtue of self-forgiveness.[13] Self-forgiveness is not sweeping problems under the rug; rather it requires confronting the issue, taking necessary steps to seek forgiveness of the harmed person, and then forgiving oneself.

Another kind of anxiety-producing uncertainty facing the health professional occurs when there are dramatic structural changes in health care that affect established practice patterns. For instance, within the last decade many health professionals were faced with the introduction of "managed care" approaches on a wide scale. Of course as you enter the health professions, this approach has largely become a norm of health care. At the same time, your generation will face, among other things, serious questions about what the movement to a completely computer-driven system of information gathering, storage, sharing, and retrieval in health care will mean for the age-old commitment to patient confidentiality. You will also face changes in the form of the health professional and patient relationship occasioned by reliance on genetic information. And there will be other dramatic changes, each carrying a high degree of uncertainty about their effects as they are introduced.[14]

What these examples highlight is that old paths up the mountain, however deeply worn by those before us, are not ensured routes to success in uncertain moments. Given the uncertainty that characterizes large areas of the practice of the health professions, health professionals necessarily must be risk takers, innovators.

However, most readers know that Pandora is not remembered mostly for her vitality, optimism, and ingeniousness, but rather for her mistake. Impulsively, she opened a box—the wrong box—and let all human blessings escape and be lost, leaving only hope. Clearly, the Pandora mode needs "tempering." Therefore, flexibility and a wide range of resources will be needed for you to find an appropriate response that will still preserve your equanimity when challenged by new approaches. Pandora and Sisyphus present two extremes of approach. Ideally, you will avoid the detrimental effects while capitalizing on the considerable strengths of each, thereby using your resources of generativity to provide high-quality care effectively.

Respect for Your Need for Solitude

No matter how wisely you choose a lifestyle that allows ample doses of both Sisyphean and Pandoran traits, you still deserve to claim time to be alone. A vital strategy for survival is solitude.

Solitude is a positive, active state of being, although the experience of solitude is not identical to happiness and may even be "bittersweet" (accompanied by sorrow or anger); nonetheless, it is *sought out* as a need in itself, not foisted upon one as a result of feeling rejected or "out of contact."[15] It is respecting your need to not always be responding to other people. Unlike loneliness, which is a form of suffering, solitude can be wonderful.

Pooh Bear, the most philosophical and reflective member of Winnie-the-Pooh's community, sought solitude often, as was said of him by his neighbors.[16]

In short, solitude is a time to be *with oneself only,* not with others, and to engage in activities that can better prepare one for relationships. Some people are active in their solitude, finding walking, jogging, biking, or other solitary activities a time for reflection. Others prefer the stillness of meditation or just sitting and staring Pooh Bear style. Yet, many health professionals do not in fact respect their need for time alone enough. Do you? If not, now is a good time to begin building such time into your daily routine.

Many professionals find that the structure of most institutions tends to create barriers to the important work of solitude. Health care institutions, like other bureaucratic systems, have efficiency as an overriding value. For efficiency to be realized, schedules, policies, and routines must be implemented and followed.

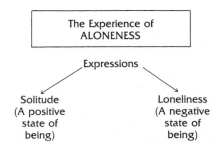

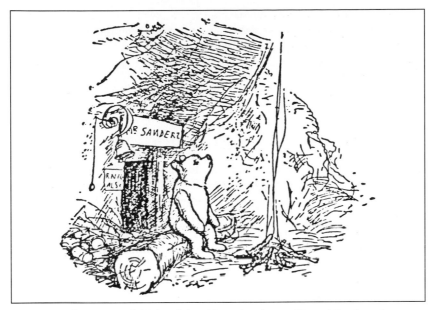

"And He sits and thinks of the things they know; He and the Forest,
alone together . . ."

From *Winnie-The-Pooh* by A. A. Milne, illustrated by E. H. Shepard, copyright 1926
by E. P. Dutton, renewed 1954 by A. A. Milne. Used by permission of Dutton
Children's Books, an imprint of Penguin Books for Young Readers, a division of Penguin
Putnam Inc.

Therefore, former routines of work are replaced by the new, usually more
rigorous demands of institutional schedules and operations, and there is little
encouragement from one's employer to stop and reflect, take time off for a jog,
or in other ways take time quietly alone!

From a psychological viewpoint, the inward-looking process of solitude can
be taxing in itself, and procrastination can keep you from ever being with
yourself. Work in solitude can lead you into aspects of your existence that have
been carefully kept hidden. Furthermore, when a health professional sees a
colleague who needs some time alone he or she sees someone who seems aloof.
While sometimes persons who withdraw are in trouble, it is difficult to
distinguish that situation from a desperate need to have some "alone time."

Therefore, you can begin to get a fuller picture: neither the structures of
health care nor one's closest colleagues and friends will automatically know how
to support your solitude since it *also* requires that you be free of them from time
to time.

Some ideas to help you make time for yourself include the following:

1. Set a time and place and rigorously adhere to it.
2. Become bold in identifying to others what you are doing.

3. Take notes on your reflections.

4. Remind yourself often that the basic minimum requirement upon which most or all other health-supporting activity depends is to take time to be with yourself.

In addition, you can help others to have their own time alone by learning to recognize this need in colleagues and encouraging it.

SHOWING RESPECT FOR EACH OTHER

It is not enough to cultivate character traits for survival in your work or to make time for yourself. Also needed for success and satisfaction in your career are persons with whom you can share joys, dreams, fun, and frustrations. Family and friends outside of your work environment are at risk of being left out of your life in very important ways unless you make conscious efforts to include them. They are your most precious and immediate source of support, but often are taken for granted and may get the leftover part of your day, the majority of which is spent in professional activities. This excerpt from a day in the life of a physician reflects a routine that many health professionals will identify with regarding the amount and quality of time spent with their family (and his may be an optimistic account):

> It is now seven o'clock. I drive home. The day of work is finished. I know that I shall not have any more calls as I sign my phone out to the telephone answering service. I sit down to dinner with my wife and three school-age children. I listen to the children recount the activities of the day. It is March, and my wife and I begin to talk about possible vacation sites for this summer. After dinner I go to my study and take a journal from a pile of unread periodicals. I thumb through it, unable to concentrate enough to get interested in any one article. I turn on the television and begin to watch an NBA game. Later, my wife wakens me.[17]

What do you find encouraging about this scene as you think about your own professional life? Troubling? Your job is to establish habits early that will reflect the rhythms needed for your family unit and friends to be *able* to support you when you need it. A young lawyer recounts the choices he began to exercise when he felt himself being consumed by his work:

> There were a few things that helped to restore my sense of equilibrium. The first was to make a conscious effort to spend time with my wife. In the beginning, I resisted when my wife would plead, cajole, and sometimes push me out the door of our apartment so that we could spend a few hours watching a movie or going to dinner. Eventually, I realized how important this time was. It strengthened our relationship by keeping the lines of communication open between us. Not only that, it also made me a *better* worker by giving my anxious mind a much needed rest.
>   A second source of balance came from getting together with other people who were facing similar pressures at work. Two or three times a month I would meet

with a few friends from law school who were working in other firms around town. Our get-togethers were combination lunches and b.s. sessions. These meetings did wonders for my perspective. I found myself becoming less anxious and self-absorbed as I discovered that my friends were dealing with the same worries and concerns I was facing. We helped ourselves by helping each other.

Another thing that helped was to take ten or fifteen minutes during my morning commute to sit quietly, reflect about my life, and say a few prayers. This helped center me for the day. It gave me a sense of perspective. It allowed me to see the ways in which my work was an integral part of my spiritual life. . . .

Together, these small things helped bring my life and my work back into balance. They let me see my work more realistically. They stopped me from investing too much of myself in my work. And they reminded me that I was more than a worker and that my work was only work.[18]

In short, this young professional utilized the resources of family, colleagues, and his own form of spiritual reflection to create the balance he felt slipping from him. In the process he created a support network. He just mentions the potential one can find close at hand in one's immediate professional colleagues. It is so important that we will examine it in more detail.

The Ties That Bind

One source of support, often overlooked, is that persons working in a health care situation have several common bonds, all of which help to establish rapport and support among them.

The Bond of Caring. Health professionals share the motivation to express caring—about the patient's problems, prognosis, and progress; about the department; about what is happening in their field; and about health services in general. The discussions of helping in Chapters 4 and 5 illustrate the avenues down which your caring takes you. You voluntarily place yourself in the mainstream of human suffering, thereby showing that you care. No neon lights beckon you in. No one commits you to this role. There are no locked doors preventing your departure. You choose to be there because you care enough about human well-being and the relief of suffering to want to effect certain changes by the use of professional skills.

Sometimes overlooked, and to the detriment of everyone involved, health professionals may take less time telling each other directly that they care about each other than they do sharing their concerns about patients, policies, or other external factors. Creating an atmosphere of shared care transforms a workplace from a site only to a true community.

Technical Language as a Bond. Another silver thread that creates a bond among health professionals is the technical language of each specific profession and the shared language of health care. Although this may seem irrelevant at first glance, it should not be overlooked as a means whereby potential tensions can be diverted. For example, an older professional who feels she has nothing in common with a young recent graduate may see him in a much different light after discussing with him newer approaches to the treatment of diabetes mellitus or a better method of analyzing cholesterol levels. Similarly, the younger professional probably will gain new respect for the older one who bothers to explain a new piece of evaluative equipment or the value of an interesting technique. Cross-cultural encounters occasioned by movement of health professionals across national and other cultural boundaries depend on this shared language too. You will have opportunities to attend international meetings or be host to professionals in your workplace who bring cultural characteristics entirely new to you. The silver threads of professional—including technical—language are the foundation for the bonds that bring, and keep, you together.

The Bond of Gratitude. Gratitude or appreciation is expressed too seldom by persons working together. A simple word of thanks can create more good will than months of competent work together during which neither person makes an effort to express appreciation to the other. There are many ways to say "thank you," from an affirming smile or nod to placing a small surprise on your colleague's desk as a way to show your gratitude. Remembering another person's birthday or the anniversary of a special event and performing other "random acts of kindness" creates a general environment of congeniality in which the language of mutual respect for the efforts and gifts of each other's presence can flourish.

Finding Mechanisms That Support Support

The three bonds—of caring, technical language, and gratitude—can help to reduce tensions among co-workers and foster a sense of "belongingness" among them. Together they can encourage the realization of mutually shared goals and values. However, as you learned in Chapter 2, it is not enough for individuals to have a desire to create a supportive environment—it must also be reflected in the entire structure and values of those who have policy authority. In other words, each person must help create mechanisms that will maintain supportive interactions.

It is a good idea, then, when you look for a position in a new setting, to seek at least one person who appears to be a potential source of support. If no one person promises to be such a resource, it is better to look elsewhere. In addition, you should be bold in asking questions that will allow you to gain some understanding of how support is expressed within the department and larger institution. To make an assessment, the following guidelines may be useful:

1. Inquire of your future employer whether there are meetings or other sessions where problems associated with the everyday stresses of health care delivery are discussed.

2. Ask some of the people you will be working with what they believe to be the sources of the most intense stress in that environment and how *the group* handles them.

3. Ask some of the people you will be working with how each as an individual deals with the stress of his or her position, and whether, as a whole, the environment is a supportive or divisive one.

4. Make a mental note of those who appear to be potential sources of support, or if no one appears to be. If everyone denies that problems exist or becomes defensive about such questions when they are tactfully posed, this probably signals a setting in which stresses are dealt with alone, without the support of one's colleagues.[19]

Fortunately, only in rare situations are no support mechanisms available. In fact, being a support to others often is the key to finding support from them when it is needed. The old adage, "To have a friend is to be one," holds true in the workplace.

Play: Enjoying Each Other's Company

If you were to complete this section on support systems with what the authors have said so far you would probably conclude that the work environment is heavy with tension and problems 24 hours a day. No one could—or should—put up with constant doom and gloom. In fact, health professionals are fortunate to be in a line of work in which they know that their work usually is making a positive difference in patients' and clients' lives. That in itself is reason to take the opportunity to enjoy the work setting.

One colleague said that for him work and play were the same thing. He called it "plork." Although it is a good thing to enjoy one's job and the work entailed in doing it well, in our estimation this is shortchanging the joy that can come from remembering to put some levity and fun into the environment, too. Pressures on health professionals to use their time well clearly create stresses at times, but the curse of stress is that one sometimes forgets to use the time still available to take advantage of a cartoon, a good joke, a lighthearted story that a colleague or patient is trying to tell, or some other type of pleasure. One author, himself a health professional, observes:

> Joy is only possible for persons who are attentive to the present. One cannot be happy if one is continually ruminating about what might have been or fretting over whether wishes will come to pass. Americans have a tough time with real joy. Americans are oriented toward outcomes, expectations, and the future; toward ever more competition in proving that they deliver the best results, and anxiously pondering how things might have turned out if only they had chosen differently. This makes it hard to be happy. In health care, these tendencies are exaggerated. Worries about what will happen next to the patient and worries about their own future careers blot out the possibility of joy for many health care professionals. Joy is a present tense phenomenon. It is possible only if one attends to the moment.[20]

Sometimes activities outside of work hours enhance the ability to enjoy each other in a more relaxed environment. There are the usual afternoon coffees or parties or sports teams, but the activities need not stop there. For instance, the authors are part of a writing group. We meet regularly with several other health professions colleagues after work. We write about our work experiences in the form of short stories, poetry, and essays. At first all of us were scared to share anything, believing it would not be good enough. However, as we became more comfortable with each other, we started looking forward to hearing each other's stories. In addition to writing about some very serious problems, we find our gathering to be a great vehicle for laughing at ourselves and good-naturedly at each other, as well as an "excuse" to get to know each other better. One delightful outcome was that we were able to publish some of our work for others to share too.

In your own search for finding a congenial group you can use some of the same approaches that we suggested above to assess the type of situation you are getting into. Ask yourself:

- Does everyone look like they have just heard the worst news of their lives as they rush around?
- Are there cartoons, lighthearted comments, funny pictures anywhere?
- Do you see any photos of the group having a good time together at a picnic or some other event? (In our present work situation the group has an annual "day away together" as well as tea for all members of the group on Thursday afternoons.)
- What kind of response do you get when you ask if the group has fun together? Is it treated as a good question? An inappropriate one?
- Is there a common area where colleagues and staff can relax when they do get a moment? Is there a congenial place away from the patient care or other professional areas for conversation, relaxation, or a snack?
- Do the people who are interviewing you seem to have good dispositions?

Obviously the professional who substitutes a good time for good work is not one who will, or should, last long in a position. However, finding and helping to further create a positive work environment can do much to enrich the situation for everyone involved, and not the least important, for yourself.

SUMMARY

Having thought about yourself as a *person* in your professional roles, now is a good time to reflect again on the values that you bring to your choice of profession. Some values and conduct may warrant reexamination in light of the opportunities you have to adopt an optimal lifestyle for your health throughout the duration of your career.

We hope the ideas in this chapter emphasize to you that your career as a health professional can include self-respectful attitudes and activities as well as support systems that will sustain you and give you an opportunity to help sustain others. You have at your disposal your past experiences, many sources of external suggestions such as those offered through self-help books, family, and friends, and—last, but not least—your professional colleagues. Showing respect for yourself over your professional lifetime finally will fall primarily on your shoulders, but it is a process worth the undertaking and one in which you will find many other means of support to break your fall if you ever feel like you are losing your footing.

REFERENCES

1. Nelson, M.J.: Authenticity: fabric of ethical nursing practice. In Chinn, P.L. (ed.): *Ethical Issues in Nursing*. Rockville, MD, Royal Tunbridge Wells, 1986, p. 91.
2. Goethe, J.W.: *Elective Affinities*. New York, Penguin Books, 1978.
3. Pinsent, J.: *Greek Mythology*. London, Hamlyn Publishers Group, 1969, p. 69.
4. National Association of Social Workers, Inc.: *Code of Ethics of the National Association of Social Workers*. Washington, DC, 1993.
5. Griffith, J.: Substance abuse disorders in nurses. *Nurs. Forum* 34(4).19–28, 1999.
6. Hughes, P.H., Storr, C.L., Brandenburg, N. A., et al.: Physician substance abuse by medical specialty. *J. Addict. Dis.* 18:23–27, 1999.
7. Voth, E.A.: Self-prescribing by physicians. *JAMA* 281:1489–1490, 1999.
8. Scofield, G.R.: Impaired professionals. In Reich, W.T. (ed.): *Encyclopedia of Bioethics*. 2nd ed. New York, Macmillan, 1995, pp. 1191–1194.
9. Pinsent, J.: *Greek Mythology*. London, Hamlyn Publishers Group, 1969, p. 48.
10. Hilfiker, D.: *Healing the Wounds*. New York, Pantheon Books, 1985. Reprinted with annotations, Omaha, NE, Creighton University Press, 1999, pp. 58–71.
11. Berefords, E.B.: Uncertainty and the shaping of medical decisions. *Hastings Cent. Rep.* 21(4):6–11, 1991.
12. Purtilo, R.B., and O'Donohue, W.J.: Resources for medical decision making in situations of high uncertainty. *Nebr. Med. J.* 70(1):277–280, 1992.
13. Blustein, J.: Doctoring and the (neglected) virtue of self-forgiveness. In Thomasma, D.C. and Kissell, J.L. (eds.): *The Health Care Professional as Friend and Healer*. Washington, DC, Georgetown University Press, 2000, pp. 87–105.
14. Purtilo, R.B.: Thirty-First Mary McMillan Lecture: A time to harvest, a time to sow: ethics for a shifting landscape. *Phys. Ther.* 80:1112–1119, 2000.
15. Purtilo, R.B.: Loneliness, the need for solitude and compliance. In Withersty, D.J. (ed.): *Communication and Compliance in a Hospital Setting*. Springfield, IL, Charles C Thomas, 1981, pp. 91–115.
16. Milne, A.A.: *Now We Are Six*. New York, E.P. Dutton and Company, 1927.
17. Reynolds, R.C. and Stone, J. (eds.): In *On Doctoring: Stories, Poems, Essays*. New York, Simon and Schuster, 1995, p .276. © Robert Wood Johnson Foundation.
18. Allegretti, J.: *Loving Your Job, Finding Your Passion: Work and the Spiritual Life*. Mahwah, NJ, Paulist Press, 2000, pp. 162–163.
19. Purtilo, R.B.: *Ethical Dimensions in the Health Professions*. 3rd ed. Philadelphia, W.B. Saunders, 1999, p. 123.
20. Sulmasy, D.P.: *The Healer's Calling: A Spirituality for Physicians and Other Health Care Professionals*. Mahwah, NJ, Paulist Press, 1997, p. 128.

PART TWO

Questions for Thought and Discussion

1. What are some skills that are important to all health professionals?

2. What are some skills that are more important to your particular profession than to the health professions as a group?

3. You go to a patient's bedside to perform a procedure. Before entering his room, you read his clinical record. Then you go in, greet the patient, ask how he feels, explain the procedure, make certain he is comfortable, carry out the procedure, get him a drink of water that he requests, bid him good-bye, and make notations in the record.
   a. What components of this interaction could be classified as social helping? Why?
   b. What components could be classified as therapeutic helping? Why?

4. You have been asked by members of your class to be the class president. You are already very busy with schoolwork and your personal commitments. List your most important priorities and decide what would be compromised the most by taking on this new position. What values will determine whether you will choose to accept your class-mates' offer?

5. John B. has been diagnosed as having AIDS and is a patient on the unit where you are working. What characteristics of the team approach can help to ensure that John receives the high-quality treatment he requires for this serious condition?

6. Barbara S. and Joan B. are two health professionals who work together in a large busy neighborhood health clinic. Both are in their late 20s and have worked together for the last 3 years. Although they enjoy a friendship at work, their personal lives are so different they do not often socialize outside of work.

   During the month of March, Barbara notices an aloofness in Joan. Whereas they used to share coffee breaks and lunch, Joan now makes excuses. Joan seems "too busy" to talk to Barbara. Barbara is upset and approaches Joan regarding the matter. During the conversation, Joan begins to cry. She confides to Barbara that her husband has been fired from his job. Joan is embarrassed and very worried. The bills are mounting fast, and the tension in her married life is increasing. Joan is terrified that the others will find out and asks Barbara not to tell. Barbara reassures her. She tells her that her secret is safe and offers to help in any way she can.

During the first 2 weeks in April, things get worse. Joan calls in sick several times, and Barbara covers for her. Several times Joan is late, and, on two occasions, she leaves immediately after lunch. Joan's work is being left undone, and others are bearing the brunt of her errors. Barbara feels she is being taken advantage of. She has done Joan's work and even lied to the director regarding Joan's whereabouts.

One day, over lunch, two of the others in the center start complaining about Joan. They say they are tired of her getting away with things. One has recently had to cover Joan's work on a sick day and says that things were a mess. They tell Barbara that they are going to talk to the director that afternoon.

Barbara is upset. What should she do?

PART THREE

Respect for the Patient's Situation

CHAPTER 7: Challenges to Patients

CHAPTER 8: Respect for the Patient's Personal
Relationships

Part Three examines closely the person who seeks professional help—the patient. Almost every person becomes a patient at some time, and you can undoubtedly recall some of the fears and problems you experienced as a patient, as well as the sympathy and special attention you received during that experience. Obviously understanding the patient's predicament helps you respond more respectfully.

In most cases, a person's role in society during a period of illness or incapacity differs significantly from that he or she held before becoming ill or injured. Part Three examines how the condition experienced by the patient affects him or her and how the health professional plays a role in the patient's remaining well or the patient's recovery, adjustment, incapacity, or preparation for death. Chapter 7 discusses special challenges faced by patients. Chapter 8 examines the patient as a member of the larger society and some ongoing issues the person may face, whether or not recovery occurs.

Ask yourself the following questions as you read about the patient as a person:

- How do my professional attitudes and conduct convey respect toward a patient?
- What goals should a patient strive to attain?
- What should I look for in a patient's responses to give me a clue to his or her own set of values and the extent to which they are constructive tools for building a patient's future?

CHAPTER 7

Challenges to Patients

CHAPTER OBJECTIVES

The student will be able to

- Describe conditions under which maintaining wellness becomes a challenge for a person
- List the most important changes experienced as losses by persons who become inpatients, and some challenges of reckoning with such changes in health care facilities
- Compare some challenges facing inpatients, ambulatory care patients, and patients who are treated in their homes
- Discuss the challenges facing patients as they interact with health professionals
- Identify why many patients try to act "brave"
- Name three "advantages" of staying in the patient role
- Describe the characteristics of (Molière's) *Imaginary Invalid* that are similar to patients today who benefit more from remaining ill than from working to recover or adjusting in other ways

Ten years ago, if I were setting out to make a film about catastrophic illness and subsequent disability, I would not have cast myself in the lead role. In my pre-stroke ignorance, I probably would have looked for someone stronger and braver than I—not yet knowing that we are all capable of much more bravery than we think.

B.S. Klein[1]

Most challenges facing patients are related to the altered role of sick persons in society and to the physical and mental changes a patient experiences in the transition from everyday routine. Fortunately, these challenges have received considerable attention in recent years, so it is likely that you will have one or more courses in which they are discussed. Some common themes are presented here as a basis for your ongoing thought and reflection.

MAINTAINING WELLNESS

It is fitting that a chapter on challenges to patients begin with some reflections on maintaining wellness. Most would agree that, if possible, the most desirable approach for an individual is to avoid becoming a patient at all.

In recent years much emphasis has been placed on maintaining and fostering a healthy lifestyle, that is, on staying well. Staying well seems to be to everyone's advantage—the individual, his or her loved ones, and society. Wellness ensues from maintaining health-supporting habits. Today some health professionals build practices based on preventive approaches—teaching people how to remain healthy. For example, dietitians are involved in school nutrition programs, nurses may work in perinatal clinics, and occupational and physical therapists often are involved in teaching wellness maintenance in the workplace, health spas, or sports settings.

A healthy life, however, depends on the individual, supported by a safe and health-inducing environment. Good eating, sleeping, exercise, and other health-fostering habits are essential. Freedom from basic want and violence are too. Maintaining a high level of emotional health can be optimized by many means, such as experiencing security, having fun with friends, engaging in activities one enjoys, and learning new skills.

At the same time, almost everyone would agree that health is not a goal completely within an individual's own control. Almost weekly there are discoveries of new genetic predispositions to illness; scientists have identified scores of environmental hazards and new viruses; some people live in conditions of poverty where basic public health and safety conditions are missing; many people suffer from work-related stress symptoms; and accidents and other misfortunes beset some people, dashing their dreams, altering their possibilities, and modifying their relationships. Moreover, most of us today have periods of less wellness or more wellness. For example, a person with mild pneumonia or late-onset diabetes or severe heart disease may function mostly as a healthy person but still may need the intervention of a health professional for some symptoms related to the condition. At best, each of us moves through life on a continuum between maximum health and life-threatening sickness or death.

RECKONING WITH CHANGE

The transition from being relatively well to becoming ill or sustaining an injury almost inevitably entails losses. The loss may be in the form of decreased physical or mental function:

> The depression I refer to comes from a sense of loss of a cherished possession. It may be the death of a loved one, an object stolen, or a fantasy dispelled—such as not getting a job one wanted, a date, or a publisher for a book. In my case the loss was a significant part of my body's ability to function. . . .

> Since depression is a sense of loss, I'm mostly set off by some disappointment in my physical improvement. There are many. Either some symptom reappears after I thought I was over it or I'm aware of another physical limitation, such as the inability to repair items needing delicate hand control. . . .[2]

Persons who lose their sight or other senses, those who lose control of movement or vital body functions, and those who through illness become incapable of making competent judgments may experience a similar sense of loss. The loss may also involve a change in physical appearance, such as the person who undergoes an amputation or is scarred after a severe burn.

The significance of these changes for each person is determined by a complex interweaving of several factors, including the physical and emotional effects of the pathological process itself, the alteration in the person's environment or social roles, and the coping mechanisms the patient has developed throughout his or her life. The concert pianist who loses an index finger will have a more profound loss than most of us, illustrating that actual loss will be more disabling for some persons than for others.

Patients react to health professionals in ways that express their concern about their losses. For example, upon entering a patient's room, the phlebotomist may catch the brunt of the patient's anxiety through comments such as "Here comes the vampire!" "Are you people selling my blood?" or "Do you have a license to take my blood?" The radiological technologist may be accused of destroying cells with her or his equipment. Professionals whose diagnostic and treatment procedures require patients to engage in physical or emotional exertion can be accused of sapping a patient's strength. All of these comments reflect the challenge the patient is facing in preserving his or her body from further loss while needing to express fear or anger about what is happening.

Loss of Former Self-Image

A natural extension of loss of function or previous physical appearance is the belief by some that one has literally lost one's old self. This is especially likely when the change promises to be extended or permanent. You have probably had the feeling sometime that you just "weren't yourself" that day or that what you did in a particular situation was not typical of the "real you." For most people, this sense of self-alienation is temporary; however, it may become more lasting for a person experiencing continuing changes associated with injury or illness.[3]

A patient's feeling of having lost herself or himself may result in part from the conviction that what one *is* is determined by what one looks like: *Self-image* depends to a large extent on body image (what one perceives oneself to look like).

A recent advertisement for women's clothing notes, "Her clothes become her; she does not become her clothes." Contrary to this marketing attempt, people do "become" their clothes, and, despite the proverb's bidding, most of us still do "judge a book by its cover." Painful sanctions are imposed on those whose appearance deviates too far from some societally determined standard of normality. Approval and acceptance are given for normal appearance only. There is a close relationship between appearance, accompanying body image, and sense of self-worth.[4]

Have you seen anyone today who you thought was exceptionally fit, or beautiful or graceful in the way that he or she moved? Our stereotypes of success and assurance of acceptance often depend on appearance. To be faced daily with changes that are the opposite from these stereotypes is at the core of the challenge for people facing many types of illness or disability.

One challenge facing many patients, then, is to reckon with changes that have taken place, to accept in some instances that things are never again going to be just as they were, and to find a realistic new body image. Only then will the person be able to fully believe that he or she is still the worthwhile human being that he or she was before the trauma. The work that accompanies developing a

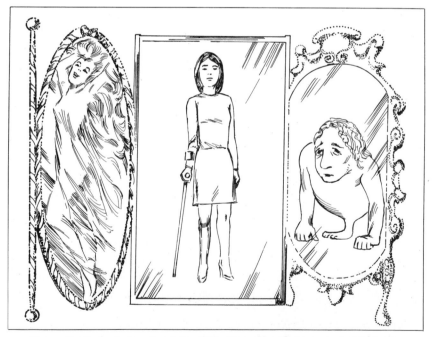

The patient's fantasies about the distortion of her former appearance may override what she sees in the mirror.

new sense of one's physical self after surgery or injury has been explored by one of the authors through poetry:

French Weaving

I piece together the tattered edges
with illusion net,
laying just the right size squares
over the gaping holes.
Carefully,
arduously
embroider the net to the original.
Trying to match the pattern,
tie up loose ends,
mimic the original curve and detail.
I pick up a thread
of who I once was,
try and attach it,
here,
here,
and here.
My clumsy attempts
only approximate the intricacy of the design.
Yet the untrained eye
cannot see my repair.
Run your fingers over my skin
to feel the flaws.

        — *Amy Haddad, 2001*[5]

The title of the poem, "French Weaving," is an embroidery technique used to repair damaged lace or crochet work. If done by an expert hand, it is hard to see areas of repair. How does this apply to the work patients do to "repair" themselves?

As you may expect, part of the health professional's success depends upon an adeptness at helping the patient either reclaim his or her old image as recovery occurs or, when necessary, discover a realistic and satisfactory new body image. An important element in your work with patients who are adjusting to changes in body image is timing. There is no preestablished time frame for a patient to accept a colostomy or look at the scar where her breast used to be. Each patient will move in his or her own way and at his or her own pace.

SPECIAL CHALLENGES OF INPATIENTS

Although not all people who become ill or injured spend time in hospitals or other health care institutions, the large number admitted as inpatients and the seriousness of their conditions warrant your consideration.

The necessity for spending time confined in a health care facility may significantly disrupt an individual's personal life, as well as the lives of family, occupational associates, and friends. The challenges associated with the disruption may be primarily social, but it is likely that they will also be economic owing to loss of work, health care-related expenses, or both. The economic burden is especially acute for a person who is self-supporting or is the breadwinner in a family. A single parent has the burden of finding and paying for suitable caretakers for children. A child, teenager, or other student loses valuable instruction and may fall behind or have to drop out of school. A professional person may have to forego participation in an important project. Whatever the individual's personal responsibilities, he or she is likely to be affected both socially and economically.

In addition to the disruption, a person is often aware that entering the hospital signals that he or she is not winning the battle of coping with an illness. This psychological defeat can be as deleterious to her or his welfare as the physical manifestations of the illness itself. In submitting to confinement in an institution, the person finally is admitting openly that the problem is "out of control" and that people professionally qualified to provide certain services are needed. The patient understandably is anxious about leaving his or her health, and perhaps life, in the hands of strangers, but judges that there are no other good alternatives.

Losses Associated with Institutional Life

The disruption of normal life patterns and coping mechanisms that may accompany patients' admissions is exacerbated by the fact that suddenly they are robbed of both home and privacy. Therefore, having met the basic challenge of admitting to illness or injury, patients now have to face other challenges.

Home. Most people view their home as a safe haven in a complex, fast-paced world. Of course, there are some exceptions, notably people for whom home is a place of loneliness, strife, or boredom. Occasionally, a person will feign illness to be admitted to a health care facility just to escape threats to their well-being. These patients require special consideration by health professionals and are discussed later in this chapter.

What makes home so desirable for most people when they are away from it and so much taken for granted when they are there? The physical and psychological comforts of home are missed by most patients in health care facilities.

Physical comforts take a number of forms. You have undoubtedly walked into someone's room or home where there was incredible chaos and disarray. In the midst of the pandemonium, the person or family members appear perfectly at ease; this is their idea of "really living!" Undoubtedly, you have also entered a home where even the teacups seem to sit primly on shelves, where dust *dares* not settle, and curtains never ruffle. In the midst of this porcelain perfection, these family members also appear perfectly at ease!

The physical comfort of home may best be described as freedom to extend oneself naturally and completely into one's immediate environment: to do (or not do) what one wishes, when one wishes, and how one wishes. The environment within the home, whether it contains 1 or 40 rooms, can be changed to conform to one's own needs, habits, and desires.

The bed is a good example of how health care facilities often are unable to adequately accommodate the needs and habits of a person. Almost anyone would agree that a good night's rest greatly determines one's outlook on life the next day, and most people acknowledge that their own bed is one of the most important comforts of home. The standard hospital bed is of a given height, width, length, and firmness. Although the hospital personnel stop short of treating patients in the manner of Procrustes, the culprit in Greek mythology who invited his guests to sleep in his guest bed and responded by chopping off the legs of those who were too tall, institutions usually are limited to offering a standard "hospital bed."

The obvious difficulties of totally personalizing the patient's health care environment are readily apparent. Nevertheless, the more that can be done to maximize physical comfort for the patient who is away from home, the more readily he or she will be able to direct energies toward healing, toward adjusting to dying from a life threatening illness, or toward living with a disability.

The *psychological comforts* of familiar surroundings also are sacrificed. A favorite chair for relaxation, a magnifying mirror for applying makeup, a family picture, or a ragged toy may all be symbols of security to the person. The mere arrangement of furniture in a room or the sight of a tree or birdbath in the yard may give a person a sense of well-being. These familiar objects are left behind when the person goes to a health care facility.

Psychological comfort also may be experienced in the routine associated with being "at home." It is not at all unusual for a patient who enters a health care facility to become confused about what day of the week it is because important regularly scheduled events are missing. The person who likes to start the day with a cup of coffee and the morning paper will be unsettled when, in a health care facility, the coffee is served with breakfast and the morning paper arrives just before he or she is scheduled to undergo the first diagnostic test or treatment session of the day. A child who is used to a bedtime story may have great difficulty sleeping without it.

Familiarity is most significantly embodied by people and pets in the home. An older woman may literally live for the companionship of a small grand-daughter. A single person may look forward to a weekly visitor or find companionship in a pet. Children have the familiarity of family and playmates. The harsh restrictions regarding visiting hours; number of guests admitted; and, most of all, the exclusion of children or pets from the bedside of institutional-ized sick, disabled, or dying patients, may be a source of increased anxiety.

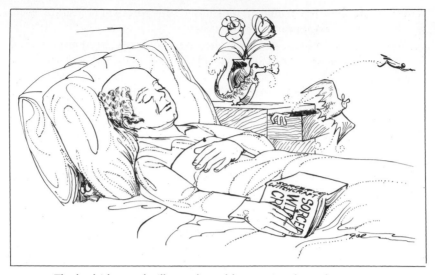

The bedside stand will reveal untold mysteries about the patient.

All of these examples highlight a basic challenge patients in health care facilities face—to find basic comforts that most have experienced in their homes. Many patients do meet the challenge of trying to retrieve a little bit of home. A remarkable sign is the contents of their rooms and bedside stands. Contents of a stand tell one as much about the patient as the contents of a small boy's pocket does about him. Generally, the tabletop is cluttered with get-well cards, flowers, candy, and stuffed animals. In the top drawer are stamps, writing paper, rosaries or religious books, yesterday's newspaper, assorted ointments, tissues, a Swiss Army knife, a Walkman, and more! One of the authors once found a smoked herring after a roommate complained that the patient in the next bed was sneaking fish into his bland diet.

Hidden caches of forbidden cigarettes and nonprescription drugs (especially sleeping pills, tranquilizers, and laxatives) are common finds, and a patient who imbibes liquor regularly will go to great lengths to maintain a supply. A health professional who has the opportunity to see into an open drawer will learn much information about the patient's personality.

You will also learn something about the patient if the room is devoid of personal objects. An empty room may indicate that the patient is not willing to be sick enough to stay too long or is too ill to have even thought about his or her surroundings. Dying patients may want to divest themselves of possessions or get rid of reminders that they will not "get well." They also may have no one to bring them anything.

You should note, however, that patients understandably may be sensitive about having a health professional snoop around the room, even if only to read a card attached to a bowl of roses or to hang up a bathrobe in the closet. Their sensitivity about these seemingly innocent gestures is due to the fact that, in addition to missing the comforts of home, the patient also is robbed of privacy in many ways and may count the invasion as inappropriate. We turn now to the issue of privacy.

Privacy. The need for individual privacy may vary from person to person depending on his or her ethnicity, age, other cultural traits, and past experience. Whatever the individual boundaries of comfort, every patient in an institutional setting will experience less control over the usual parameters of privacy. Take, for instance, the typical hospital unit. The patient who is uprooted from his or her home and placed in a hospital room (usually with at least one other person—a stranger) may be thrust into a situation in which the door to the room has no lock and "walls" are curtains through which health professionals and others can listen or intrude without warning; there is no opportunity for holding a confidential conversation, having a good cry without others hearing, or engaging in lovemaking with one's sexual partner. In most cases light switches either are out of reach or can only be controlled by persons entering the room. Except in rare circumstances, all the usual privacy "props" are removed. For some, privacy is necessary to succeed in certain activities such as sleeping or urinating. If a patient feels that he or she is being watched constantly because of monitors or windows from the hallway, it may well be impossible for him or her to conduct the most basic activities of daily living.

The hallmark of the loss of privacy is the hospital gown. Even presidents and kings are not spared the potential indignity of walking down the hall in that garment with the gaping back! You can help patients by making sure they are covered adequately to preserve their modesty.

The patient, when robbed of privacy, is likely to feel intense discomfort. Health professionals must be diligent in helping patients meet the challenge of maintaining their rightful privacy.

Loss of Independence

Challenges related to the loss of home and privacy are rooted in the far more basic loss of independence. The institutional value of efficiency, which is important so that the facility can be responsive to the many demands of its functioning, create serious problems for the patient who needs time for solitude, variety in a schedule, or other accommodations. Most health facilities impose profound restrictions on independence, many of them unnecessary. For instance, almost every minute of the day is scheduled for patients, and their choices about how and where their unscheduled time can be spent are limited. Studies have identified a phenomenon known as decision burnout or decisional stress. Patients are transported or accompanied from place to place for therapy, diagnostic procedures, and other activities, often not knowing where they are headed. In many facilities visiting hours are fixed, and the telephone switchboard may prohibit calls from going through after a certain hour at night.

Often the patient's (or other patients') safety and well-being are factors in restricting independence. However, for many patients it is a challenge to sort out when and how much restriction of their independence is merited. For example, in some cases, the patient may be on a restricted diet, may not be allowed to have a drink of an alcoholic beverage, may be required to exercise (or to rest) at given intervals, and may not leave the facility. For acutely ill patients, this is a temporary frustration. In the worst case, for some chronically ill and permanently institutionalized patients, it becomes a way of life. Fortunately, we are in a period when some health care institutions are taking a hard look at changes that can be made to enhance independence while maintaining a high level of efficiency and patient safety. You will be in a good position to help suggest changes in institutional structures that will allow its occupants to realize a maximum degree of independence.

SPECIAL CHALLENGES OF AMBULATORY SETTINGS

More and more procedures are being performed in ambulatory settings. Here institutionalization is very brief and in many cases does not even involve an overnight stay.

Ambulatory care patients are in the difficult position of sitting on the fence between two worlds. They may appear completely well and therefore not be stigmatized by the label of "sick" or "disabled." However, they are definitely *patients* for the following reasons: physical or mental function is impaired enough to produce discomfort in the person or to result in his or her inability to proceed with some activities formerly taken for granted, the symptoms are severe enough to have been openly acknowledged by the person and confirmed by a physician or other health professional, the person has agreed to participate in a treatment or diagnostic regimen that requires regular trips to the health facility, and the visit takes high enough priority in the patient's life so that other competing activities are sacrificed.

From the health professional's perspective, challenges facing such patients are in many regards indistinguishable from those facing patients who are admitted to a facility (inpatients). However, there are notable differences. For instance, ambulatory care patients or clients may suffer from the loss of self-image even more keenly than inpatients because the person in the health care facility is surrounded by others in a similar predicament and is allowed to look and act ill, whereas ambulatory care patients do not have this license. They come into the treatment setting for a brief period and then return to the world of the more well and able-bodied. The person who is ambulatory only sometimes feels excluded from the "action" that appears to be taking place in the health facility, like a spectator at a game he or she wanted to play and play well. The inpatients know each other, understand the rules, and have a better chance of "winning." Consequently, ambulatory care patients may feel jealous of those who are in closer contact with the healers and worry that they are not getting adequate attention. And there are other practical challenges. In some instances persons may have to fight for time off from work, find someone to care for children, or attend to a homebound spouse or parent. They may lose precious pay or vacation time. The trip to and from the health facility can be so arduous and expensive that the person questions the worth of the visit, especially if when they arrive there is a 2- or 3-hour wait before they are seen.

The health professional who observes that a person receiving ambulatory care is feeling socially isolated can help the person overcome this alienation, become acquainted with others, and in other ways meet the challenge of finding a sense of belonging in the health care environment. At the same time, the health professional can also help the person meet the challenge of enjoying the gains of being able to live in society rather than having to remain in a health care facility.

SPECIAL CHALLENGES OF THE HOME CARE PATIENT

Although home care patients do not have to suffer the trauma of adapting to a strange environment as inpatients do, nonetheless there are special challenges for persons receiving formal health care services in their homes. Historically, families and friends have cared for their sick and infirm in the home setting. The presence of skilled health professionals who come to provide sophisticated therapy and professional care is a relatively recent phenomenon. Thus, there is always tension between the true purpose of the home, a refuge from the outside world, and the home as a site where patients receive technical interventions and care from strangers. Furthermore, homes are not hospitals and are not designed to be mini–intensive care units or rehabilitation centers.

The presence of health care professionals in the home is received with mixed emotions on the part of patients and families. On the one hand, there is a sense of relief that there will be assistance with foreign equipment and procedures and help with the burden of continuous care. On the other, there is a feeling of intrusion into personal space and behaviors that accompanies professional care in the home. Patients may not know how to treat health care professionals in their homes. Should they treat them as guests and afford them social courtesies such as coffee and cookies? Or should they treat them as hired help, much as one would treat a plumber or electrician who comes to the home to perform a specific task and then departs without the demand for pleasantries?

Home care is clearly unique in that professional services are carried out on the patient's turf. Here, the rules and dynamics of a household are the standards for behavior rather than the rules of a bureaucratic organization. Patients and their family members may feel that they can never truly relax or be themselves when professional staff are in the home. Thus, the challenge of maintaining privacy takes a different form in the home care setting than it presents in institutions. Patients and their families may not appreciate the long-term stress this invasion of privacy can cause because they are initially so elated to be out of an institution and back home. For example:

> A family with a 20-year-old quadriplegic, ventilator-dependent son decided that they wanted him to be a part of the family's life when he returned home. They did not want him placed away in a second-story bedroom, so they cleared the dining room of furniture to make room for the bed and equipment. After 2 months with this arrangement, the family decided this was a poor decision. The family had little privacy when professional caregivers were in attendance. The patient felt like he had no privacy at all. The solution was to move the son to the lower-level recreation room where he could still be a part of the family life but not the center of all activity.

Home care personnel should work with the family and patient to plan their schedule and care delivery so that the patient can have some privacy and the family can develop a sense of appropriate psychological, if not physical, distance between themselves and the caregivers in their home.

WEIGHING LOSSES AND PRIVILEGES

It sounds curious to talk of patients as having "privileges," especially in light of the previous sections in which you were introduced to serious challenges that patients face during illness or injury. At the same time, other members of society usually make some accommodations for a person who has become ill or injured by relieving him or her of certain roles and responsibilities. In Chapters 2 and 3 you were introduced to how respect for the patient has been embodied in various rights, laws, and social policies and practices. Even so, some people— though they are rare—experience more gains from being patients than when they are well. Each of these situations presents a different set of issues to you and your colleagues.

Certain accommodations are reserved for anyone who temporarily is struck down by physical or mental impairment. Recall the privileges you had as a child when you were sick. What changes did you experience? Common answers include the following:

- Meals were brought to me in bed.
- I didn't have to go to school.
- I had first choice of the toys.
- I was exempt from doing the dishes.
- I had the television or radio or a video brought to my room.

- I was given a cold washcloth for my forehead.
- I had fresh orange juice or chicken soup (or some other special food or home remedy).

Support for the stricken person is part of the accommodation being extended to him or her out of respect for the difficulties that attend being sick or injured. However, inherent in the granting of such privileges is a message that they are also an encouragement to keep up the good fight back to health. In other words, the privilege does not convey permission to remain in the patient role indefinitely.

The increasing emphasis on the patient's role as an active agent in the healing process and not just as a passive recipient of the health professional's ministrations was noted at the beginning of this chapter. Patients correctly believe that some of the "help" they need is to seek professional intervention, but also that they have information about their own lives that can assist in the process of healing.[6]

Part of this "taking responsibility for their own illness" is crucial to patients' healing. However, the authors have observed a kind of "braveness" in many patients that at first appears to be an example of "taking the bull by the horns" and assuming full responsibility for the course of treatment. At some juncture in the course of the illness, however, the braveness dissipates, leaving the patient feeling fully out of control and frightened. A woman who previously had been treated for adenocarcinoma of the lung, and who was now undergoing new tests because of a persistent cough, lends insight into the dynamics of "bravery" among patients in the following excerpt:

> Bending over the table as a doctor inserted a needle into my back to extract some fluid, I started to think about what I would do if a presumably innocent cough turned out to be the sound of the other shoe dropping. I had once had a good reason to listen for that other shoe; I'd had malignant lymph nodes in my mediastinum—the middle of my chest—as well as a tumor in my lung. I had always been amazed at how little time I'd spent listening for it, and what I most disliked about having the needle stuck into my back was that it began to awaken what I'd come to think of as the dragon that sleeps inside anyone who has had cancer. I'd written once that we can never kill this dragon, but we go about the business of our daily lives—giving our children breakfast, putting more mulch on our gardens—in the hope that it will stay asleep for a while longer. What I hadn't said was what I'd do if the dragon woke up. But, even as I braced myself for the insertion of the needle, it seemed unlikely that lung cancer, a notoriously aggressive disease, would hang around for so long only to reassert itself in the guise of a cough that interfered with my dreams of seeing the Bosporus.[7]

This type of bravery is useful at times as a means of maintaining hope. It may also be a means of dealing with the awareness that the accommodations by other people usually are short lived and that new methods of coping with the illness or injury must be brought into play.

SOME ADVANTAGES OF REMAINING IN THE PATIENT ROLE

Society is willing to grant at least temporary accommodation to a person who is ill or injured. The inability to recover completely presents the patient with many challenges and opportunities. However, we focus our attention here on the rare person who could—but does not want to—recover. Clearly, for these people, the privileges they receive while they are ill outweigh those granted them when they were well. One way a person remains in the patient role is to feign symptoms long after they are gone or to fabricate them if they never existed at all. Such a patient is engaged in malingering.

Sometimes the problem is complex in other ways. The patient may have symptoms of organic illness in the absence of organic pathological signs. This patient is said to have a "hysterical symptom" or to have undergone a conversion reaction (i.e., a psychological problem has been converted into an organic, or physical, symptom). Of course, sometimes the organic basis is very difficult to diagnose, and the person may be treated as a "malingerer" only to later find the cause. A third kind of patient may refuse to take the necessary measures to relieve the symptoms, thus destroying his or her chances of ever returning to society as a healthy, responsible person.

Escape

One may wonder what such patients gain by their behavior, considering the advantages of a healthy, independent, and active life. They see protection from the threatening outside world as one advantage of remaining in the patient role. This may be especially true of a person who has been hospitalized or institutionalized and is suddenly faced with discharge. Uncertainty about the future, which will be discussed in the next chapter, becomes a paralyzing fear for some. Their response to the fear is to avoid the moment of release.

Financial Gain

Financial gain is also an advantage for some. Malingering patients are seen often in clinics that treat industrial work-related injuries, which cost society millions of dollars each year in labor losses. Their situation has resulted in an increasing number of programs in the workplace, such as "work hardening" and other approaches, with the goal of slowly returning persons to work after they have been absent because of illness or injury. This is accomplished through positive incentives to stay at or return to work. Many of these patients have jobs that are boring or arduous or offer no opportunity for advancement; therefore, they welcome any means of escape from the job as long as workers' compensation or some other form of disability insurance subsidizes them. In the United States, similar attempts to gain early retirement or to receive extensive disability often are settled through the court system. The solutions to these issues are complicated and require thoughtful approaches by governments, the health care system, employers, and workers.

Social Gain

Social gain is a third advantage realized by some persons who choose to remain in the patient role and receive the privileges afforded to people in that role. Some people are able to manipulate the attention of family and friends through dependence when they perceive that this approach is successful. If the results are rewarding enough, an individual may decide that it is not worthwhile to be restored to his or her former symptom-free life.

Argan, Molière's malingering imaginary invalid, is a perfect example of such a person. He manipulates everyone in his life by virtue of his weakened condition. When his daughter Angélique is old enough to be married, he chooses a physician as her husband. Toinnette, the maid, asks Argan why the physician has been chosen when Angélique is obviously in love with someone else.

> **Argan:** My reason is that, in view of the feeble and poorly state that I'm in I want to marry my daughter into the medical profession so that I can assure myself of help in my illness and have a supply of the remedies I need within the family and be in a position to have consultations and prescriptions whenever I want them.
>
> **Toinnette,** boldly: Well that's certainly a reason and it's nice to be discussing it so calmly. But master, with your hand on your heart, now, *are* you ill?
>
> **Argan:** What, you jade! Am I ill! You impudent creature! *Am I ill?*
>
> **Toinnette:** All right then, you *are* ill. Don't let's quarrel about that. You *are* ill. Very ill. I agree with you there. More ill than you think. That's settled. But your daughter should marry to suit herself. *She* isn't ill so there's no need to give *her* a doctor.
>
> **Argan:** It's for my own sake that I'm marrying her to a doctor. A daughter with any proper feeling ought to be only too pleased to marry someone who will be of service to her father's health.[8]

The world thus revolves around Argan's medicines and body functions. His emotional dependency is revealed in his continual tattling to his wife about the annoying Toinnette, who confronts him with his hypocrisy. His brother Béralde observes, "One proof that there's nothing wrong with you and that your health is perfectly sound is that in spite of all your efforts you haven't managed to damage your constitution and you've survived all the medicines they've given you to swallow."

Argan quickly counters, "But don't you know, brother, that that's just what's keeping me going. Mr. Purgon [the physician] says that if he left off attending me for three days I shouldn't survive it."[9]

Audiences for 300 years have been laughing at Argan's obvious self-deluding rationalizations. They laugh, of course, because they can identify with Argan's reluctance to give up the privileges of the patient's position in society. However, most differ from Argan in that they do not enjoy these privileges enough to create a lifestyle around their symptoms and debilitating disorders.

RESPECTFUL RESPONSES TO MALINGERING

You will occasionally meet an Argan and should be prepared to respond constructively and respectfully to him or her. It is understandable that most health professionals become frustrated when confronted with a patient who apparently does not want to get well, but who wants the attention of treatment, often at the price of attention that you and your colleagues judge should be giving to other patients. The following case will help you reflect on what you can do:

> Marilyn Siegler is a 19-year-old woman who has long had "family problems." Her father is a successful businessman, and her mother is very much involved in the charitable and social activities of the large city in which they live. Marilyn has felt, from the time she was a child, that her parents favored her older brother, who now has decided to become a partner in their parents' business.
>
> Marilyn has been seen by numerous counselors and psychiatrists since her teen years, when she made a suicide attempt. All agree that her feelings of rejection are the basis for her unhappiness. Several attempts have been made to bring the parents in for family counseling, but they have always been too busy.
>
> Marilyn is now a junior in college. She went from boarding school to a college dormitory, where she has been living for three years. During the past six months she has developed a progressive weakness in her legs. She is now confined to a wheelchair. Extensive tests have revealed no physical basis for the disabling symptoms. Recently her parents have decided it would be best for Marilyn to return home, where they plan to employ a private tutor for her.
>
> You are living in the dormitory where Marilyn lives. She has been a patient in the clinic where you are currently working as part of your professional on-site preparation. You know much more about Marilyn's clinical history than any of the other people in the dorm.
>
> Early one morning, about 1 A.M., you go out in the corridor. Much to your astonishment you see Marilyn walking into her dorm room. The door closes quickly, before you can call out to her.

What should you do now? What can be done to help such a person? Obviously, she will benefit from professional help, yet you have seen something in a social situation! Whenever such a thing happens, the following suggestions may assist you when confronted with a person believed to be malingering. First, believe the patient until all reasonable evidence that he or she is ill has been legitimately discounted. Every member of the health professions who is in contact with the person can assist in this process. For instance, if the patient is hospitalized, a dietitian or radiologist, who often is in briefer contact with a patient than, say, a nurse or occupational therapist, may provide helpful information by sharing his or her observations. Second, discuss the issue in staff meetings to alert a large number of people to the problem. If the patient is not receiving ambulatory care, one can sometimes tactfully employ the assistance of family and friends.

In all cases, such fact-finding must be carried out with the idea that the patient's complaints of symptoms are legitimate until evidence shows otherwise. Sometimes collecting information about a patient can take on the aura of a witch-hunt, and the patient understandably grows to distrust or even despise the health care professionals. In fact, the focus of therapy can turn into attempts to prove patients wrong or find them out. This attitude, almost one of retribution, is often seen in the treatment of patients with pain for which no objective cause can be found. In these cases, patients are given placebos instead of analgesics to prove that the pain is illusory. If patients find out about this deception they are invariably angry and hurt. To avoid the development of an adversarial relationship, the patient's report must be accepted until there is well-documented evidence of malingering, to which one is willing to testify under oath in court.

Once a case of malingering is proved, it may occasionally be worthwhile to talk with the patient privately. In most cases, however, it is better to recommend that he or she see a professional counselor. The patient cannot be coerced into wanting to return to society or previous roles and responsibilities until his or her underlying problems are solved. Health professionals often become involved in this problem-solving process by working closely with the psychologist or psychiatrist and by reinforcing conduct that contributes to reclaiming the degree of healthfulness available to the person.

SUMMARY

In this chapter you have had an opportunity to focus squarely on some peculiarities of the patient's challenges during changes that virtually everyone finds difficult in one way or another. Whether the transition involves real and perceived losses or the adjustment to a change in roles and responsibilities that others view as privileges or accommodations, they involve some degree of disruption from long-established patterns. Some things will be viewed with disdain, distrust, or impatience by persons who make up the fabric of the patient's life. Your role and skills cannot be divorced from this larger real-life picture that the patient brings to your doorstep. Their challenge then becomes your challenge too—and one worth meeting well.

REFERENCES

1. Klein, B.S.: *Slow Dance: A Story of Stroke, Love, and Disability.* Berkeley, CA, Page Mill Press, 1998, p. 5.
2. Dahlberg, C.C. and Jaffe, J.: *Stroke.* New York, W.W. Norton, 1977, pp. 62–63.
3. Dudzinski, D.: The diving bell meets the butterfly: identity lost and re-membered. *Theor. Med. Bioeth.* 22:33–46, 2000.
4. Wendell, S.: The rejected body: feminist philosophical reflections on disability. New York, Routledge, 1996.
5. Haddad, A. "French Weaving," 2001, unpublished. With permission of the author.
6. Purtilo, R.: Professional-patient relationship: ethical issues. In Reich, W. (ed.): *Encyclopedia of Bioethics,* Vol. 4. 2nd ed. New York, Macmillan, 1995, pp. 2094–2101.
7. Trillin, A.S.: Betting your life. *The New Yorker* Jan. 29, 2001, p. 38.
8. Molière, J.B.: *The Misanthrope and Other Plays,* Wood, J. (trans.). London, Penguin Books, 1959, p. 218.
9. Ibid, p. 257.

CHAPTER 8

Respect for the Patient's Personal Relationships

CHAPTER OBJECTIVES

The student will be able to

- Describe three circumstances that may account for a patient's difficulty in sustaining important relationships during a period of illness or injury
- Describe how family relationships are strained during serious illness or injury
- Identify several key challenges that family caregivers face
- Explain how uncertainty creates anxiety in the patient and family and describe the health professional's role in attempting to alleviate anxiety
- List sources of support that can help minimize the deleterious effects of stigma for patients and caregivers
- Discuss how costs can add to the patient's personal problems.

> We stop being people and start being patients. . . . Our identity as people and the world we once knew both are relinquished; we become their patients and we live in their hospital.
>
> *D. Gottleib[1]*

The personal life of the patient consists of the relationships, experiences, and values that a person brings to the health professional and patient relationship. Respect for this fact is all that matters ultimately in your goal of maintaining the patient's dignity for the duration of your professional relationship with her or him. This chapter is a reflection on the important but fragile nature of many relationships, with an emphasis on some ways the patient's personal relationships might be affected by her or his clinical status and condition.

FACING THE FRAGILITY OF RELATIONSHIPS

Inpatients, those receiving ambulatory care, and home care patients—all come into contact with the health care system as people who have families, neighborhoods, churches, clubs, and workplaces and as members of the larger society. These relationships have a profound bearing on their responses and adjustment to the conditions that brought them to you for your professional services. Often you will hear, "I could have never made it through this ordeal without Mary (or John, or my church group)," and it makes good sense that this is so!

Some ways patients' personal relationships are affected can be guessed from the topics addressed in the previous chapter: loss of familiar surroundings in which relationships are most easily nurtured, loss of independence so that the patient may not be able to participate in his or her usual fashion, privileges granted by others but with conditions attached, and expectations by others that the patient will return to former roles. Illness has the power to alter the patient's status and role in the various communities he or she enjoys or at least knows, so that the new position may seem awkward at best. Recall, for instance, the young man who was put into the family dining room initially when he went home because the family wanted him to be a part of the family action, only to learn that for all of them this arrangement was too disruptive. In fact, when one person in a relationship changes, the others must too. Like a mobile, every piece necessarily moves when an outside force causes one to move. The fragility of relationships is brought into focus by subtle factors such as the time the person had to spend away from loved ones or the fact that the patient was too ill to participate in the ongoing life of the family or that she incurred a blow that permanently changed her capabilities. Patients often express concerns of abandonment or that they will be unable to contribute to the relationship. We discuss some important aspects of each of these situations.

"Will Others Lose Interest?"

We all hope that our families, friends, and associates will take our problems to heart, and fortunately often they do. However, sometimes a patient is surprised by the degree of indifference they feel many people show to the struggle the person went—or is going—through. You know from your own experience that this feeling is not limited to persons who become patients. More generally speaking, it is dismaying to realize that, no matter what momentous event you have been through or are still experiencing, the majority of people in your life do not want to know very much about it!

There may be a lot of reasons for others' apparent lack of interest. For instance, when there is good news to share some might be jealous of your good fortune or feel that their security is threatened by your success; when the news is bad some may be threatened by it, too, thinking, "There but for the grace of God go I." For that matter, some really do not care much in the first place, even though it was easy and enjoyable to show interest when things were going well.

Sometimes the patient becomes extremely boring or demanding. In extreme circumstances most people do turn more inward and become self-absorbed,

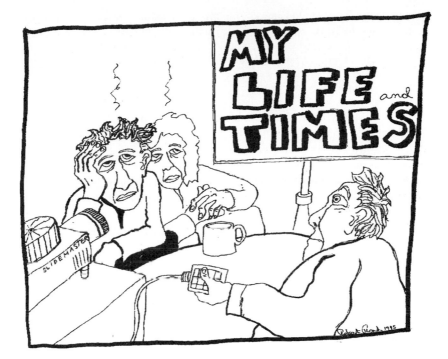

and patients are no exception. Friends and loved ones may assume that the patient no longer really cares about them either and lose interest in maintaining the relationship for that reason.

The truth is that most people expect at least their family and friends to be there for them when difficult times arise. However, these usually reliable sources of support are not always willing to abide a person in difficulty. A physical therapist recounts the moment when her 20-year-old patient named David, who was quadriplegic as a result of diving into a shallow pond when he was 19, told her the bad news about his beloved older brother Jim and David's fiancée, Jane. She noticed that something was wrong this particular Monday morning. Trying to get David into conversation she asked if he had been "on a weekend binge or something."

"No. But I need a drink."

"What do you mean, you need a drink?"

"It doesn't matter anymore. All those weights. The pulleys. Just get me outta here."

He couldn't move any part of his body, but I felt as if he had physically thrown something at the wall or at me. The alarms went off in my spirit.

"David! *What's the matter?*"

His shoulders sagged lower and I saw the flaps of skin on his chin and belly . . .

Eighty pounds lighter too quickly for his young skin to keep up with his diminishing bulk. He raised his head, barely, and whispered hoarsely from somewhere way back in his throat, or life, "Jane is going to marry Jim."

For the first time ever, I was without words with David. He looked straight into my eyes, locked in that moment of recognition that we had both lost our footing and were falling.[2]

Sometimes an event in a patient's life really hits you and, like the therapist in this excerpt, you do not know what to say or do. She probably did the right thing just by acknowledging that this event was too grave for a quick response. Fortunately most patients do not have blows to absorb like those David endured, but health professionals never should be surprised when a patient suffers an emotional blow. However difficult, it is always worthwhile to try to offer comfort and hope in such situations. For instance, you can try to prospectively help prepare patients for a disappointment they might encounter in their expectations if you see it coming and make suggestions for renewed participation in their communities. Just by talking directly to the patient about an obvious absence of people who once were or should be present during his or her stay in a health care facility sometimes helps relieve the patient's suffering. Of course, to pry deeply into the particulars of a relationship (or increasing absence of one) can be an intrusion into the patient's privacy if the timing is not right. An untimely intrusion may even increase the suffering for the patient. Gentle probing may lead to an opportunity for the patient to talk through and think more expansively about a situation. Sometimes asking a patient about family, friends, or other social contacts will help him or her start remembering things about the relationships that are treasured and allow him or her to focus on strengthening the relationship even during this time.

"Will We Weather the Winds of Change?"

Patients justifiably worry about the long haul when the illness or injury is serious. Recall from Chapter 1, the poet and playwright T. S. Eliot was aware of how timid most of us are when faced with a disruption in the status quo. In *Murder in the Cathedral,* the townspeople learn that the Archbishop Thomas Becket is coming to their small village. They plead with the heavens to deliver them from this new presence in their lives, besieging the powers that be to let them continue in their state of not living and not dying, expecting nothing and receiving nothing. The title of the play suggests their response; this stranger cannot be incorporated into their existing relationships, no matter how unsatisfactory they presently might be. He had to be expunged from their midst, even though his message was of hope for relief from their doldrums.

An irony is that the change a person undergoes during illness or injury may cause the person to become almost a stranger to those around him or her.[3] In the most extreme cases, the original form of old relationships becomes unrecognizable in the present ones: a spouse who sustains a traumatic brain injury may become like a child; a trusted business partner who becomes mentally ill may become suspicious or violent toward others; or a young man known for his bravado may become fearful of hanging out with the guys after a heart attack, thinking they will see him as a has-been. However, usually the changes are more subtle, like a chill wind brushing through an otherwise refreshing fall breeze. They can send an unexpected shiver of worry across all those in the relationship. One of the authors, who was helping to prepare a family to take their brain-injured husband and father home, was struck by the wife's comment: "I'm not sure we can take him home. We don't know *him*," she said, pointing to her husband.

Ethicists, psychologists, and others slowly are recognizing the importance of exploring the challenge of continuing commitment in a significant relationship when one person in it is changed by illness or injury. This recognition is extremely important because all too often the health of family or other caregivers has been ignored to the detriment of everyone involved, especially when the new situation requires an intense, long-term (or even lifelong) commitment. At the time this book is being written the U.S. Census Bureau estimates that approximately 23 million family caregivers in the United States are providing ongoing care to seriously ill, injured, or disabled family members and that the period of time of caring for each person has increased significantly over that of even a decade ago.[4]

Most family caregivers rise to the occasion with remarkable courage, good spiritedness, and, if all else fails, resignation. Still, study after study reveals that the everyday reality of life for most family caregivers begins with the belief that they are saddled with *unbounded obligation* by virtue of their wedding vows and commitments as parent, spouse/partner, son or daughter, or "only living relative."

The high incidence of stress-related disorders among family caregivers is understandable and extremely disquieting. The rising incidence of serious physical injury from lifting or lack of good judgment because of exhaustion are rarely considered by policy makers.[5] This problem is so serious that one recent study shows caregiving itself as an independent risk factor for death among elderly caregivers or spouses, 75% of whom are women.[6] Family members who "drop out" because they literally cannot "take it anymore" are faced with acute guilt feelings for abandoning their loved one and often are rewarded with banishment from their own dwindling sources of family and community support. With these data it is not surprising that persons facing care-giving situations often do so with trepidation and that those needing the care are anxious about what is ahead for everyone.

ABIDING UNCERTAINTY

At some time in every recovery or adjustment process, a person's uncertainties about the future loom before him or her. For instance, some conditions are characterized by roller coaster-like remissions and exacerbations. As a young child put it to one of the authors, "My sickness is like a ghost. You're doing OK, then it can creep up on you and 'Pow!' because you can't see it coming." Family caregivers often have similar responses.

The disquieting effects of uncertainty are manifested in many ways during the time the patient is receiving health care and afterward. For instance, a woman may express reticence to undergo a follow-up test to show that she is now free of cancer. A man who has received good care in the past suddenly may doubt the health professional's competence when there is no rational basis to do so.

In Chapter 4 we discussed your own anxiety as a student, and how uncertainty may cause people who have been relatively carefree to become rigid and fearful. Most people would rather know that the news is bad news than not to know at all and live with uncertainty. What about you?

You will encounter patients who ask, "Do you think I'm improving?" or "Do you think it will ever recur?" Sometimes it is hard to know what to say. In a sincere effort to encourage such persons you should provide as much certainty about their status as your own information and role allow. At the

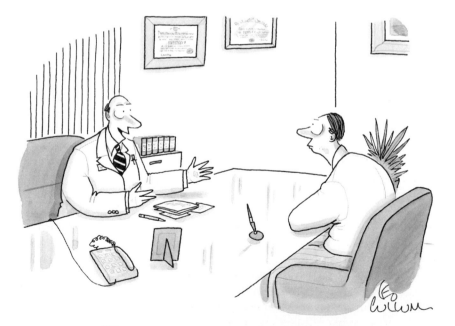

"There are many questions, of course, that won't be answered till the autopsy."

same time you should exercise care not to give false information or instill false hope. The wise health professional does not try to "play God" and pretend to see into the future when it is unknown. In this situation the desire to comfort the patient or family by providing false certainty will lead to a feeling of distrust or betrayal in the long run, compounding the person's suffering. However, patients may ask a different question, although not always as directly as we will state it here: "Will you be present to see me through this situation, whatever the outcome?" To this you can respond by assuring that everything possible will be done for the patient by you and your colleagues, if in fact you are confident it is true. If you yourself are unsure of whether the patient will be neglected or outright abandoned by the health care professionals or system, the challenge is to work toward improving the conditions that led to that type of situation.

We discuss some examples of when a patient's fears might be totally realistic. For example, later in this chapter reimbursement policies that may make it impossible for you to continue to treat the patient will be addressed briefly. In Chapter 2 we address relationship issues between you and the patient that may lead you to try to refer this person to someone else. However, a good general rule is to reassure patients that you will not abandon them.

FIGHTING STIGMA

The idea of stigma was introduced in Chapter 3, and we raise it again here with a focus on its effects on the personal life of the patient. A stigma is an attribute that makes a person possessing it different from others in a negative way. It is, therefore, a deeply discrediting feature.[7] Recall that people suffer the stigma of age, skin color, or ethnicity. Poverty is stigmatizing in our society. People who have AIDS are prime examples of a highly stigmatized group of people: by virtue of their illness they may lose their job, friends, and health insurance. Often they find themselves unwanted in their neighborhoods or shunned by acquaintances.

One of the most damaging elements of being a stigmatized person in society is the social expectation that he or she will feel personal *shame* for the predicament. The range of conditions for which a patient may be led to believe he or she "should" feel shame will vary according to the social values of the patient's culture and subculture. In Christina Lee's excellent book, *Women's Health, Psychological and Social Perspectives,* she points out that women may be expected to be ashamed of reproductive conditions such as premenstrual syndrome, menopause symptoms or infertility, postpartum depression, excess weight or physically "disfiguring" conditions that lay outside the norms of beauty, and age-related symptoms.[8] Not only the patient but caregivers also often become stigmatized and may even be blamed for the loved one's difficulties.[9] A colleague was teaching a 3-week summer course in another city when her husband had a serious heart attack. She recalls the following conversation upon hearing the news that her husband was in the cardiac intensive care unit:

> **Cardiologist:** Your husband has had a serious heart attack and is in the cardiac care unit.
> **Woman:** Oh my God. What happened?
> **Cardiologist:** [Explains some medical details.] Was he well when you left? Has he been ill?
> **Woman:** He was very well! To my knowledge there's no history of any problem whatsoever! [More questions about his condition.]
> **Cardiologist:** Has he been eating well?
> **Woman** (still shaken): I think so! I've been gone for three weeks but. . .
> **Cardiologist:** Husbands often don't eat well when their wives are gone. . .

The woman said that although she knew the doctor was not intentionally blaming her for her husband's heart attack, it took her a long time to get over a feeling of shame that somehow she was to blame because of the cardiologist's comment.

The rise of grassroots support groups for both patients and caregivers can be of some help, but stigmatizing responses from others remain a problem for many who unnecessarily are made to feel disrespected or blamed for their experience. Patients make significantly better adaptations to catastrophic illness when placed in contact with other similarly affected persons who have learned of ways to succeed in a stigmatizing society. Peer counseling programs can be effective: a "veteran" patient or caregiver introduces a new person with the same situation into the group. The process sometimes is coordinated by a member of the health care team.

Some church and civic groups provide means of support for people in times of crisis. A church in our city has a system that ensures that no one is ever left alone in a time of sickness or at the death of a loved one. By dividing their time, the members of the group are able to give around-the-clock support if the patient or family wishes it.

However it is provided, one of the most important elements in a patient's successful continued participation in society is the support of friends and loved ones as well as health professionals and the accompanying knowledge that the person has a place. A professional colleague who was seriously injured in a car accident as a result of being hit by a drunk driver reflected in his Christmas letter that year:

> If you are one of those too busy to ponder my fate, take care that you do not join me. The journey back is a difficult one, and not everyone, I think, has a Jane (his wife) to lead the way or so many good friends to mark his progress.

The presence of loved ones and professionals is exactly the type of encouragement we have observed as being one key to a patient's successful recovery or adjustment. Any time you can speak up to counter stigma, and any way you can act to increase the patient's support systems, is time well spent.

DISCOVERING VALUES: OLD AND NEW

If you learned that you had a serious condition that would likely lead to your death in the near future, would you do anything different from what you are doing now? Would you continue as a student? Would you decide to spend more time with a particular relative or friend or project? Would you spend your money differently? Are there things you would like to say to someone? Are there responsibilities you would like to shed? Places you would visit?

Many people faced with illness or injury ponder these types of questions. You will sometimes be brought into the patient's thoughts as the person reflects about those things she or he has done and left undone. Sometimes he or she will ask your advice. At times you will be faced with a real dilemma about what to say to a patient, but again, your considered and nonjudgmental attempts may be of value.

Sometimes the weight of a condition is so heavy that a patient or family member never seems to fully recover from a trauma. In a previous chapter you learned about malingering and secondary gain. You will work with some people who do recover physically but seem to retreat and never again emerge emotionally from their condition. A patient who suffered a severe back injury from a car accident, but recovered completely, told one of the authors, "The pain's gone, but I can't get over the feeling of being shell shocked." Recently the idea of a delayed response to a serious earlier trauma ("posttraumatic syndrome") has been explored, and its power to hinder or delay recovery and adjustment has been acknowledged.

At the same time, most people do recover or adjust emotionally and, during their illness, take the opportunity to reassess what is really important in their lives so that they might begin to act on those aspects more fully. A man who felt he was too busy to enjoy his family may decide to take every opportunity to do so, a young couple may decide to reconcile their differences and try to make a new life together, or an older woman may go to college for the first time. The stories of a difficult situation becoming the springboard to a new release into life are legion. Often you will have the satisfaction of watching patients or former patients use their condition as an opportunity to think things over and start afresh.

Religious Values and Practices

In Chapter 3 you were reminded of the rich diversity of religious beliefs and practices among the patients and others with whom you will interact. Showing respect requires that you be sensitive to the ways in which religious beliefs, rituals, and images help provide meaning to the experience and aid in healing or adjustment. We believe the following is an apt example for your consideration. You may know Psalm 23 in the Hebrew-Christian scriptures. There is a passage that reads, "He [God] makes me lie down in green pastures. He leads me beside still waters; he restores my soul." One middle-aged man with colon cancer said that this was God's way of getting him to "lie down" so that his soul could be restored. The health professional present said he had a hard time thinking of colon cancer as a "restoring moment," but he took the opportunity to learn how to look at this man's religious interpretation and used this image to support the patient through trying periods. Some patients may want you to pray with or for them or help them honor certain rituals necessary for the practice of their religion.

Religious beliefs that are far removed from mainstream Western religious traditions may challenge health care professionals' tolerance and willingness to make accommodations. Consider the following case:

> A 30-year-old Hmong male was dying of hepatic cancer. The patient was well known in the Hmong community (that had been transplanted from Laos to this large Midwestern city) and had a very large family. As many as 30 visitors occupied the visitor lounges and filled the patient's room to capacity at any given time. The health professionals were having a difficult time getting the family to make a decision about whether the patient should be resuscitated if he stopped breathing or his heart stopped. The family appeared to be unable to make a decision as the patient's status deteriorated.
>
> When the patient became short of breath, the family became quite agitated. The health professionals tried to explain again that the patient was dying. The family said they wanted to be present when the patient died. At this point, the primary physician decided to make the patient a "no code," meaning that the patient would *not* be resuscitated. As he lay dying the family began chanting, lit candles, and performed various rituals around the body.

The health professionals involved with this patient were uneasy about many things, such as the number of people in the room, who should make decisions about life-sustaining treatment, and the unusual rituals surrounding death. They were unsure how to honor the religious beliefs of the family and still provide safe, quality care. What would you like to know about the Hmong culture that might help you in caring for the patient? Make a list of these items in one column on a sheet of paper. In a second column next to each item you have listed indicate how you would go about getting the information. Who might be a resource? Although there is certainly room for improvement in how the health professionals handled this particular case by maintaining a respectful openness to beliefs the health professionals did not share, the patient and family were not deprived of powerfully symbolic expressions of their religious beliefs.

You will benefit from discussion with your colleagues and others about how to show respect even if you are not comfortable personally with honoring a patient's request for participation in a religious activity such as prayer. At the very least it is always appropriate to work through the religious care office of your institution or even make a direct call to a patient's or family's religious advisor so that spiritual values and needs can be addressed respectfully.

Paying for Care

In today's health care arena, at least in the United States, many patients' situations will be affected by the high cost of health care. Therefore, a chapter examining key aspects of a patient's relationships would be incomplete without at least a brief discussion of the burden of costs, whether for the individual or, if ongoing care is required, for the caregiver. For example, whereas an adult's values may include that of being a good provider for the family, the loss of opportunity to earn money for a time (or permanently) may be compounded by the high cost of his or her medical and other health care bills. The person who decides to make a highly desirable change in life direction or lifestyle may be prevented from doing so by the reality of the desperate financial distress it may mean for others in the family or community. One of the things you can do is to be attentive to the possibility of stress that patients and caregivers are experiencing from this source. Their stress may express itself in depression, or a person may make health care choices you do not understand. For instance, it is well known that many instances of so-called "noncompliance" on the part of patients is occasioned by the cost of medications, treatments, devices, or services that the individual or family cannot begin to pay for. Your sympathy—and at times your intervention—can make a difference in their situation.

Some health professionals, discouraged by the high costs of health care, recognize that they are in a position to intervene on behalf of patients and in their own interests. Therefore, this chapter on the patient's personal relationships ends with his or her link to you in your role as an advocate in policy arenas that are sometimes less accessible to patients and families themselves. The following five activities are constructive suggestions for helping to address cost problems and reject compromises that are inconsistent with their needs. You may be able to think of others:

1. You must become aware of the basic language and concepts of economics and health policy so that you can contribute to the discussions when you have an opportunity to do so.

2. You can assume responsibility for documenting instances in which being forced to say "no" on the basis of cost constraints or policies compromises good clinical judgment. For example, in the United States, Medicaid, Medicare, or private insurance reimbursement practices that control the number of days the

patient is eligible for treatment sometimes place professionals in such a position. Judiciously gathering empirical data regarding treatment effectiveness and patient outcomes can assist policy makers in creating the most cost-effective approaches to care.

3. You can work directly with institutional and governmental administrations through legislation or input into other policy-making mechanisms.

4. Innovations at the departmental level should be used to assess the strengths and weaknesses of cost-containment policies.

5. Conferences and in-service sessions similar to those held in clinical departments can highlight themes that are ongoing problems. At these conferences, health professionals as a group may have the resources to face the challenge of good stewardship regarding costs that individual professionals may lack.[10]

SUMMARY

The personal life of the patient consists not only of him or her, but also of the many relationships that help to provide meaning, support, and a sense of belongingness to this person. The most immediate relationship for most people is their family; therefore, showing respect for the patient and assessing the challenges facing the patient means thinking about how his or her predicament affects the family and vice versa. This chapter addresses the fragility of relationships in general and, more specifically, highlights several areas of the patient's personal life that are at highest risk vis-à-vis his or her personal relationships. The final section turns to the need for patients to reexamine old values and assess which ones are the most viable within their new situation. Families, too, bring their values and beliefs to the situation and part of your job is to try to show respect for everyone in the patient's circle of key relationships.

REFERENCES

1. Gottlieb, D.: Patients must insist that doctors see the face behind the ailment. In Frank, A.W. (ed.): *The Wounded Storyteller. Body, Illness and Ethics.* Chicago, University of Chicago Press, 1995, p. 10.
2. Purtilo, R.: The story of David. In Haddad, A.M. and Brown, K.H. (eds.): *The Arduous Touch: Women's Voices in Health Care.* West Lafayette, IN, NotaBell Books/Purdue University Press, 1999, p. 76.
3. Akin, C.: *The Long Road Called Goodbye: Tracing the Course of Alzheimer's.* Omaha, NE, Creighton University Press, 2000.
4. Harrington, M.: *Care and Equality.* New York, Knopf, 1999, pp. 37–40.
5. Levine, C.: The loneliness of the long-term care giver. *N. Engl. J. Med.* 340:1587–1590, 1999.

6. Schulz, R. and Beach, S.: Caregiving as a risk factor for mortality. *JAMA* 282(23): 2215–2219, 1999.

7. Goffman, E.: *Stigma: Notes on the Management of Spoiled Identity.* Englewood Cliffs, NJ, Prentice-Hall, 1963, p. 3.

8. Lee, C.: *Women's Health: Psychological and Social Perspectives.* London, Sage Publications, Inc., 1998.

9. Zuckerman, C.: 'Til death do us part: family caregiving at the end of life. In Levine, C. (ed.): *Always on Call. When Illness Turns Family into Caregivers.* New York, United Hospital Fund of New York, 2000, pp. 159–176.

10. Purtilo, R.B.: Thirty-first Mary McMillan Lecture: a time to harvest, a time to sow: ethics for a shifting landscape. *Phys. Ther.* 80:1112–1119, 2000.

PART THREE

Questions for Thought and Discussion

1. If you sustained an injury that required you to be in various health care institutions for 7 weeks, what aspects of home do you think you would miss most? What would be your greatest frustration? What would you find to be the most difficult adjustment to make in returning to your old role and friends?

2. If you were to lose the use of your lower extremities in an automobile accident, what would be the most difficult aspects of adjusting to this permanent change? What do you hope people would do to respect your situation?

3. Name some technologies and procedures that your profession uses to evaluate or treat patients. Do they enhance a patient's dignity or demean it? For those that might have demeaning aspects, what can you do to help maintain respect toward the patient during the application of these procedures?

4. Here is an awkward situation that you might find yourself in at some time:

   A patient asks you if she can bring her friend to treatment with her. You know that this patient has been asking a lot of questions and seems to be very anxious. When the friend comes, she is very angry with you for the terrible way you have treated the patient. You are confused. You have no idea what the woman is talking about, but you begin to feel hostility toward her.

   What can you do in this situation to sort out what is going on? What steps can you take to show this patient and her friend respect in spite of your feelings?

5. A single woman in her 60s comes to you with symptoms you know are related to the stress of her position as caregiver for an elderly parent who has Alzheimer's disease. You know the best thing for her is to have some time away from her ailing father. You first ask her about other family members who might share her responsibility, but she claims to have none who are willing or able to help share her burden. Her situation seems perilous to you, and you begin to think of a perfect society where she would not be stuck in this seemingly endless and intense situation. List all the things you can think of to design an environment for her and her father so that both are able to realize the respect they deserve.

PART FOUR

Respect through Communication

Just as history does not exist in nature, but is created in the telling, so, too, autobiography and the patient's case history emerge out of interactions, which mean that they are at the same time both less and more than the "facts" of the case.[1] Chapter 9 focuses on how we understand our patients by examining the ways the patients' stories are created. Illness and injury are milestones in patients' lives. The clinical record is one place where the experience of the patient is set into words, words that are shared with the whole health care team. The format, syntax, perspective, and language we use to tell the patient's story deserve your attention as much as the content. It becomes apparent that it is not enough to merely describe the chronology of events that bring patients to us. You will want to understand why things happened the way they did, what meaning the patient gives to the experience, and what the patient expects from you.

To come closer to understanding the meaning your patients give to their experience, you will depend on your ability to communicate. The most immediate "tool" you have available to you for respectful interaction is your own communication, whether that tool is used verbally or nonverbally. What you say, how and when you say it, and how you communicate nonverbally through gestures and other types of physical messages will set the tone for everything else that happens in the relationship.

Chapter 10 focuses on components of respectful interaction in verbal and nonverbal aspects of communication. As you read and reflect on all the types of messages you give and receive, think back to Part One, especially to the parts of those chapters addressing values and culture. It is almost certain that you will work with colleagues and patients from countries and backgrounds different from your own. These differences are evident as we listen to what patients choose to include in their stories and what is left unsaid. Consider how the challenge of communicating both verbally and nonverbally is enhanced and influenced by these factors.

REFERENCE

1. Greenhalgh, T., and Hurwitz, B.: Why study narrative? In Greenhalgh, T., and Hurwirtz, B. (eds.): *Narrative Based Medicine: Dialogue and Discourse in Clinical Practice.* London, BMJ Books, 1998, pp. 3-17, citation from p. 5.

CHAPTER 9

The Patient's Story

CHAPTER OBJECTIVES

The student will be able to

- Distinguish between the different "voices" encountered in the telling of a patient's story

- Identify some of the literary forms used in health care communications

- Describe two of the contributions of the study of narrative to respectful health professional and patient interaction

- Discuss how a patient might express the experience of illness or injury in a poem, short story, or pathography

- Relate a patient's narrative to his or her own experiences, values, and beliefs

- Discuss how literary narratives such as poems, short stories, and drama about patients' and health professionals' experiences apply to actual clinical practice.

When you have mouth sores you think very carefully before even trying to take a bite of food; even something as innocuous as a yogurt smoothie is like swallowing a handful of nettles. This also happened to be the time when my hair truly fell out. Because I couldn't eat my weight had dropped alarmingly. I happen to be one of those people who look a wreck when I have a mere head cold; I look horrible out of all proportion to my symptoms. This time when I looked in the mirror I was truly alarmed. This was not a case that the Look Good-Feel Better people could solve.

J. Hooper[1]

Human beings experience illness, injury, pain, suffering, and loss within a *narrative,* or story, which shapes and gives meaning to what they are feeling moment to moment.[2] One may say that our whole lives are an "enacted narrative." Another way to understand this is to think about life as an unfolding story. Narration is the forward movement of the description of actions and events that makes it possible to later look back on what happened. And it is through that backward action that we are able to engage in self-reflection and self-understanding.[3] Illness and injury are milestones in a patient's life story. Much of this book has emphasized that health professionals are called into a particular relationship with patients because of the importance of the illness experience. The medium of that relationship is the patient's story.

This chapter will help you grasp the importance of paying attention to the unique and personal story of a particular patient's life beyond the more general suggestions we have offered so far. In other words, we focus here on the idea of enacted narrative. Because the final focus of all of our efforts in health care is the patient, the insights that narrative analysis can offer to health professionals is important. We highlight how different voices or perspectives offer different stories of the patient's predicament. We briefly explore some of the basics of narrative theory and apply it to health care communications, such as textbooks, scientific journal articles, and the medical record. We include some examples of narrative literature to give you an opportunity to read and think about poetry and short stories that speak to patients' and health professionals' experiences. The chapter closes with a reminder that you also bring a unique and personal story to the professional and patient encounter and that you both participate in the creation of the continuing story of your lives.

WHO'S TELLING THE STORY?

When a patient enters the health care system, regardless of the place of entry, an exchange of stories begins. It might be hard for you to consider the patient's "history" portion of the history and physical examination to be a kind of story, but it is. So are the entries in a medical record and the scientific explanation of a particular pathologic condition in a textbook. Even within the medical record, for example, a "diverse collection of individual voices as well as interactions or viewpoints" exists that constitutes the single entity of the chart.[4]

Montgomery has convincingly argued that all knowledge is narrative in structure. She claims that medicine is not as much science as it perceives itself to be,[5] but this could easily apply to all of the health professions. She views the physician and patient encounter in terms of a story. The patient tells the story of an illness or injury, which she notes is an interpretive act in that the patient chooses certain words and not others and reports some incidents and not others. The physician then interprets the story and translates it into a list of possible diagnoses. Frank suggests that the physician's story is guided by the notion of "getting it right." "Diagnostic stories are about getting patients to the appropriate treatment as quickly as possible."[6] Getting it right may or may not be what counts for the patient. For example, a patient who has a chronic illness such as multiple sclerosis might have a story that is guided by figuring out how to cope with the unpredictable nature of the disease. So, at a minimum, we have two different notions of what the physician's response should be in terms of the patient's hopes and expectations.

The Patient's Story

One way to highlight the different ways that the same story can be viewed is to look at it from various perspectives. For example, how is a cerebral vascular accident (CVA) seen from the perspective of the patient, the medical record, and a medical textbook? We will begin with a personal account of a patient who had a CVA. He recounts his experience in the past tense. This is common since most patient stories are recollections.[7] The following is an excerpt from a much longer account of the CVA that changed this person's life:

> . . . all I knew was that I had a raging headache, and then, the next morning, I could hardly move.
>
> It was just another Saturday morning when I found myself in bed, alone and unable to get up at home in Islington, north London. My wife, Sarah Lyall, a journalist, was in San Francisco. It was odd to be on my own and odder still to be so helpless, but I was in no pain, and, in retrospect, I realise that I was barely conscious. Downstairs, the grandfather clock was chiming the hour: 8 o'clock. I could see that beyond the heavy maroon curtains it was a lovely day. I was supposed to drive to Cambridge to visit my parents. So, it was time to get up. But I could not move my left side. My body had become a dead weight of nearly 15 stone. I thrashed about in bed trying to sit upright, and wishing Sarah were with me. I experienced no anxiety—just irritation and puzzlement.[8]

Obviously, the patient/author is English, so some of the language may be unfamiliar such as his reference to his weight as "15 stone." A stone, a measure of weight, is approximately 14 pounds, so at the time he had his stroke he weighed 210 pounds. Weight can also be measured in kilograms. Thus, we have an immediate example about the differences in words and terms that all mean fundamentally the same thing. Besides the obvious differences in language, what did you notice first about the patient's story? He claims he was not anxious, just irritated and puzzled. Would you expect this type of reaction? What sorts of emotional reaction, if any, did you have to the story? It is probable that this is not the first time the patient told the story of his stroke, although it could be the first time that he actually wrote about his experience. In the telling and retelling of landmark experiences such as the trauma associated with a stroke, "the narrative provides meaning, context, and perspective for the patient's predicament. It defines how, why, and in what way he or she is ill. It offers in short, a possibility of *understanding* which cannot be arrived at by any other means."[9] When a patient begins to tell you the story of his or her illness, you might be able to discern whether this is a familiar, often told story or if the patient is still trying to figure out what happened and make sense of the experience.

The Medical Record

Beginning with the patient's direct experience of the trauma that he has undergone, let us move forward in time to a different setting and interpretation of what is happening to him. We will assume that the patient was eventually discovered and taken to a hospital. In a hospital, one of the vehicles for communication between health professionals who care for a specific patient is the medical record, or chart. The "chart" might be handwritten or can be a file on the computer. How might the patient's story continue in the medical record? Here are two types of entries, the first from the nurses' notes and the second from the medical progress notes. Assume that they were written on the day after the patient was admitted to the hospital.

Nurses' Notes—7/18/01: Impaired verbal communication R/T aphasia 2° to cardiovascular accident.[10]
  9:00 A.M.
  S: "Where's my book? Where's my book?"
  O: Pt. tearful and keeps repeating above statement. No books found in bedside stand. Pt. then picked up wallet from over-bed table and opened it to a picture of him and his wife. Pt. pointed to picture and repeated the above phrase. Calmed down when reassured wife was on way to hospital. Pt. unable to use L arm. Ate breakfast independently.
  A: Pt. appears frustrated and stressed due to inability to find the right words to express himself.
  P: Continue to support pt.; consult with speech, occupational, and physical therapy as needed; encourage as much independence as possible; remind pt. to attend to L arm and leg affected by sensory alteration.

Physician's Progress Notes—7/18/01: Dx: R hemisphere hemorrhagic infarct.; Pt. stable; echo, CXR, MRI; contact speech/OT/PT for rehabilitation.

What do you notice first about this version of the patient's story? Clearly, there is a difference in how the patient and health professionals describe what is going on. In Chapter 10 we discuss the use of jargon in health care and how it serves a useful purpose of facilitating communication between health professionals but also works to distance patients from caregivers. The jargon in these sample entries from a fictitious medical record almost becomes impenetrable to a novice in the official language of health care. Did you understand all of the terms and abbreviations? What is "aphasia"? Did you know that "R/T" means "related to," that "echo" is shorthand for echocardiogram, and that "CXR" is an acronym for "chest x-ray"? Although the patient describes his experience of having a stroke in the first person, the medical record refers to him in the third person. We will discuss point of view in more detail later in this chapter. It is sufficient here to note the type of voice used in writing and the implications of using a particular voice. Third-person voice distances us from what is going on in the narrative.

Consider one more version of the patient's story, this one even further removed from the personal experience of a CVA. In the classic medical tome *Textbook of Medicine,* a cerebral infarction is described as follows:

> The pattern of onset of neurological symptoms and signs in a cerebral infarction often suggests the cause. Cerebral embolism causes an abrupt onset of symptoms, and headache often precedes other neurological symptoms by several hours. When infarction is limited to the cerebral hemisphere, there is weakness or paralysis in the extremities contralateral to the infarction. Patients may also be aware that sensory perception on the side of weakness is impaired and may complain of heaviness or numbness in the arm or leg.[11]

What does this final version of the patient's story tell us? The author of the medical text is not concerned with a specific patient who has a CVA. The description is general, one that can be applied to all patients who suffer a stroke. The symptoms are described as a matter of clinical, scientific fact, not of personal experience. You might be thinking, "Perhaps this is not all bad. A general description helps a health professional learn what to expect when a patient has had a CVA." The danger lies in accepting the textbook description as "fact" or the truth as opposed to just one more interpretation of what a CVA is and means to individual patients. To assist you in scrutinizing the narratives you encounter in clinical practice, turn now to some basic concepts from narrative theory.

AWARENESS OF LITERARY FORM IN YOUR COMMUNICATION

When you see a poem on a page, even if you do not know anything about poetry, you recognize it as a poem because of its form and structure, i.e., the way it looks on the page. Because it is a poem, you also know that the particular words the poet chose are important. In poetry, every word matters. It is unlikely that you look at the writing in your textbooks, even this one, in the same way. Yet, any type of written communication has a form and structure, subtle or obvious. By paying attention to these aspects of the various types of writing you encounter in clinical practice, you can develop an appreciation for how language is used and its impact on your thinking and behavior. Two assumptions from narrative theory applicable to narratives encountered in health care are that narrative language is not transparent and does not reflect the whole reality of what is going on.

Narrative Language Is Not Transparent

The language of narrative does not function like a clear glass that lets messages be directly sent from sender to receiver. In other words, it is not transparent.[12] No language is neutral or "colorless." This is true of any narrative whether it is a story, a case study, or an article in a scholarly, professional journal. Scientific writing (this includes the writing on a patient's medical record) does not call attention to itself the way language does in a poem or novel. As you saw in the sample entries in the medical record of the patient who had the CVA, there were no metaphors, similes, or figures of speech. The nurse did not write, "I walked into the room and found the patient sobbing his heart out." Yet, professional writing is based on and created in a particular context. The closest we get to an emotion in the nurses' notes is in the phrase "Pt. found tearful," but there is no mention of grief, loss, or the depth of his sadness, just a statement of fact or observation.

As Chapter 10 mentions, one skill you must learn in your professional preparation is to write in this manner to communicate as a professional. Robert Coles describes an interaction with one of his teachers when he was in medical school. Although it involves physicians-in-training it is applicable to all health professions. "He remarked that first-year medical students often obtain textured and subtle autobiographical accounts from patients and offer them to others with enthusiasm and pleasure, whereas fourth-year medical students or house officers are apt to present cryptic, dryly condensed, and, yes, all too 'structured' presentations, full of abbreviations, not to mention medical or psychiatric jargon. No question: the farther one climbs the ladder of medical education, the less time one has for relaxed, storytelling reflection."[13]

Language Creates Reality

Rather than reflecting reality, language creates reality.[14] For example, without thinking very much about it, most health professionals would say that a patient's history in a medical record states the case as it is. In other words, the history is simply recorded observation. Yet, the language used actually creates the reality of the case in so far as it frames the kinds of questions we ask about it, how we seek answers, and how we interpret what we find and limits what we observe or even consider. Refer back to the structure of the nurses' notes. Did you know what the letters "S," "O," "A," and "P" that preceded the nurse's entries meant? The SOAP charting method is a common way to record information in clinical records. The words being abbreviated by SOAP are *subjective* (usually a direct quotation from the patient), *objective* (the health professional's observations or description of the situation), *assessment* (the health professional's interpretation of the situation), and *plan* (actions to be taken to solve the problem presented).[15] The opening step in SOAP charting, subjective, is a rare occurrence in the medical chart. The health professional seems to actually record what the patient said at a particular point in time. But even the inclusion of a direct quote from a patient is filled with interpretation. The health professional chooses which quotes to include and then proceeds to use the quote as a springboard for the rest of the entry. Furthermore, the whole structure of SOAP charting requires one to think of patients as individuals with problems that need professional resolution.

Language can also be used to exclude others. A clinical ethicist noted this manipulation of language on medical rounds:

> As I began to watch this process more carefully, it became apparent that the physicians spoke a language which was quite understandable when they thought the ethical issues were fairly clear and where there would probably be some consensus but resorted to high code when they felt uncomfortable with the decision(s) before them or when there was dissent in the group.[16]

So when things were easy and comfortable, everyone spoke the same language. When things got tough, the physicians switched to a language that allowed them to distance themselves from the discussion and allowed them to dominate it as well.

Extremely technical language, or high code (as Rogers calls it), creates a different sort of reality in clinical practice than everyday, lay language. In addition, scientific language and information are more highly valued than what the patient has to say. "Witness the time devoted on rounds to discussing serum magnesium levels as compared to the time spent discussing the patient's experiences. When the patient's narrative (variously called 'subjective,' 'qualitative,' or 'soft' data) conflicts with laboratory or radiographic findings (considered 'objective,' 'quantitative,' 'hard' data), the narrative is usually given the lesser weight; it might well be ignored or minimized and the patient attacked for being a 'poor historian.' "[17] Although the language may vary from profession to profession, generally speaking the health professional's language will prevail.

CONTRIBUTIONS OF NARRATIVE TO RESPECTFUL INTERACTION

Health care practice is a rich metaphor for so many archetypal human dramas, featuring such riveting themes as life and death, loss and hope, and love and hate. All play out in different scripts, some meaningful and others trivial, each experience providing its own opportunity for wonder at the infinite capacity for human invention. There is an increasing emphasis on the use of literature, a specific type of narrative, in health professional education. The premise is that studying literature about illness, death, or caregiving will help you, the student, relate more personally to patients, hear patients' stories more clearly, and make decisions that reflect a humane appreciation of patients' situations.[18] Reading novels, stories, and poetry is a means of participating imaginatively in other lives; it encourages you to construct your own stories in relation to the ones you are reading. Consequently, you will come to know yourself better, too.

Literary Tools

Narrative literature, and by this we mean language used in an intensified, artistic manner, can be used to offer a fresh way for you to understand the encounter between health professional and patient. You can use some simple literary tools such as point of view, characterization, plot, and motivation to examine narrative literature, and as you have seen, the usual types of narrative writing in health care communication, such as the patient's chart.

Point of View. This is a good place to begin because it gives you an immediate sense of who is speaking to you through the poem or story. As you think about point of view, here is a simple question to get you started: Who is the narrator of the piece? In a medical record, the point of view is always third person. Health professionals talk about the patient in the third person, even avoiding pronouns whenever possible; that is, the patient is referred to as "Pt." not as "him" or "her." In the excerpt from the *Textbook of Medicine*, the point of view is that of an omniscient narrator, but one who is almost invisible. The personal voice is deeply hidden in scientific and professional writing, yet it is there.

Characterization. Also in good narrative, characters bring their whole intricate selves to the story. For instance, if the character in a story or a drama is a physical therapist, you will also learn that he is a son, maybe a husband and father, a friend, a softball coach, and a religious man. As the narrative unfolds, you appreciate how multiple, often conflicting, interests and identities figure in the twists and turns of his motivations and decisions. You follow along, getting the feel of his prejudices, fears, passions, and pains. Then, if you are lucky, the magic of transference will take you on a journey into his story and eventually into the byways of your own life, but from some new and different angle. The lived quality of narrative is what makes it plausible. "I could be him," feels the reader, "I've been there, too."[19]

Plot and Motivation. Narratives of clinical interest tend toward plot in their structure rather than the more basic narrative of a simple story. In his oft-cited work, *Aspects of the Novel,* E. M. Forster explains the difference between a simple story and a plot: ". . . in a story we say 'and then—and then' . . . in a plot we say 'why?' "[20] Why do the people in a particular clinical narrative make certain choices and act in specific ways? You can examine the motives of the individuals in clinical narratives in the same way that you can those of characters in a short story or novel. Once again, you may have to try harder to find motivation in clinical narratives because so much work goes into hiding the feelings or emotional reactions of health professionals. Even emotional outbursts by patients are written to appear objective and "clinical."

Poetry

The following poem explores the patient's experience with a colostomy. We suggest that you read the poem at least twice before reading the questions to help you analyze it.

A Rare and Still Scandalous Subject
From Susan Sontag's Illness as Metaphor

The title of my confession
is "Colostomy." The word,
cured and salted,
sizzles on my tongue.

This is shame:
standing naked at the sink,
unsnapping the adhesive flange
from my abdomen.

I couldn't have imagined
the stoma, the opening,
red glistening intestine.
Peristalsis moves it like a caterpillar, hatched
from a visceral cocoon.

My life depends on the stoma,
which insists on gratitude,
gurgling, "Listen to me,"
but I place my hand over it,
even now when I am alone.

— *R. Solly*[21]

After you have read through the poem, you should be able to recognize who is speaking, what his situation is, and to whom he is speaking. Take each stanza in turn. What mood or tone is the author trying to convey? Refer to poem's title, "A Rare and Still Scandalous Subject." What does the author mean by this title? How does this poem affect your understanding of what it means to have a colostomy? These are just a few questions to help you begin to analyze the poem.

Short Stories

The same literary tools that apply to poetry also apply to fiction. It is important to understand that the narrator in both poetry and fiction is not necessarily the author. Authors can create narrators who are more or less involved in the story. Consider the following short, short story about a nurse and a patient on an intensive care unit in psychiatry.

NADINE'S SECRET

The women in the adult intensive care unit for psychiatric patients slept down one hallway of the L-shaped unit, the men down the other. At the point where the two hallways converged, the night shift staff usually pulled a card table out of the day room so they could sit in the intersection and monitor both hallways. The first patients to arise in the morning were usually the smokers who would walk down to the card table to get a light. Sometimes the patients would pull a chair out from the day room and sit in silence while they smoked their first cigarette of the day.

As head nurse of this unit, I was often there very early and very late. One particular morning I arrived early to meet with one of the night staff before she went home for the day. As I stood exchanging whispered small talk with the night staff, a door opened down the women's hallway. Nadine emerged from her room and slowly made her way down the hallway to us. Nadine was a middle-aged woman who had been diagnosed with manic-depressive psychosis. On admission, she was in a full-blown, flamboyant manic phase. She had run all of her credit cards to the limit, hadn't slept for days and was picked up for disorderly conduct when she refused to leave a bar at closing time. When the police brought her to the emergency room, still dressed in a red sequined cocktail dress, she was singing at breakneck speed as loudly as she could. Now with medication she was subdued, at least in demeanor. However, she still wore the vestiges of her former outrageous self by applying make-up every morning as though she was going to appear on stage.

For a moment, it looked as if Nadine was naked as she walked towards us, but as she got closer I could see the faint outline of a flame-orange baby-doll nightgown. The nylon was so thin that it was essentially transparent except for ruffles around the low-cut neckline and arms. She wore gossamer orange panties that were no more than two triangles connected by string. As Nadine leaned forward with a cigarette hanging from her mouth she said, "Got a light?" I was momentarily speechless as I lit her cigarette.

"Nadine," I began, "I'm afraid you won't be able to wear that nightgown around here."

"Why?"

"It's just not appropriate. You cannot wear it here. You'll have to wear something else that's not so sheer."

"*All* my nighties are like this. I like them bright, cool, and sexy."

"If all your nighties are like this then you will have to wear a patient gown."

Nadine paused and smoked. She leaned against the door and seemed to be completely at ease, even though the two psychiatric technicians and I could see everything—her sagging, ample breasts, the pouch of her stomach over the top of the bikini pants, her pubic hair. Nadine rolled her eyes and sighed. She ran her fingers through her disheveled hair that was dark at the roots and bright red on the ends from the dye she used during her manic phase.

"Those patient gowns are ugly. Come on. I'm not hurting anyone. Besides, my butt will hang out in the back," Nadine countered.

I was ready for this argument. "You can wear two patient gowns. Put one on the regular way and the other like a coat to cover your backside."

I heard some of the male patients rousing from sleep so I followed my words with action. I did not want Nadine standing out in the hallway dressed like that when the male patients came out of their rooms. I opened the linen closet and got out two gowns. "Here," I said in my most professional voice. "Put out your cigarette and put these on in the bathroom."

"You know what?" Nadine said over her shoulder as she walked to the bathroom. "You're no fun."

The next morning, Nadine was again the first one up. I was pleased to see that she had on the requisite patient gowns, front and back. She pulled a chair out of the day room, sat down, yawned loudly. A few minutes later, three male patients made their way down the hall to the communal bathroom. The noise of the toilets flushing and water running inevitably woke the rest of the patients on the unit. As the women patients awoke and opened their doors, the scene down their hallway was like some badly colorized version of *Night of the Living Dead.* One by one, every female patient shuffled down the hall in various stages of drug or sleep-induced stupor decked out in neon shades of green, red, purple, yellow, fuchsia, blue, and orange, transparent baby-doll nighties and matching bikini pants. Although the nighties were of similar style and size, the women were not. Some of the women barely fit into the flimsy gowns, others swam in them, the bikini pants held up by a hand.

Some of the early risers on the men's side of the hall ran back to their rooms and pulled their roommates out of bed to come see the sight. Eventually, the staff and all of the male patients stood at the end of the hallway and dumbly watched this garish procession. Nadine smiled slightly and said, "Got a light?"[22]

From this short story, what do you know about the narrator of the story? Can you trust that the narrator is telling the truth? What emotions and reactions is the author trying to evoke in you and how is this accomplished? Do you have any insights into what the main characters are thinking? Would it change the story if you had specific knowledge about what Nadine is thinking? How?

Illness Stories/Pathographies

A third type of literary narrative is the pathography, a form of autobiography or biography that describes personal experiences of illness, treatment, and sometimes death. "What it is like to have cancer" or "How I survived my heart attack" or "What it means to have AIDS" are examples of the typical subjects of pathography.[23]

Refer to Judith Hooper's description of her experience with chemotherapy after breast cancer surgery, which opened this chapter. Hooper's pathography would probably be characterized as an "angry pathography," even though it is laced with sarcastic humor. In angry pathographies, the author expresses frustrations and disappointments with the health care system in general and with particular programs or health professionals. Most pathographies are of the testimonial type in that they offer advice and guidance to others who are faced with the same disorder or problem. Pathographies offer you yet another type of narrative to help you understand your patients and their struggles.

WHERE THE STORIES INTERSECT

After exploring all the various ways a story can be told, you might wonder: "What is the true story?" The health professional must listen carefully to the patient's story but also understand that the patient does not know the "truth" either; the patient is not always accurate. There are clearly differences between the patient's experience and the health care professional's explanation of the experience. So how do we get coherence, if not the true story? "The patient and physician [health professional] are writing the story of the clinical encounter together."[24] Frank affirms the dialogical nature of narrative: "We tell stories that sound like our own, but we do not make up or tell our stories by ourselves; they are always co-constructions. Stories we call our own draw variously on cultural narratives and on other people's stories; these stories are then reshaped through multiple retellings. The responses to these retellings further mold the story until its shape is a history of the relationships in which it has been told."[25]

SUMMARY

Literary explorations of the subjective and interpersonal responses of patients, family members, and health professionals to the tensions encountered in health care settings can engage you in your own personal questions and reflections about your response to similar situations in your clinical practice. Narrative, in all of its forms, offers a way of seeing the deeper, subtle nuances involved in your interactions with patients, families, and peers, thereby improving the chances that the opportunities for showing them due respect are not missed or behaviors misguided.

Your role in your patients' stories will vary from assisting them to recover to witnessing their deaths. Whatever roles you take, recall that you also bring your own unfolding story to the relationship. You will build a story, with each patient you encounter, that then becomes another moment forming the narrative of both of your lives.

REFERENCES

1. Hooper, J.: Beauty tips for the dead. In Foster, P. (ed.): *Minding the Body: Women Writers on Body and Soul.* New York, Anchor Books, 1994, p. 117.
2. Donald, A.: The words we live in. In Greenhalgh, T., and Hurwirtz, B. (eds.): *Narrative Based Medicine: Dialogue and Discourse in Clinical Practice.* London, BMJ Books, 1998, p. 17.
3. Churchill, L.R. and Churchill, S.W.: Storytelling in the medical arenas: the art of self-determination. *Lit. Med.* 1:73–79, 1982.
4. Poirier, S., et al.: Charting the chart—an exercise in interpretation(s). *Lit. Med.* 11(1):1–22, 1992, quote p. 1.
5. Montgomery Hunter, K.: *Doctors' Stories: The Narrative Structure of Medical Knowledge.* Princeton, NJ, Princeton University Press, 1991.
6. Frank, A.W.: From suspicion to dialogue: relations of storytelling in clinical encounters. *Med. Humanit. Rev.* 14(1):24–34, 2000, quote p. 26.
7. Robinson, J.A., and Hawpe, L.: Narrative thinking as a heuristic process. In Sarbin, T.R. (ed.): *Narrative Psychology: The Storied Nature of Human Conduct.* New York, Praeger, 1986, p. 111.
8. McCrum, R.: The night my life changed. In Greenhalgh, T., and Hurwirtz, B. (eds.): *Narrative Based Medicine: Dialogue and Discourse in Clinical Practice.* London, BMJ Books, 1998, p. 34.
9. Greenhalgh, T., and Hurwitz, B.: Why study narrative? In Greenhalgh, T., and Hurwirtz, B. (eds.): *Narrative Based Medicine: Dialogue and Discourse in Clinical Practice.* London, BMJ Books, 1998, p. 6.
10. North American Nursing Diagnosis Association: *NANDA Nursing Diagnoses: Definitions and Classifications 1995–1996.* Philadelphia, NANDA, 1996.
11. McDowell, F.H.: Section eleven: cerebrovascular diseases. In Beeson, P.B., and McDermott, W. (eds.): *Textbook of Medicine.* 12th ed. Philadelphia, Saunders, 1967, pp. 646–669, quote p. 655.
12. Donley, C.: Whose story is it anyway? The roles of narratives in health care. *Trends Health Care Law Ethics* 10(4):27–31, 39–40, 1995.
13. Coles, R.: *The Call of Stories: Teaching and the Moral Imagination.* Boston, Houghton Mifflin Co., 1989, p. 24.
14. Donley, C.: Whose story is it anyway? The roles of narratives in health care. *Trends Health Care Law Ethics* 10(4):27–31, 39–40, 1995.
15. Weed, L.L.: Medical records that guide and teach. *N. Engl. J. Med.* 278:593–600, 652–657, 1998.
16. Rogers, J.: Being skeptical about medical humanities. *J Med. Humanit.* 16(4):265–277, 1995, quote p. 274.
17. Coulehan, J.: Pearls, pith, and provocation: teaching the patient's story. *Qual. Health Res.* 2(3):358–366, 1992, quote p. 361.
18. Davis, C.: Poetry about patients: hearing the nurse's voice. *J. Med. Humanit.* 18(2):111–125, 1997.
19. Brown, K.: Using narrative in reflection and practice. Unpublished manuscript, June 17, 1994.
20. Forster, E.M.: *Aspects of the Novel.* New York, Harcourt, Brace and Co., 1927, p. 130.

21. Solly, R.: "A rare and still scandalous subject." (Unpublished. Reprinted with permission of the author.)

22. Haddad, A.: Nadine's secret. In Haddad, A., and Brown, K. (eds.): *The Arduous Touch: Women's Voices in Health Care.* West Lafayette, IN, Purdue University Press, 1999, pp. 22–24.

23. Hawkins, A.H.: *Reconstructing Illness: Studies in Pathography.* West Lafayette, IN, Purdue University Press, 1993, p.1.

24. Bishop, J.B.: Creating narratives in the clinical encounter. *Med. Humanit. Rev.* 14(1):10–23, 2000, p.19.

25. Frank, A.W.: From suspicion to dialogue: relations of storytelling in clinical encounters. *Med. Humanit. Rev.* 14(1):24–34, 2000, quote p. 32.

CHAPTER 10

Respectful Communication in an Information Age

CHAPTER OBJECTIVES

The student will be able to

- Compare and contrast models of communication
- Describe basic differences between one-to-one communication and working with groups
- Identify four important factors in achieving successful verbal communication
- Assess three problems that arise because of the failure to use appropriate vocabulary in communicating with patients
- Discuss two voice qualities that influence the meaning of spoken words
- Identify two types of nonverbal communication and describe the importance of each
- Describe how attitudes such as fear and humor affect communication
- Give some examples of ways in which time and space awareness differ from culture to culture
- Discuss ways to show respect through effective distance communication
- Identify seven levels of listening and describe their relevance to the health professional and patient interaction

---

After surgery last May, my first memory upon awakening in the ICU was a feeling as if I were choking on the ventilator, and of desperately wanting someone to help me. I could hear the nurse behind the curtain. I lifted my hand to summon her, only to realize I was in restraints, immobilized. I felt as if I were being buried alive. Lacking an alternative, I decided to kick my legs until someone came. This worked. The nurse came and suctioned me briefly, then disappeared behind the curtain. Still afraid and still feeling as if I needed more suctioning and the presence of another near me, I kicked again. She returned, this time to lecture me on how I mustn't kick my legs. And then she left.

S.G. Jaquette[1]

TALKING TOGETHER

By about the age of 2 years, a child makes all possible phonetic sounds. He or she clucks, coos, chirps, and gurgles, and the audience, totally captivated, provides encouragement. However, by the age of 4 years, a child knows that only certain sounds evoke a response from adults. The child thus begins to repress some sounds and mimic adults in combining sounds to form words. In this way, the highly complex, intricate skill of language is acquired, and an important bridge to relationship is built.

Patients rely on verbal communication to try to explain what is wrong or seek comfort or encouragement from health professionals. Yet they may have difficulty with the language itself, with finding the right words, or they may literally be unable to speak and have to resort to gestures, such as the woman in the opening scenario of this chapter. Health professionals rely on verbal, nonverbal, written, and electronic communication to share information, plan care, and collaborate with others on the health care team.

The greater responsibility for respectful communication between you and a patient lies with you, although both must assume responsibility. By examining interdependent components of effective communication, you will gain insight into this critical area of human interaction.

In your work as a health professional you will be required to communicate verbally with a patient to (1) establish rapport, (2) obtain information concerning his or her condition and progress, (3) confirm understanding, (4) relay pertinent information to other health professionals and support personnel, and (5) give instructions to the patient and his or her family. Periodically, you are expected to offer encouragement and support, to give rewards as incentives for further effort, to convey bad news, to report technical data to a patient or colleague, to interpret information, to teach the patient, and to act as consultant. Naturally, you will be more comfortable with some activities than with others, according to your own specific abilities and experiences. Nevertheless, all health professionals should be prepared to perform the entire gamut of communication activities.

Verbal communication is instrumental in creating better understanding between you and a patient. However, this is not always the result. You will often be able to trace the cause of a misunderstanding to something you said; it was probably the wrong thing to say, or it was said in the wrong way or at the wrong time. The way words travel back and forth between individuals has been the subject of a great deal of study in the communication field. Several models have been proposed to graphically describe what happens when two people exchange the simplest of words.

MODELS OF COMMUNICATION

Although the following quotation focuses on the exchange of information between the physician and patient, the same can be said of all health professionals as they communicate with patients.

> It is revealing to examine how this flow back and forth between physician and patient is shaped, what is revealed or requested, when, by whom, at whose request or command, and whether there is reciprocal revelation of reasons, doubts, and anxieties. When we look at the medical context, instead of a free exchange of speech acts we find a highly structured discourse situation in which the physician is very much in control. Some patients perceive this sharply. Others more vaguely sense time constraints and a sequence structured by physician questions and terminated by signals of closure, such as writing prescriptions.[2]

Communication understood in this way involves the transfer of information from the patient to the health professional so that a diagnosis or plan for treatment can be made. The focus is on the "facts" and generally begins with a question about what brought the patient to the health professional. However, once the initial complaint is stated, there appears to be little time or attention devoted to other patient-centered concerns.[3]

Think of some reasons this is problematic. For example, the first complaint that a patient mentions may not be the most significant. More important, the patient may take an abrupt closure after discussion of the first complaint as an overt sign of disrespect. As one older patient mused, "The doctor acted the whole time like he was double parked on the busy street outside his office."

Most interactions with patients take the form of "interviews" rather than a conversation or dialogue. Health profession students take great pains to learn this interview technique designed to reveal, by the process of data gathering and elimination, the patient's health problem. The interview becomes a means to an end, the end being a diagnosis and treatment plan. This end may not be the one the patient is seeking. It could be that the patient's primary goal is for a knowledgeable person to really listen and understand. This variance in goals is nowhere more evident than when the patient is terminally ill: often when health professionals interact with patients to plan for end-of-life care, the idea of an interview does not seem appropriate, but the need for "end-of-life conversations" does.[4]

Furthermore, by strictly following the interview model of communication, the health professional effectively controls the introduction and progression of topics. This pattern of communication involves the use of power and authority but remains largely hidden from awareness. Patients may literally be unable to get a word in edgewise during the time they have to speak with health professionals.

Imagine yourself changing your view of communication to one of a dialogue or conversation so that you can focus your attention on different aspects of the process such as minimizing the disparities in power and creating opportunities for true understanding between you and the patient. Figure 10–1 conceptualizes communication, both verbal and nonverbal, as the bridge between you and a patient. The model also includes some of the primary and secondary cultural characteristics introduced in Chapter 3 that influence what each party brings to the dialogue. All of these factors (and others not listed in the figure) have an impact on the interaction.

THE CONTEXT OF COMMUNICATION

Figure 10–1 places the two parties who are communicating within an environmental context. Where, with whom, and under what circumstances the dialogue or conversation takes place can have a profound influence on the process and outcomes of the interaction. Clinical encounters between you and your patients are, according to Arthur Frank, a particular form of dialogue:

> Most of the particularities generate tensions: stakes are often high for both parties, time is often limited, intimate matters are being broached between comparative

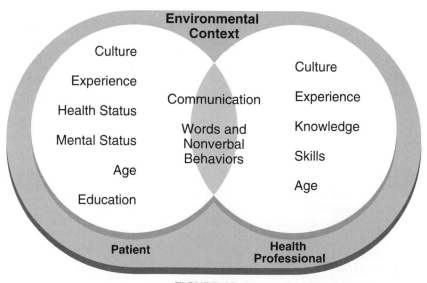

FIGURE 10–1
Essential and influencing variables of the communication environment.

Adapted from Keltner, N.L., Schweke, L.H., and Bostrom, C.E.: *Psychiatric Nursing.* 3rd ed. St. Louis, Mosby, 1999, p. 115.

strangers, power differentials intrude, and—not last but enough—both parties often have idealized expectations for what should take place.[5]

Thus, the internal context of this exchange between you and the patient sets it apart from everyday conversations. The external environment also has an impact on the process and outcome of your dialogue. Because of technology, you may find yourself communicating with the same patient in a variety of contexts (e.g., face-to-face in a clinical setting, talking on the telephone, or corresponding via e-mail).

Face-to-Face or Distant

If someone is standing or sitting right in front of you, the type of interaction you will have is very different from what occurs on the telephone or through an e-mail message. What varies most between face-to-face interactions and those that occur across distances is proximity and anonymity. When we are in direct personal contact with another person, there are fewer places to hide our fears and discomforts. In fact, knowing this, some health professionals specifically choose areas of practice in which they will have little direct contact with patients.

When you have the opportunity to meet face to face with a patient, all of the possible ways of communicating can be engaged. Each sense can be a source of information about the other. This explains, in part, why the exchange is that much richer and, to some, more frightening than those that take place from a distance.

We will discuss various forms of "distant" communication tools later in this chapter. During your career there is a good chance you will use all sorts of devices to communicate with patients. Perhaps at some time in the future, a holographic, computer-generated version of yourself will "interact" with the patient. For the time being, there is some evidence that patients are more satisfied with face-to-face interactions with health professionals than with other forms of communication, even when the information involved is exactly the same.[6]

Furthermore, studies also show that face-to-face interaction promotes the greatest trust, followed by phone, then text-chat, then e-mail. It is interesting to note that when test subjects use e-mail they behave mostly in self-serving ways; in other words, they communicate in a single direction that is directed toward meeting their own needs.[7, 8]

One-to-One or Group

Before you begin any type of interaction with a patient, you should make sure the patient knows who you are and what you do. This sounds so basic that it hardly seems worth mentioning. However, some health professionals are so focused on getting on with the diagnostic examination or asking questions that they forget the introductions. Of course this is not necessary if you are seeing a patient often. If you have met before, but there has been some time between your interactions, it does not hurt to reintroduce yourself and explain your role.

If you are meeting a patient for the first time, be sure to use his or her full name. Do not presume to address a patient, unless the patient is a child, by his or her first name until the patient gives you explicit permission. Ask the patient how to pronounce his or her name if there is any doubt about the correct pronunciation. The 6-year-old niece of one of the authors was highly insulted when her pediatrician continually mispronounced her first name after being corrected. The child said, "How would she like it if I kept saying her name the wrong way?" So even children notice this lapse in respect.

After you introduce yourself, tell the patient what you do in a few sentences. It is helpful to practice this explanation with a sympathetic audience such as relatives or friends who will tell you if you are being too technical or confusing.

Having established this initial rapport, you can now devote your attention to the patient before you and vice versa. We will address matters such as facial expression, gestures, and touch later in this chapter. All of these nonverbal forms of communication may override verbal messages, and this is especially obvious in a face-to-face interaction.

Working with an individual patient is far different from working with a group of patients. Most health professionals will often interact with groups of patients rather than a single patient. Thus, it is important to become knowledgeable about group functioning because much of what you plan for and deliver may be accomplished through a group process. To have a constructive effect in a group setting you must be familiar with how a group influences individual behavior and the forces that operate in any group. The groups you interact with as a health professional may be spontaneously formed for a short period of time, such as a group of diabetic patients currently on the unit who come together for instruction about their diet, or they may be groups that will interact for longer periods of time, such as a support or therapy group in a rehabilitation setting. We focus here on the behavior that occurs when any group interacts and how you can improve the functioning of a group process whether you are the facilitator or a group member.

There are two major aspects of group functioning: the work orientation and the social orientation. Most groups share both. For example, you may socialize with members of your work group over coffee or during lunch breaks. In addition, all groups appear to go through various stages of development. The first stage of group development is called the "orientation," or "groping," stage. Members ask: What are we doing here? What is our purpose? If you are working with a group of patients, it is important to identify the specific goal of the group or what is to be accomplished in a specific time frame. In this initial phase of the group process, members are usually highly reliant on the leader. When you are in the leadership or facilitator role, you can do a lot to increase the effectiveness and decrease the anxiety and confusion of the group by clearly providing structure.

The second stage is called the "griping," or "war," stage. Members of the group express, either openly or covertly, frustration and anger with the group process. This phenomenon seems to symbolize the group members' struggles to maintain their own identity and still be part of the group process. Much of this irritability will be directed at the group leader, so if you are in this role, be prepared. It is important to remember that this hostility is not personal, but part of the normal growth of the group.

If the group survives the second stage intact, members will move on to the "grouping," or "we," stage of group process. They will identify with each other and the task of the group. They will begin to feel a sense of togetherness and shared purpose. The group is then able to move to the fourth stage of performance, the "grinding" stage, and actually work on the task at hand. This fourth stage is marked by problem-solving behavior and cooperation to achieve the goal.

Of course, not all groups will move through these stages in such a straightforward manner. Group composition can change, disrupting the growth process. Also, in the frantic pace of contemporary health care, groups come and go quickly; therefore, many times, little cohesion can be achieved. In other words, you may find yourself constantly working in the "groping" stage of group development with your role remaining one of providing guidance and structure.

Institution or Home

In Chapter 2 we discussed a variety of environments in which patients receive care today. Whatever the environment in which you encounter patients, for social, psychological, and financial reasons, there is a strong tendency to medicalize the setting. So even in settings such as a skilled nursing facility or the patient's home, medical props and devices shape the atmosphere. It is evident to health professionals who work in patients' homes that they are viewed as guests, at best, or intrusive strangers, at worst. Home care places the health professional on the patient's turf. Communication in the home care setting is shaped by that environment. Health professionals are more deferential, more attuned to asking before doing. Other health care environments, such as intensive care units or an emergency department, do not even pretend to be "home-like" or welcoming to patients. The sights, sounds, smells, and urgency of these high-tech environments have a profound impact on patients, particularly because this environment is often foreign and threatening. Consider this excerpt from a poem involving a mother who gets her first glimpse of her child in critical care in a hospital.

Intensive Care
I am called.
But nothing prepares me for what I see, my child

in her body of pain, hooked to machines. Grief
comes up like floodwater. Her body floats on a sea

of air that is her bed, a force field of sorrow
that pulls me to her side. I touch pain I know

I have never felt, move into a new land
of nightmare. She is so still. Only one hand

moves, fingers oscillate like water plants risking
the air. Machines line the desks,

the floor, the walls, confirm the deep pink
of her skin in rapidly ascending numbers. One eye blinks.
— *L.C. Getsi*[9]

If you were to enter this patient's room and come upon this mother, what would your first words be? How would this institutional environment impact communication? What might you do to minimize the strangeness of the surroundings? Sensitive communication depends on an appreciation of the effect of the environment on what transpires between you and the patient.

CHOOSING THE RIGHT WORDS

The success of verbal communication depends on several important factors: (1) the way material is presented, that is, the vocabulary used, the clarity of voice, and organization; and (2) the tone and volume of the voice.

Vocabulary and Jargon

As we note in Chapter 9, the descriptive vocabulary of the health professional is a two-edged sword. A student must learn to offer precise, accurate descriptions and must be able to communicate to other professionals in that mode.

Technical language is one of the bonds shared by health professionals among themselves. In contrast, highly technical professional jargon is almost never appropriate in direct conversation with the patient. It is imperative that you learn to translate technical jargon into terms understandable to patients when discussing their condition or conversing with their families. Only in the rarest instances are patients schooled in the technical language of health care

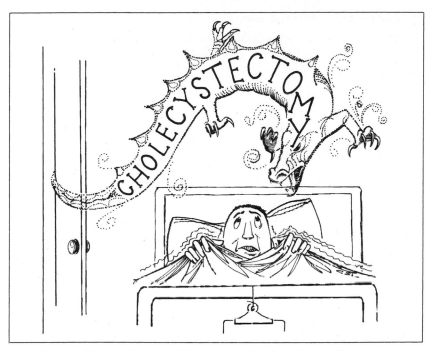

Mastery of appropriate vocabulary means knowing when and how to use professional jargon and to translate it into lay terms.

sufficiently to understand its jargon, even in today's world of the Internet, television, and other health care–related resources. Even when the patient happens to be a health professional, it is important to use the patient's language when talking about what is happening with him or her. Do not assume that the therapist or nurse who is your patient is conversant in all areas of health care.

Although we have been stressing that a dialogue or conversation model of communication is preferable, there are some distinct cases in which direct, simple questions are more appropriate. In a study of caregivers who worked with patients with Alzheimer's disease, a "yes/no" or forced choice type of question (e.g., "Do you want to go outside?") rather than an open-ended question (e.g., "What would you like to do?") resulted in more successful communication.[10]

Thus, as always, the general rule has exceptions, and you will have to assess what types of questions work best with each patient. Of course, the way to respectful communication is to try as much as possible to talk to patients as equals (because that is what the majority of patients want) while remaining flexible in your style to meet individual patients' needs.

Problems from Miscommunication

Several problems arise when miscommunication occurs because the health professional is unable to communicate with the patient in terms understandable to him or her:

Desired Results Are Lost. The health professional attempts to receive the patient's complaints verbally. Often the descriptions are too vague or too difficult to classify. Rather than continue to work to understand the symptoms and their significance for the patient, the health professional immediately turns to the more objective criteria of laboratory and other diagnostic findings and bases treatment programs on experience described in the literature or derived from a large number of other patients. This "miss" in communication all too often inhibits the results the health professional wished to achieve and could have achieved, had effective communication with the patient been established.[11] Once again, by the health professional taking the interaction with the patient as merely the transfer of information, the opportunity for true discourse was lost.

Confused Meanings. Another common area for miscommunication is when the health professional and patient are both using the same word but ascribe different meanings to it. In a qualitative study of diabetic patients and their physicians, it was found that different conceptions of the term "control" affected the ability of patients and their physicians to communicate effectively.[12] Although the physicians in the study acknowledged the numerous physical, psychological, and social obstacles to treatment, they did not focus on these aspects of the disease when they interacted with patients. Rather, they focused almost entirely on managing blood glucose numbers. This led to a great degree of frustration on the part of the patients.

Disbelief in the Health Professional's Interest. Another problem that can result from using technical language is that the person to whom you are speaking will not be convinced that you really want to know how he or she feels. Additionally, your choice of words can unintentionally hurt the patient. For example, after her first prenatal visit to the doctor a pregnant teenager reported to her friends, "The doctor wanted to know about my 'menstrual history.' I didn't know what that was. Finally, I figured out she was talking about my periods. Why didn't she just say that? I felt so stupid."

When the health professional persists in using "big words" or technical language, the patient may interpret this as a sign that his or her problems are not important. The complexity and impersonality of a health facility will undoubtedly be communicated to the patient if health professionals are unwilling to explain carefully to the patient, in understandable terms, his or her condition and its treatment. The amount that is accomplished within any allotted period of time, rather than the actual amount of time spent, will convince the patient

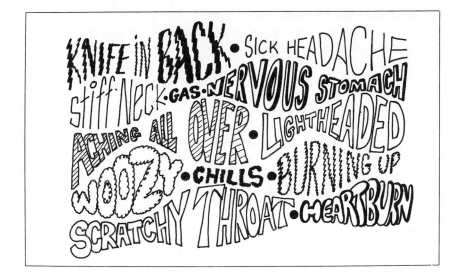

that the health professional really cares. If the patient cannot understand what is being said, very little will be accomplished.

The mastery of appropriate vocabulary, then, includes being able to communicate with your colleagues but at the same time being willing to converse with patients in words they can understand. You will, in essence, need to become "bilingual," translating from professional terms to common everyday language. When this is accomplished, the patient will be able to do what is requested, will respond accurately to your questions, and will more likely be convinced that you care about him or her.

Clarity

In addition to using overly sophisticated language, a health professional may not be able to speak with clarity. What is the difference between the two? Lack of clarity occurs when you launch into a lengthy, rambling description of the diagnosis and proposed tests, not even realizing that the patient was lost at the outset. Furthermore, a highly organized, technically correct, and very meaningful sentence loses its impact when it is poorly articulated or spoken too softly or hurriedly. Patients can often be preoccupied with one particular facet of a problem and, consequently, interpret everything else you say in light of that preoccupation.

It is surprising to some students that patients may be too embarrassed to ask them to repeat something, and so patients rely on what they think they heard. Patients are sometimes hesitant because they are a bit awed by you as the health professional and so try to act sophisticated instead of asking you to repeat what you said. Patients may be awed primarily because they realize that health professionals have skills that can determine their future welfare and that, regardless of their influence in the business or social world, they are at your mercy in this situation.

Explanation of the Purpose.   Clarity is also necessary to establish the purpose of your interaction. As was mentioned earlier in this chapter, you first establish the purpose of your interaction when you introduce yourself and explain your role. This general introduction should be followed by a statement of the purpose of this particular encounter (i.e., what is going to take place at this time and why). Thus, you and the patient know what the goal of the interaction is from the start. Because the patient may be tired or uncomfortable, it is also helpful to state at the outset how long the interaction will take. Then the patient can decide if he or she is up to it or needs to have the encounter broken down into smaller periods of time.

Organization of Ideas.   A health professional often has to explain a procedure to a patient. A health professional who rambles confuses a patient by jumping from one topic to the next, inserting last-minute ideas, and then failing to summarize or to ask the patient to do so. Failure to progress from one step to the next to reach a logical conclusion is usually caused by (1) a lack of understanding of the subject or of the steps in the procedure or (2) ironically, a too-thorough knowledge of the subject or procedure. The former causes the patient to grope for all the facts, whereas the latter causes the speaker to overlook points that are obvious to him or her but not to the listener. In either case, it is advisable to organize the description of a procedure or test into its component parts and then to practice describing it to a friend who is not familiar with the procedure. That person will be able to identify any obvious steps that have been omitted. Complicated information should be broken down into manageable chunks so that the patient is not overwhelmed by everything that follows. This is especially true when the information involves bad news.

Verbal information and instructions alone are not always adequate to assure clarity. Written notes or instructions, diagrams, videotapes, and nonverbal illustrations are highly desirable adjuncts to the spoken word because they may help the person organize the ideas and information more fully.

Tone and Volume

Paralinguistics is the study of all cues in verbal speech other than the content of the words spoken. Although paralinguistics is considered part of the realm of nonverbal communication, we will discuss tone and volume here because they are so closely connected to the content of speech. Sometimes a person's voice or volume belie his or her words. Any vocalized sound a person makes could be interpreted as verbal communication, so besides your words you will communicate "volumes" with the tone, inflection, speed, and loudness of the words you use.

Tone. Give several meanings to the simple question "What are you doing?" by varying the tone in which it is spoken. Compare the tones of the following people: (1) a man telephoning his wife at midday; (2) the man's wife, who has just caught their 2-year-old son writing on the living room wall with a purple crayon; and (3) the 2-year-old son trying to make up to the mother after his scolding and spanking. Each is trying to communicate more than the literal content of the same spoken message. An expression as short as "oh" can be used to express anger, pity, disappointment, teasing, pleasure, gratitude, exuberance, terror, superiority, disbelief, uncertainty, compassion, insult, awe, and many more. Try this exercise with "no," "yes," and other simple words or phrases to fully grasp the rich variety of meanings a word can convey.

Tone is a voice quality that can actually reverse the meaning of the spoken word. When the patient's response is puzzling to the health professional, the latter should be alert to the tone in which the patient communicated a message or reacted to a statement. For example, if the patient asks, "Am I going to get better?" the health professional can inadvertently confirm the patient's worst fears by answering in a not-too-convincing tone, "Yes, of *course* you will."

Volume. Tone and volume are closely related voice qualities. An angry person may not only spit out the words indignantly but may also alter the volume of the message. For instance, it is possible to communicate anger either by whispering words through gritted teeth or by shouting them.

Voice volume controls interaction in subtle ways. For instance, if one person stands close to another and speaks in an inordinately loud voice, the listener invariably backs away. On the other hand, a soft whisper automatically causes the listener to move closer. Thus, literally and symbolically, the volume of the voice does control distance between people.

Whatever you say, you must make certain that the patient can hear you. An easy way to assess if you are speaking loudly enough is to ask the patient to repeat instructions rather than just solicit "yes" or "no" responses. Make sure the patient can see your face when you speak, as some patients need the physical cues of your expression and the movement of your lips to understand what is being said.

CHOOSING THE WAY TO SAY IT

Your educational experience will provide you with the right words, but you will send many other messages to patients in addition to the spoken word. The most basic of nonverbal forms of communication is the manner in which you think, feel, or act—your attitude. We will begin our discussion of attitudes by presuming the inherent good in each other. We presume an attitude of mutual trust and respect. Most health professionals maintain a caring attitude toward patients, and their way of speaking to them helps to communicate this genuine concern. On rare occasions, however, you may feel anger or disdain for a patient. In Chapter 19 we address some types of patients who present a challenge in this regard.

Attitudes

One variable that is frequently overlooked and has considerable impact on the exchange of information is the patient's emotional and mental state and attitudes. Examples are anger or fear that complicate communication and the management of his or her condition. If you want to effectively communicate with a patient, you must be knowledgeable about his or her mental state. You do not have to perform an exhaustive mental status examination to determine a patient's ability to comprehend, his or her orientation to the task at hand, or his or her ability to follow directions. You can obtain this information as you interact with the patient. If there is any doubt as to the patient's mental state, you can use one of the screening tools to assess general mental functions such as the Mini-Mental State Examination developed by Folstein et al.[13]

The attitude or feeling that a health professional has toward the patient will help to determine the effectiveness of spoken interaction, too. Two attitudes that are commonly encountered among health professionals are fear and a sense of humor.

Fear. Patients are often afraid for many reasons. Fear may present itself as stony silence, clenched fists, profuse sweating, or an angry outburst. Patients may not recognize the emotion that they are experiencing as fear, so you must be watchful for the signs of fear and do your best to help reassure the patient.

The specific situations in which health professionals' fears arise are numerous. How will your fear manifest itself during spoken communication? Fear can arise when the health professional is inexperienced or the patient is threatening in some way. In the following exchange from Samuel Shem's satire "Mount Misery," a new psychiatric resident interviews just such a patient:

> "So, Dr. Dickhead, tell me about yourself," Thorny said.
> Uh-oh. Surely this was backward—*I* was supposed to be asking about *him.* "I'm the new resident." I felt a sharp pain in my palm. I was clutching my key ring so hard the keys were biting into my flesh. "You?"
> "Got here a month ago from New Orleans. My daddy's rich, made a fortune burnin' trash down Cancer Alley. Calls himself the Burn King of the Bayous. I did okay till I was eighteen, 'n' got sent north to Princeton. Lasted about three months. You look kinda tentative, Doc. Scareda me?"
> I was, but I wasn't going to let *him* know it. "Nope."[14]

The patient, Thorny, began this exchange by putting the physician on the defensive. No one likes to be called an obscene, derogatory name. Furthermore, the patient took control of the interview process. Finally, the patient brought direct attention to the fact that the physician was scared. Here was an opportunity for the physician to be honest with the patient and acknowledge his fear. By denying his fear, he amplified its presence, and it remained a roadblock to communication. Of course, it is not prudent to announce to all patients when you are fearful. Patients count on the confidence and courage of health professionals. So as with all things, you must consider your relationship with the patient and the circumstances that would suggest disclosure of fear and other emotions.

Humor. A subtler, often effective way of dealing with a problem or hiding fear is through the use of humor. Health care settings can be full of banter, laughter, and jokes, some of which serve useful purposes, whereas others are destructive. Humor can be used wisely to help patients cope with stress related to their illness and accompanying problems.

In communication between the patient and the health professional, joking and teasing can be used constructively to (1) allow the person to express hostility and anxiety, (2) permit exploration of the humor and irony of the condition in which he or she is placed by illness or injury, and (3) reduce tension. Shared humor and a good laugh can often defuse anxiety in tense situations and open up connections between you and the patient. The following story by a psychiatrist highlights the mutual benefits of humor.

> I had one patient in therapy for a year who was completely bogged down in inappropriate guilt, always ready to take the blame for anything that happened to anybody anywhere in the world. She was, as usual, castigating herself, when I interrupted with, "You know, I don't mind the things you have done to the economy. I don't even mind the fact that you're responsible for high inflation. I don't even mind the taxes you cause me to pay. But I'm just madder than hell at you for causing it to rain the past three days."
>
> There had been a sharp intake of breath when I started. Her worst fears had been realized: *I* blamed her too! The seconds ticked by. First there was a small smile—just a twitch of the lips, really—then a grin, followed soon by a giggle, then a guffaw—which I joined. We literally laughed until we cried.[15]

In the preceding situation, the psychiatrist was an experienced health professional and knew the patient well. Both of the components, experience and familiarity or a bond with the patient, and good timing need to be present for humor to be therapeutic and not destructive. The same psychiatrist compared humor to nitroglycerin: in the proper hands it serves a useful purpose, but in the wrong hands it can cause great harm.

The inexperienced health professional and the lay person are often shocked by the openness with which patients joke about themselves. For instance, patients whose legs are paralyzed often joke about rubber crutches and icy surfaces, both of which are real threats in their present situations. Persons with disfiguring injuries call themselves "freaks." Their joking helps to alleviate their anxiety about these problems. Patients with temporary or permanent sexual impotence also joke a lot about sex. It is helpful to recognize their joking as one means of expressing very difficult thoughts and emotions.

The use to which humor is put will determine whether it fosters respectful interaction or is a poor substitute for direct confrontation. "When used appropriately, humor can have positive psychological, communication and social benefits, as well as positive physiological effects."[16]

COMMUNICATING BEYOND WORDS

In this section we turn our attention beyond vocal utterances designed to engage us in dialogue and conversation to consider all the additional (or substitute) ways we enter into communication with patients and others. Collectively these means are often referred to as nonverbal communication.

Facial Expression

Earlier in this chapter, you were asked to consider the variety of messages conveyed by altering the tone and volume of the spoken word "oh." It is possible to omit the word altogether and, with only a facial message, convey a variety of emotions.

Eye contact generally communicates a positive message. There is a powerful, immediate effect when we gaze directly at another person. If two people genuinely like each other, they will position themselves so that they look into each other's eyes. The distance between them as they face each other further communicates how they feel about each other. Distance as a form of nonverbal communication is discussed later in this chapter.

Even without eye contact, the rest of the face reveals many things. The presence or absence of a smile and the genuineness of a smile are all clues to a person's emotional state. Grimaces from pain, the vacant stare of a child with a fever, or the bland affect of a depressed patient provides important information that speaks volumes without the use of any words. Your own facial expression need not be somber, but should be friendly and open. This is preferable to an overly cheerful demeanor that does not permit a patient to express his or her true feelings.

Facial expressions are reinforced by other information. Nonverbal messages meant to show the health professional's authority are enhanced if the health professional is standing over the patient, a point not lost by satirist-cartoonist James Thurber. Since our facial expression is "connected" to the rest of what we are trying to convey, the patient looks at it all as one configuration of messages.

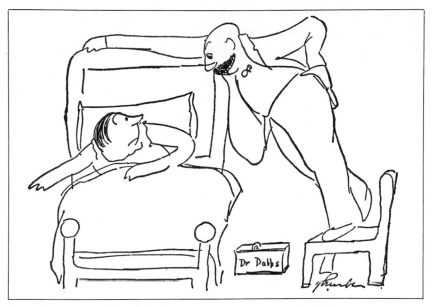

"You're Not My Patient, You're My Meat, Mrs. Quist!"

Copyright © James Thurber. Copyright © 1973 Helen W. Thurber and Rosemary T. Sauers. From *The Thurber Carnival*, published by Harper & Row.

Gestures and Body Language

Gestures involving the extremities, even one finger, can suggest the meanings of a message. Consider the mother who folds her arms when a child begins to sputter an excuse for coming home late, the man who clenches his fist, the thumb roller, the shoulder shrugger, and the foot shuffler. What unspoken messages are they sending? Refer to the patient scenario that opened this chapter. Because the patient had no other way of communicating her fears and her need for the presence of the nurse, she kicked her legs. The nurse misinterpreted the patient's gesture and left her alone not only feeling like she was suffocating but also chastised like a recalcitrant child.

Unlike the nurse in the opening scenario, many health professionals develop the skill of truly reading the meaning of the gestures and behaviors of patients. For example, a study involving nursing assistants in a nursing home setting explored their observations of changes in patient behavior and whether or not it was predictive of the development of acute illness. The nursing assistants used a 12-item instrument to help guide their observations of behavioral and functional status of a group of elderly residents. The study found that the nursing assistants' documentation of signs of illness preceded chart documentation of acute illness by an average of 5 days.[17] Understanding subtle and obvious gestures is an important component of good communication.

Physical Appearance

Stereotypes are formed from outward appearances. In some instances, a person tries to adopt a stereotyped manner of dressing or speaking in the hope of being identified with a particular group.

Some health professionals adopt a stereotyped manner of dress (the uniform) to be identified easily within the world of health care. The "uniform" may include clothing, a patch, a pin, a cap, or a name tag or badge. Certain instruments also identify the person: the nurse's or physician's stethoscope dangling from the neck or the laboratory technologist's tray.

However, some health professionals today are engaged in a controversy over uniforms. One group prefers to shed the symbols of their profession and to approach each patient on a more person-to-person basis. This group bases its argument partially on studies suggesting that patients, especially children, react negatively to a uniform. The other group defends the traditional uniform, arguing that it is a quick means of identification and serves as a positive stereotype in matters as simple as gaining admittance to a patient's room. Some patients actually feel more comfortable with a uniformed health professional who is about to begin a procedure that would be inappropriate in a social setting. Further, the uniform is often designed for durability and movement and may therefore be more desirable than clothing designed for less rigorous wear. Finally, it is a relatively efficient, economical mode of dress. Those on both sides of the argument agree that it is not the uniform alone but what the person in the uniform does that ultimately determines how a patient interprets the health professional's actions.

Besides clothes, other factors contribute to a person's physical appearance. Grooming is often a controversial subject because hairstyles and facial hair, the amount and type of makeup worn by women, and body piercings are so dependent on current styles. Some professional people resist rigid rules that define physical appearance because they feel it is very important to express their individuality through their appearance. Others are less concerned that compliance with regulations governing physical appearance will damage their individuality. What do you think is most likely to convey to patients your respect for them?

Touch

For a child, a touch holds great significance: Aladdin produces a genie by touching the magic lamp; Cinderella's coach appeared at the touch of her fairy godmother's wand; and handsome princes awaken beautiful, bewitched princesses with their kisses. Adults, too, give touch great symbolic meaning in everyday conversation. They promise to "keep in touch," are "touched" by a tender scene in a film, and accredit the hostess with having "a special touch" for hospitality. Despite all this, most of us come from a predominantly nontouching society.

In all societies, individuals come into physical contact with each other all the time, but the context is crucial; that is, they tend not to put their hands on each other except in well-defined rituals. However, upon entering a health facility a person who dislikes physical contact may have to allow himself or herself to be palpated, punctured with needles, squeezed, rubbed, cut, and lifted.

These unusual touching privileges are granted to health professionals by society. Licensing of health professionals is primarily a protection against the charge of unconsented touching (battery). In Chapter 12 you will learn about the boundaries that must be maintained, even when legitimate touching is recognizable as part of the therapeutic or diagnostic procedure.

Fortunately, the comforting touch is usually regarded as legitimate, and you have in it a powerful tool for communicating caring. The effects of a caring touch are sometimes observable in the patient. For example, you may observe one or more of the following: a lowering of the patient's voice, a slowing and deepening of the patient's breathing, or a spontaneous verbal response like a sigh or "I feel relaxed."

People pick up signals conveyed by your manner of touching. This is often related to your appearance, the speed and ease with which you move, and the quality of your touch. The sensation received by the patient when his or her arm is lifted by the health professional's cold, clammy hand sends quite a different message from the gentle support of a warm, dry hand. The reassuring hand resting on a patient's shoulder sometimes speaks more loudly than the kindest words. Patients should be touched with respect for the person who lives inside the body being manipulated. Even if our touch is less than perfect, perhaps a bit clumsy, patients are generally deeply grateful for being handled with care by another.

Patients will be much more aware of this touching than the health professional, who has become used to touching patients. The experienced health professional probably has so firm a concept of his or her good intentions that the question of inappropriateness or improper familiarity never arises. However, touch, as one form of nonverbal communication, does involve risk. It may be a threat because it invades an otherwise private space, or it may be misunderstood, but the risk, properly undertaken, should yield favorable results.

Proxemics

Proxemics is the study of how space is used in human interactions. For example, authority can be communicated by the height from which one person interacts with another. If one stands while the other sits or lays, the person standing has placed himself or herself in a position of authority (recall the Thurber illustration earlier in this chapter).

Height is sometimes an unwitting message to a patient when the person is confined to a bed, a treatment table, or a wheelchair. In many instances, the relationship would be improved if the health professional would move down to the patient's level. An important rule for respectful interaction whenever you are talking to a patient is to sit down. This signals to the patient your willingness to listen and gives the impression, even if this is not true, that you are not going to rush through your time together.

Another aspect of proxemics is the distance maintained between people when they are communicating. In his now classic *The Hidden Dimension,* an intriguing book that explains the difference in distance awareness among many different cultural groups, anthropologist Edward T. Hall defines four distance zones maintained by healthy, adult, middle-class Americans.[18] In examining these zones, you may also be better able to understand how they differ from those of other cultural and socioeconomic groups. Dr. Hall stresses that "how people are feeling toward each other at the time is a decisive factor in the distance used." The four distance zones are:

1. Intimate distance, involving direct contact, such as that of lovemaking, comforting, protecting, and playing football or wrestling.

2. Personal distance, ranging from 1 to 4 feet. At arm's length, subjects of personal interest can be discussed while physical contact, such as holding hands or hitting the other person in the nose, is still possible.

3. Social distance, ranging from 4 to 12 feet. At this distance, more formal business and social discourse takes place.

4. Public distance, ranging from 12 to 25 feet or more. No physical contact and very little direct eye contact are possible. Shopping centers, airports, and city sidewalks are designed to maintain this type of distance.[19]

Health professionals perform many diagnostic or treatment procedures within the personal and intimate distance zones. You may have to invade the patient's culturally derived boundaries of interaction, sometimes with little warning. Consider, for instance, the weak or debilitated patient who comes for treatment and must be helped to a treatment table. To get the patient on the treatment table, you might have to "embrace" the patient and, in some cases, actually lift the patient to the table, deeply invading his or her intimate zone.

When you work with an ethnic or cultural subgroup outside of your own experience or travel to other parts of the world, culturally defined uses of space readily become apparent. It can be disconcerting to the average untraveled American abroad to be given hotel directions by a stranger who nearly embraces him or her or to observe men kissing and hugging and women strolling along arm-in-arm.

However, you need not travel abroad to experience uneasiness about distance zones; you will encounter members of the global village, with distance zones different from your own, in the health facility in your own community. The patient who clings to you or refuses to talk unless he or she is nearly in your lap may be confused or insulted if you unwittingly withdraw. In addition, you may become aware of some things that you did not expect to be part of the interaction. For instance, body odors become more apparent when you are working at close range. In a society in which a man or woman is supposed to smell like a deodorant, a mouthwash, a hair spray, or a cologne, but *not* a body, it is not surprising that some health professionals find the patient's body odor offensive, sometimes nauseous; some admit that it so repulses them that they try to hurry through the test or treatment.

Patients will respond to the health professional's odors, too. An x-ray technologist confided to one of the authors that one of her biggest shocks while working in a mission hospital in India came when her assistant reluctantly admitted that patients were failing to keep their appointments because she "smelled funny," making them sick. The "funny" smell turned out to be that of the popular American soap she was using for her bath.

Bad breath is a problem. What constitutes "bad breath"? It is *not* necessarily the smell of garlic, onion, tobacco, or alcohol. Its definition depends on who is asked the question. The health professional who is unwilling to try to go beyond his or her own culturally derived bias of distance awareness (with its accompanying distance zones for interaction) will have difficulty in communicating with many patients. While working at close range, your reaction to body and breath odors will affect interaction. Most patients are far too ill or preoccupied with their problems to have sweet-smelling breath, and others are not aware that they are being hustled out quickly because of the salami sandwich they had at noon.

Adhering to a patient's need to maintain an appropriate distance reinforces the patient's ability to feel secure in the strange new world of health care institutions. By handling distance needs respectfully, you are helping the patient to find himself or herself in the sometimes frightening vastness of the unknown health care environment into which he or she has been cast.

Differing Concepts of Time

A culturally derived difference that affects nonverbal communication is how people interpret time. The right time and the correct amount of time are relative, depending on one's cultural perspective. One aspect of the time dimension that directly affects the patient and health professional interaction is the scheduling and maintaining of appointments with patients. Most health professionals are punctual and expect their patients to be the same. In fact, the health facility operates each day on a schedule. Harrison points out that "punctuality communicates respect while tardiness is an insult." However, "in some other cultures to arrive exactly on time is an insult (it says, 'You are such an unimportant fellow that you can arrange your affairs very easily; you really have nothing else to do.'). Rather, an appropriate amount of tardiness is expected."[20] You may find that a patient is scheduled to arrive at "10 o'clock health-professional time" but arrives instead at "10 o'clock patient time," feeling no need at all to explain or apologize.

The amount of time spent in rendering professional service may also vary from one culture to another. How should a given amount of time (one-half hour) be spent so that the patient benefits most? By middle-class American standards, you should greet the patient briefly and begin treatment or a test without delay. If you rush in setting up equipment, the patient may interpret it to mean you care enough to hurry. When the treatment is over, the patient usually leaves immediately.

However, in some cultures, if the treatment does not begin as soon as the patient arrives, it does not matter as long as it will eventually be done. Rather than rush into the procedure itself, you should first inquire about the weather, the family, and other things that may be important to the patient, sometimes spending ten minutes in this way. During the actual treatment or test, you may hurry, but good-byes must not be short and rushed. One of the authors worked in an African village where she was expected to slowly enter the room, then greet the patient for a few minutes. The treatment or test could begin immediately after that, but at no time could she rush around the room. To rush while the patient remained seated was an unspeakable insult that could only mean that the health professional believed herself more important than the patient.

These examples give you an idea of the rich variety of ways in which time may have to be organized within different cultural contexts to convey respect toward the patient and others.

Other problems arise for the American health professional. We practice in a culture in which the idea of organizing patients' time on a "first come, first served" basis seems correct. However, in some cultures, this time-dependent criterion is not considered a just method for determining priority among patients who arrive for treatment. Who should be treated first if the patients with 9:15, 10:00, and 10:15 appointments all arrive at 9:15? Should the man scheduled for 9:15 be first? Or should the oldest of the three be first? The man or woman? The sickest or the highest-ranking official of the three in that tribe or community? The way in which you handle this situation will greatly determine your success in cultures other than those that are considered mainstream.

Ways of operating within and indicating time, then, are highly relative. The few examples presented only skim the surface of differences in time awareness among different cultures. As mentioned in Chapter 3, you should always take possible differences into consideration when working with people whose cultural backgrounds are different from your own, recognizing that both distance and time awareness are deep seated and culturally derived. A person usually is not consciously aware of how he or she interprets time and distance, and so neither factor is easily identified as the cause of misunderstanding. Clearly, culture influences the interpretation of verbal and nonverbal communication in terms of time or distance.

COMMUNICATING ACROSS DISTANCES

Much of the literature regarding communication between the patient and health professional has taken for granted that the two parties are within close

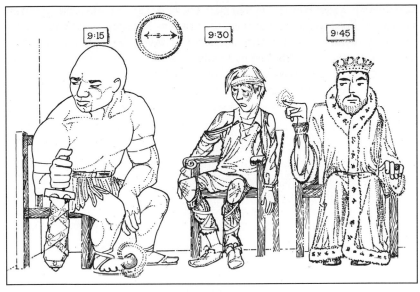

Who's first?

proximity of one another. In many cases today, because of the mobility of society and technological developments, health professionals and patients can communicate across great distances. In addition, you may work with colleagues on the same complex patient problem and yet geographically be in two different cities. All of the techniques to enhance communication in general apply to communication across distances, but they must be adapted to the special demands created by miles between a patient and health professional instead of inches.

Written Tools

Written communication includes information about diagnostic tests, instructions to patients to perform activities, informed consent documents for surgery, and surveys to obtain information from patients about services rendered. Whatever the reason for the written communication, there are distinct advantages to its use over verbal communication. Written communication has the advantage of visual cues. The reader has control over the pace of absorbing the information and can reread the information any number of times. However, written communication demands a high degree of accuracy. All written communication should clearly state and define the reason it is being sent. The content should be well organized. Clarity and brevity are also hallmarks of good written communication. The vocabulary must be fitting for the recipient. Studies of informed consent forms indicate that these forms generally do not give patients a clear understanding of the proposed treatment. A review of the readability of consent forms used in pediatric research found that they typically require reading skills at the advanced college level and have an average ease of readability comparable to that of the *New England Journal of Medicine.*[21] In other words, they are *not* fitting for the intended recipient. Clear, concise written messages will be more easily understood and problems prevented if both verbal and written forms of communication can be used.

Voice and Electronic Tools

Since the telephone has become so much a part of our lives, you may not even notice how much you use it to communicate with patients. In an ambulatory setting, the phone may be your only contact with a patient between visits. It is best not to rely solely on this communication modality. It is especially important not to give bad news over the phone or try to explain a complicated diagnosis or treatment plan. However, exchanging information or data such as blood glucose levels or electrocardiogram printouts electronically is an effective and efficient adjunct to other forms of communication.

Voice mail is another capability of the telephone and has been used with mixed results. When you order a sweater from a catalogue over the phone or check your savings account balance, you generally do so with automated voice mail. But what is appropriate for some activities may not be with others. Patients may find it odd to call a clinic and receive an automated voice mail response that asks them to press certain numbers to leave a message. The person-to-person communication that is so necessary to compassionate care is clearly missing when a computerized voice is on the other end of the telephone. However, a benefit of voice mail is the opportunity for a patient to leave a detailed message about a question or problem and avoid playing "phone tag" with busy health professionals. The professional can then call back at a less hectic time to talk directly to the patient.

Telephones can also be used to triage patient care. "Telephone triage is the process by which a health care provider communicates with a client via the telephone and, thereby, assesses the presenting concerns, develops a working diagnosis, and determines a suitable plan of management. Determination of the seriousness of the situation will dictate whether the client can be cared for at a distance or whether a more comprehensive in-person evaluation is in order."[22] Of course, use of the telephone to render care must be done cautiously, particularly when the health professional determines what follow-up is needed.

E-mail is another form of electronic communication that is just now becoming a part of health care practice. Although the following quotation describes the possible advantages of e-mail use in a physician's practice, the same applies to all health professionals.

> E-mail between physicians and patients holds much promise and clearly has the potential to enhance the medical professional relationship. E-mail has the advantage of speed and convenience for both parties ... at the same time [it]

allows correspondents to compose careful and structured responses. It is self-documenting. Used in conjunction with office visits, e-mail might allow patients and physicians to augment information or advice that was overlooked during a previous office consultation.[23]

Although e-mail may assist in communication, its use depends on the availability of a personal computer. Needless to say, not everyone has access to a computer. In fact, U.N. Secretary General Kofi Annan (in his "Millennium Report") pondered what the world would be like if it were truly a global village: "Say this village has 1,000 individuals with all the characteristics of today's human race distributed in exactly the same proportions. What would it look like? Fewer than 60 people would own a computer and only 24 would have access to the Internet."[24]

Even though it might appear at times that everyone in the world is on the Internet, the reality is that most people do not have access to this sophisticated technology.

According to proponents of computers and related technology in health care, the goal is to move to a "paperless" environment. As yet, this has not happened. "Despite the enormous popularity of computers and personal digital assistants, along with improvements in screen technology, mobile computing techniques, navigational and input tools, paper usage in the United States continues to increase."[25]

It seems that people still like to have a paper or hard copy of information in their hands on which to make notes or highlight important points. Although technology will continue to add new ways to communicate or complement old ones, face-to-face interactions remain critical to the success of health care and central to basic communication.

EFFECTIVE LISTENING

A considerable portion of a health professional's day is spent listening to patients and colleagues in person or over the telephone. Elizabeth Smith describes the following levels of listening and suggests that health professionals are usually involved in the more complex levels, cited first:

1. Analytical listening for specific kinds of information and arranging them into categories.
2. Directed listening to answer specific questions.
3. Attentive listening for general information to get the overall picture.
4. Exploratory listening because of one's own interest in the subject being discussed.
5. Appreciative listening for esthetic pleasure, such as listening to music.
6. Courteous listening because one feels obligated to listen.
7. Passive listening, as in overhearing something; not attentive to the matter being discussed.[26]

Most people lack the skills to listen effectively. If you do, you should have two goals: (1) to improve listening acuity so you hear the patient accurately and (2) to ascertain how accurately a patient has heard you. The first step to achieving these goals is to examine the reasons messages get distorted. Only then can you transfer this knowledge to your own experience. Besides the often-overlooked, important possibility of a hearing deficit, there are at least three reasons a health professional or patient distorts a verbal communication.

First, a mind set or frame of mind may distort meaning. It is the result of past experience. In this case, a person fails to listen to the spoken words or to note subtle individual differences because he or she is very sure of what the other person will say. A poignant example of people talking at and across each other and not really communicating in the health care environment is the following dialogue poem between members of the health care team and the mother of an infant in the neonatal intensive care unit:

THE PATIENT CARE CONFERENCE

"I just want them to show some respect for me . . . to understand that I'm her mother."

"What she has to understand is these doctors are busy; they can't stand around waiting for her to come and besides, she doesn't always understand anyway."

"I'm leaving here and I'm glad of it. I've never been anywhere they let the nurses talk back like they do here. In Alabama, the attending is the only one allowed to talk to the family and he does, so it's all coordinated. This group of nurses sides with the family and sets us up to be the bad guys."

"I don't leave often. If I go to the store, the nurses know when I'll be back. Don't they have some legal thing that requires my permission before they do things to her?"

"What you have to understand is we *have* talked to her. I heard Dr. Smith on the phone with her just the other night. He went over each of the possible outcomes. We can't help it if she forgets. Maybe she should call us to see what's going on. That might fit her schedule better. I'm sure whoever is on call could deal with her."

"Well, so the pulmonary guys said the lung was blown. We didn't ask that. Why are *we* always blamed for not telling her? She didn't ask the right service."

"He said changing her trach wasn't considered a procedure. OK. So what should I call those things I don't want them doing to her without me here?"

"What she has to understand is. . . ."[27]

Beneath the misunderstandings conveyed in the poem, what other communication issues are going on in the patient care conference? What are the attitudes of the health professionals described in the poem? The patient's mother becomes just another mother in the neonatal intensive care unit, not a unique person with her own concerns and needs. Because the listeners, the health professionals, have made up their minds about what they will and will not hear, the mother's voice gets lost.

Second, most people tend to force an idea into a familiar context so that they can understand it quickly and ignore aspects of it that do not fit this context. This tendency is, of course, related to their mind set but is also a defense against possible change. It may be that a person's inability to accept new concepts is a result of a basic lack of self-understanding. Thus, the weaker or more ill defined a person's self-image, the greater the need to resist ideas that are more complex or ambiguous.

Third, the rate at which incoming information can be processed varies significantly. This is partially but not entirely due to differences in innate ability. Overconfidence or too little confidence in predicting what will be said also determines whether a person will cease to process incoming information. If a person is overconfident, boredom settles in. If a person has too little confidence, he or she tends to become overly anxious and tune out the message. Active listening also requires undivided attention. If a person is distracted by too much sensory input, he or she will not be able to listen.

The rate and level of understanding at which you direct communication will alter the listener's ability to process the information. Thus, it is important that you have some knowledge of the patient's basic intelligence and past experience with a subject. The listener's set, the need to defend existing precepts, and the listener's innate intelligence both determine how accurately he or she will hear a message. Sometimes you will be the poor listener and at other times the patient will be.

You cannot completely control how effectively the patient listens but you can become a more effective listener. By simply restating what the patient has said, you can confirm part of a message before proceeding to the next portion of it. In addition, the following are some simple steps to more effective listening:

1. Be selective in what you listen to.
2. Concentrate on central themes rather than isolated statements. Listen in "paragraphs."
3. Judge content rather than style or delivery.
4. Listen with an open mind rather than focus on emotionally charged words.
5. Summarize in your own mind what you hear before speaking again.
6. Clarify before proceeding. Do not let vague or incomplete ideas go unattended.

The stakes are high when a patient is trying to communicate with you. Sometimes the patient's personality and fears may even cause the health professional to doubt the patient's information or dismiss it as a "somatization disorder," meaning that the patient's report of reality does not coincide with a medical explanation. This can lead to tragic results. For example, people in whom multiple sclerosis is eventually diagnosed are often first referred to psychologists for some form of somatization disorder.[28]

SUMMARY

The purpose of this chapter was to give you an overview of the numerous components of respectful communication. You will communicate in many ways with your patients: in person and across the miles, verbally and in writing. It may seem impossible to pay attention to the context of communication, the words you choose, your attitude, and the nonverbal messages you send all at the same time. However, good communication is like any skill: it takes practice. If you are willing to truly listen to your patients, they will assist you in refining and improving your communication skills throughout your career in health care.

REFERENCES

1. Jaquette, S.G.: The octopus and me: the nursing insight gleaned from a battle with cancer. *Am. J. Nurs.* 100(4):24, 2000.
2. Smith, J.F.: Communicative ethics in medicine: the physician-patient relationship. In Wolf, S. (ed.): *Feminism and Bioethics: Beyond Reproduction.* New York, Oxford University Press, 1996, pp.184–215, quote p. 187.
3. Byrne, P.S., and Long, B.E. *Doctors Talking to Patients.* London, Her Majesty's Stationery Office, 1976.
4. Larson, D.G., and Tobin, D.R.: End-of-life conversations: evolving practice and theory. *JAMA* 284(12):1573–1578, 2000.
5. Frank, A.: From suspicion to dialogue: Relations of storytelling in clinical encounters. *Med. Humanit. Rev.* 14(1):24–34, 2000, quote pp. 24–25.
6. Terry, P.E., and Healey, M.L.: The physician's role in educating patients. A comparison of mailed versus physician-delivered patient education. *J. Fam. Pract.* 49(4):314–318, 2000.
7. Jensen, C., Farnham, S., Drucker, S., and Kollock, P.: The effect of communication modality on cooperation in online environments. In *Proceedings of CHI'00* (The Hague, The Netherlands, April 1–6). New York, ACM Press, 2000, pp. 470–477.
8. Rocco, E.: Trust breaks down in electronic contexts but can be repaired by some initial face-to-face contact. In *Proceedings of CHI'98* (Los Angeles, April 18–23). New York, ACM Press, 1998, pp. 496–502.
9. Getsi, L.C.: "Intensive care." In *Intensive Care.* Minneapolis, New Rivers Press, 1992, p. 5.
10. Ripich, D.N., Siol, E., Fritsch, T., and Durand, E.J.: Training Alzheimer's disease caregivers for successful communication. *Clin. Gerontol.* 21(1):37–56, 1999.
11. Bergsma, J., and Thomasma, D.C.: *Health Care: Its Psychosocial Dimension.* Pittsburgh, Duquesne University Press, 1982, pp. 66–67.
12. Freeman, J., and Loewe, R.: Barriers to communication about diabetes mellitus. Patients' and physicians' different view of the disease. *J. Fam. Pract.* 49(6):513–542, 2000.

13. Folstein, M.F., Folstein, S., and McHugh, P.R.: Mini-Mental State: a practical method for grading the cognitive state of patients for the clinician. *J. Psychiatr. Res.* 12:189–198, 1975.

14. Shem, S.: *Mount Misery.* New York, Ballantine Publishing Group, 1997, p. 31.

15. Chance, S.: *A Voice of My Own: A Verbal Box of Chocolates.* Cleveland, SC, Bonne Chance Press, 1993, pp. 35–36.

16. Buxman, K.: Humor in critical care: no joke. *AACN Clin. Iss. Adv. Pract. Acute Crit. Care* 11(1):120–127, 2000.

17. Bookvar, K., Brodie, H.D., and Lachs, M.: Nursing assistants detect behavior changes in nursing home residents that precede acute illness: development and validation of an illness warning instrument. *J. Am. Geriatr. Soc.* 48(9):1086–1091, 2000.

18. Hall, E.T.: *The Hidden Dimension.* New York, Doubleday, 1966, pp. 108–117.

19. Ibid, p. 110.

20. Harrison, R.: Nonverbal communications: explorations into time, space, action and object. In Campbell, J.H. and Hepler, H.W. (eds.): *Dimensions in Communications: Readings.* 2nd ed. Belmont, CA, Wadsworth, 1970, pp. 260–261.

21. Tarnowski, K.J., Allen, D.M., Mayhall, C., and Kelly, P.A.: Readability of pediatric biomedical research informed consent forms. *Pediatrics* 85:58–62, 1990.

22. DeVore, N.E.: Telephone triage: a challenge for practicing midwives. *J. Midwifery* 44(5):471–479, 425–429, 1999.

23. De Ville, K.A.: Ethical and legal implications of e-mail correspondence between physicians and patients. *Ethics Health Care* 4(1):1–3, 2001.

24. Annan, K.: Millennium Report. Available at http://www.un.org/millennium/sg/report/ch1.htm.

25. Lui, Z., and Stork, D.: Is paperless really more? *Commun. ACM* 43(11):94–97, 2000.

26. Smith, E.: Improving listening effectiveness. *Tex. Med.* 71:98–100, 1975.

27. Ogborn, S.: Patient care conference. In Haddad, A., and Brown, K. (eds.): *The Arduous Touch: Women's Voices in Health Care.* West Lafayette, IN, Purdue University Press, 1999, p. 21.

28. Webster, B.: *All of a Piece: A Life with Multiple Sclerosis.* Baltimore, The Johns Hopkins University Press, 1989.

PART FOUR

Questions for Thought and Discussion

1. In groups of three, have one student act as a patient with an injury, such as a fall off a ladder, have the second act as the interviewer trying to find out how the client was injured, and have the third student critique the interview process. Change roles three times so that all get to play each part. What works well and what does not?

2. Write out instructions for a simple procedure that a patient might carry out at home. Share the instructions with a classmate and see if he or she

is unclear about any of the written instructions. Work together to improve clarity.

3. Dennis is a 24-year-old man who has a rare form of dementia. His mother brings him to your department and you can see his anxiety. You must perform some tests on him that will not hurt him but will require his cooperation.

   a. What parts of this setting may be causing his anxiety?
   b. What aspects of your appearance may be causing his anxiety?
   c. What steps will you take to establish communication with him?
   d. How may his mother be helpful in facilitating effective "dialogue" between you and Dennis?

4. You verbally instruct an intelligent young businesswoman in the use of a home-treatment device and ask her if she understands what you want her to do. She assures you that she does. The next week when she returns, you discover that she has done exactly the opposite! You are dumbfounded.

   a. How will you react and what will you say when your patient glowingly reports that she did exactly what you said and you realize that she did exactly the opposite of what you said?
   b. List the possible reasons your patient failed to do what you asked of her.
   c. What changes might you have made during the initial instruction period to decrease the likelihood of this happening?

5. Find a standard "case study" in a professional journal. Rewrite it from the patient's perspective.

6. You walk into the hospital room of a Mexican-American woman to perform a procedure. You have not seen her as a patient before, but you know that she is new to this country and cannot speak any English. What will you do in this situation?

PART FIVE

Components of Respectful Interaction

In Part Five you have an opportunity to integrate many of the concepts you have encountered in this book so far. In Part One you were introduced to the centrality of the idea of respect in the health professions. You also were encouraged to reflect on your personal values and key institutional and societal forces that make up the larger value system in which health professionals today work. Even at the outset we began to caution you that respect must be nurtured by everyone for a respectful environment to flourish. In Parts Two and Three you focused on each of the two critical people who make health care a personal phenomenon—you and the patient. Part Four provided you with an opportunity to understand how challenging it is to communicate with patients and others in a way that allows the deeper meanings of their situation and our role to emerge. In this part you will need to use everything you have learned from this book so far as the focus turns to the health professional and patient relationship itself.

Many students are quick to observe that successful health professionals seem to be able to approach and interact with their patients in a friendly manner. Recently, after an afternoon of observation in the University Hospital, a student wrote this entry in his journal: "I noticed an interesting thing happening between my clinical supervisor and her patients. They seemed to almost be friends and yet it was somehow different too. The patient always remained patient and the health professional remained health professional. . . ."

Although at the time he did not yet know quite how to interpret it, he had observed a professional person who had integrated respect into the health professional and patient relationship. Sometimes it does not appear so on the surface, but closeness between you and a patient is significantly different from a friendship. When the similarities and differentiating characteristics are carefully defined and understood, you will enjoy the satisfaction of knowing that you, too, have achieved a habit of respectfully exercising the privileges of your role.

Chapter 11 describes some foundation stones in the relationship itself: trust and trustworthiness, attention to transference and countertransference, a commitment to caring, skillful handling of dependencies in the relationship, and the desire to empower. Chapter 12 discusses the reliance of respectful interaction on maintaining appropriate boundaries and moving toward comfortable closeness in your relationships with patients. In Chapter 13 you will have a chance to consider the ideal of professional closeness, the situation in which respect is bountifully expressed.

CHAPTER 11

Professional Relatedness Built on Respect

CHAPTER OBJECTIVES

The student will be able to

- Describe how trust is a tool that gives shape to the idea of respect between patient and health professional
- Compare the main similarities and differences between Veatch's and Smith's models of the health professional and patient relationship
- Describe the role of "reassurance" in respectful health professional and patient interaction
- Explain the phenomena of transference and countertransference in the health professional and patient relationship
- Contrast casualness and genuine caring
- Describe and compare detrimental dependence and constructive dependence in the health professional and patient relationship
- Identify some signs that the patient is empowered and the health professional empowering

---

Of course the questions had to do only with illness. By the time he was through this young man would know all about her years in the sanatorium, about her hysterectomy, and about her damaged lungs—and that is all he would know. Laura was amazed to discover that she was struggling to make a connection on another level. In a hospital one is reduced to being a body, one's history is the body's history, and perhaps that is why something deep inside a person reaches out, a little like a spider trying desperately to find a corner on which to begin to hang a web, the web of personal relation.

M. Sarton[1]

In this chapter you have an opportunity to take the insights you have gained from the book so far and put them into the context of your relationship with patients or clients: knowledge about the health care system, your journey into your professional role, the patients' predicaments, and communication skills essential to your success. From time to time the authors have encouraged you to think about how you would respond to certain relationship challenges, but now you have the background to focus on the health professional and patient relationship itself.

Some characteristics described in this chapter are essential for any relationship to thrive. For example, trust and reassurance are fundamental. A psychological phenomenon called "transference" can always be a factor in how you view, and respond to, another person. At the same time, some characteristics of a professional relationship are unique, and at the end of the chapter we address professional caring, with two types of dependence and patient empowerment as foundational concepts. Having grasped the ideas presented in this chapter you will be prepared for the more in-depth exploration of this special relationship described in the rest of Part V.

BUILD TRUST BY BEING TRUSTWORTHY

Trust is a tool that gives shape to the idea of respect for persons. In the traditional physician–patient relationship, trust was thought to mean blind faith in the physician and the blind hope of the patient and family that everything would be fine if everyone did what the physician said. Until recently trust was just about all that health care providers had to offer. Until the beginning of the 20th century, a patient had less than a 50% chance of benefiting medically from an encounter with a physician. This total reliance on trust as the "glue" of the relationship meant that the doctor should be benevolent and protective toward patients.

Modern insights regarding the role of trust in human relationships are molding the understanding of the health professional and patient interaction. In the view of developmental psychologists, trust plays a central role in our developmental task of figuring out when to depend on others and when to be cautious. Erikson called this the task of intimacy and individuation.[2] Viewed from this developmental perspective, the focus shifts from the idea that Person A must learn to be blindly trusting to the idea that Person B must earn trust by being worthy of it (trustworthy). Only when there is evidence that Person B is trustworthy can Person A's trust flourish. The professional's trustworthiness should enable patients to feel secure and exercise autonomy appropriately. But what, exactly, does trust entail in the health professional and patient relationship? In an article entitled "Engendering Trust in a Pluralistic Society," Secundy and Jackson observe,

> When a patient speaks of trust in a health care setting, he or she is essentially speaking about a comfort level, a feeling of safety, a belief that he or she can rely on people with power not to hurt or exploit him or her. Maximization of those positive feelings on the part of the patient is essential to optimal recovery. Such

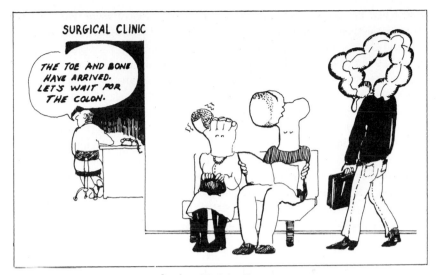

Professionals' view of patients.

From Vård, Vårdare, Vårdad.

positive feelings can ensure appropriate cooperation and compliance during the course of an illness. When such feelings are absent or ambivalent, the patient's behavior can influence outcomes negatively. There are several areas in which trust is relevant: The patient can trust or distrust the system of health care itself, the specific institution or setting in which health care services are being delivered, and the person or persons providing service or care.[3]

One basic ingredient for trust to flourish is the patient's conviction that he or she is viewed as something more than a symptom or an interesting medical case or a body part. Unfortunately health professionals and institutions sometimes are insensitive to the messages they are conveying in this regard. For example, the "bone clinic," the "allergy clinic," the "heart specialist," and the "rehabilitation nurse" all convey images of "things" rather than living, breathing human beings, and some have called this the phenomenon of "thinging" a patient by making him or her more of a thing than a person. Why should a patient trust professionals who seem more committed to the person's diagnosis or symptom than to the person?

To the extent that health care providers recognize patient perceptions of thinging they will be more likely to be successful in engendering genuine trust.

Building Trust within Different Models of Relationship

The centrality of trust behooves you to engender trustworthiness in as many forms as you have available to you. The actual behaviors may vary from patient situation to patient situation, depending on the individual as well as on the model of relationship within which you are operating at any one time. Several researchers have tried to categorize such models, and we present two that have become classical examples in the literature; the first is Veatch, summarized in Table 11–1.

Veatch interprets how the doctor–patient relationship is viewed by different patients in different situations.[4] For example, if a physician adopts the "shaman" framework and believes that it is proper to assume the role of authority figure, then he or she feels obligated to behave in a way that is consistent with that role. However, to fulfill the demands of such behavior, the physician must screen out other information and the patient must accept this authority figure as being trustworthy based on his or her actions. In the friendship framework the patient and doctor would believe the relationship was "working" (i.e., the patient was being helped) if the patient initiated activities other than those the doctor had planned. Trust would develop if the doctor accepted the patient's ideas as worthy of serious consideration. So you can see that the framework a professional adopts will have an effect on the behaviors that follow and the basis upon which trust must build. Go through each of Veatch's types and suggest ways of acting that would be consistent with that particular model. In each case, what would a patient and/or family be expected to do to demonstrate that they trusted the physician?

Viewed from a nursing perspective, Smith distinguishes three models of the nurse–patient relationship: the "surrogate mother" model in which the nurse is morally required to take full responsibility for the well-being and care of the patient, and the patient is expected to accept it willingly, somewhat similar to the shaman model; the "technician" model, which places the nurse in the role of competently applying technical knowledge and skills and requires that the patient receive them as a benefit, similar to the engineering model; and the "contracted clinician" model, in which the nurse's responsibility is defined by reference to the values and rights of the patient. The patient is assumed to be capable of determining his or her own best interests. This latter model combines aspects of Veatch's contract and friendship models but comes closer to making the professional a true advocate for the patient than adherence to the Veatch models would allow.[5] Pause and consider how trust and trustworthiness would be expressed within these models.

More recently, Emanuel and Emanuel have proposed a framework that includes many of the same important concerns of their colleagues, although their emphasis reflects the current focus on patient autonomy as the governing consideration in the relationship. They also make the important observation that at different times in a health professional–patient relationship, patients might trust different models for a time.[6]

Reassurance and Trust

You have learned in previous chapters that a patient's request for your services often is generated by the presence of a sign or symptom that manifests itself in

TABLE 11–1. Some Frameworks of Interaction in Helping Relationships*

Framework	Basis of Interaction	Characteristics		"Justifiable Expectations"
		Helper	Helpee	
Priestly (shaman)	Authority-dependence	Powerful, superior, has skills that helpee needs	Vulnerable, inferior	Health professional leads; defines, initiates, evaluates tasks; is not necessarily responsive. Patient follows; discloses much.
Engineering (engineer or architect)	Problem resolution and some authority-dependence	Designer, analytical	Flexible, has insight into own problems	Health professional defines and may initiate tasks; guides rather than leads; may be responsive, but discloses little. Patient may initiate tasks; is guided by helper; discloses little.
Contractual (business partners)	Shared benefits, fidelity, promise-keeping, and problem resolution	Decisions may be made by both as part of contract; openness to negotiation, cooperativeness		Health professional and patient: expectations vary according to contract.
Friendship (friends, buddies)	Radical equality and some shared benefits, fidelity, and promise-keeping	Few distinctions made with regard to roles; mutual interest maintained, trustworthiness		Health professional and patient: at times each defines and initiates tasks; there is much mutual disclosure.

*All four frameworks operate, at one time or another, in the health professional and patient interaction. Value assumptions about how things "ought to be" influence interactions in any of these frameworks. (Adapted from Veatch, R.M.: Models for medicine in a revolutionary age. *Hastings Cent. Rep.* 2:5–7, 1972.)

the form of pain, lack of ability to function, or some other discomfort. In these instances a patient needs assistance in learning a diagnosis, initiating and following a treatment process, and identifying desired outcomes. People also seek advice about staying healthy and preventing health-related difficulties. The relationship essentially is over when the patient's symptom disappears, the patient chooses to no longer maintain the relationship, or the health professional ascertains that no further intervention and professional care are needed or possible. In the latter case, the patient may be referred to someone else who is competent to address the type of problem he or she brings to the initial relationship or go away reassured that as much as possible or needed was done.

No matter what their differences in other regards, all patients bring the need for reassurance to the relationship. The patient may benefit from reassurance about a changing body image; about an uncertain financial, vocational, or personal future; or about resources available to help him or her adjust to the situation. To be "assured" is to have a feeling of confidence and certainty. Chapter 8 recounts some major ways that life's "slings and arrows" can shake confidence in the way the world behaves and what is reasonable to expect in the future. Reassuring requires offering information that you can stand behind with certainty yourself, however minimal it might seem to you in your current state of relative healthfulness. It may also take the form of your willingness to respond to difficult questions about areas that are causing anxiety for patients or their families. Can you think of a time when you felt reassured by another person? What did the other person do that worked? You can use your own experience when you are engaging in a relationship with a patient's or family's worries.

Occasionally, the patient's reasonable desire to be reassured creates an ambiguous situation for both the health professional and the patient. For example, consider the story of Mrs. Gleason and Sheryl Steinberg.

> Mrs. Gleason, a 70-year-old homemaker, has had amyotrophic lateral sclerosis (ALS) for just over a year. Mrs. Gleason has learned that ALS, also known as Lou Gehrig's disease, is a progressive neurological disease affecting all voluntary muscles of her body. Most patients become weaker and weaker until they die, usually of respiratory arrest. Mrs. Gleason has only a small amount of movement left in her legs but can get around in a wheelchair. She is in the hospital for treatment of pneumonia that is probably due to weakness of her swallowing muscles, allowing aspiration of her mouth contents into her lungs. Her weakness has accelerated since hospitalization, even though her pneumonia is responding to antibiotics. She is very discouraged, knowing that the aspiration will continue and that in her present state she will not be able to go home. Her family feels unable to care for her at home, and yet none of them would like to see her in a nursing home.
>
> The physician has ordered extensive occupational therapy intervention, which improves Mrs. Gleason's spirits, although no one expects

much improvement in strength, endurance, or mobility. Sheryl Steinberg, the occupational therapist who is seeing Mrs. Gleason, quickly determines that occupational therapy will have very little value as far as Mrs. Gleason's strength and endurance are concerned. However, Mrs. Gleason tells Sheryl that the daily visit is the only thing keeping her spirits up. She calls Sheryl "the sunshine girl." The physician and family are delighted that Sheryl is such a source of reassurance and tell her so.

Sheryl is ambivalent about visiting Mrs. Gleason because she knows that her department will not be reimbursed if it bills for "reassurance" sessions. Finally she decides to discuss her dilemma with Mrs. Gleason. Mrs. Gleason is ambivalent, too. She does not want to lose Sheryl's visits, yet she understands the situation that Sheryl is in. She asks Sheryl why the doctor recommended occupational therapy if it doesn't help.

Very often health professionals like Sheryl, who are sensitive to patients' needs for reassurance, find themselves in a position of having to define the comfortable limits of their own involvement. In this case, the extent to which Mrs. Gleason's "treatments" are taking away attention needed by others will be one deciding factor. Sheryl's willingness to extend her private time to do whatever is necessary to meet her other professional commitments is another. Sheryl probably enhanced her relationship with this patient by addressing their mutual problem directly.

A good basic rule is to recognize that when you first meet a patient, he or she may have far greater expectations of you than those defined simply by what your technical expertise can provide. The patient's bearing conveys an alertness stimulated both by anticipation and anxiety about what might happen next. Every sense is attuned to this new experience in much the same way that one would anticipate a vacation or be wary in a time of possible danger. That in itself creates an opportunity for reassurance that you will do whatever you can within the scope of your professional skills to serve the person well. The time and activities you devote to reassurance will be as varied as patients themselves, but it will always be worth your effort to express your respect in this manner.

TEASE OUT TRANSFERENCE AND COUNTERTRANSFERENCE

The psychotherapeutic notion of "transference" can help you understand certain kinds of behavior some people might exhibit toward you when you enter into a professional relationship with them. Transference is the process of shifting one's feeling about a person in the past to another person.[7] A young man, angry that his father "ruled with an iron hand," will think, "Here it comes again!" as soon as the health professional does anything that reminds him of his father. One of the authors knows of a male nursing student who prepared extensively and carefully to provide care to his first obstetrics-gynecology patient. Upon entering the patient's room for the first time he said, "Good morning. I'm going to be your nurse today." The patient took one look at this bearded, 6-foot-plus student and said, "Oh, no you're not! You look too much like my son, honey!" He spoke to his supervisor who judged it would be best to reassign the patient to another student nurse.

Transference can be negative or positive. The anger expressed by the young man is an example of negative transference. Positive transference, the good feelings the patient transfers to the health professional, can promote relatedness. A health professional might evoke an association of a friend, a favorite aunt, the patient's son or daughter, or a special teacher.

It is not always easy to tell whether the transference will create a problem. A young woman caught a new patient staring at her very hard. Finally he shook his head and said, "Man, I could have sworn my first wife walked in when you came in the room. The resemblance is startling!" Of course, this raised some questions—and the woman responded by saying, "Well, is that a good or bad thing?" He said, "Both!" So she was still in the woods on this one. She had no choice in this case but to continue with the patient. However, just the knowledge of the man's association allowed her to be more on the alert for any unusual behavior or comments. (There were none, and the matter never came up again.)

The patient is not the only party in the relationship who experiences transference. Countertransference takes place every bit as often. A health professional may transfer feelings to the patient on the basis of name, eye color, age, or even gestures. Any one of these can increase the chance of countertransference. It is up to you to be self-aware about such associations and adapt your behavior to correct for any negative or other troubling responses you think might be issuing from your mental association of the patient with someone in your past or present relationships.

At the same time, total neutrality is not required. If you have served on a jury, you know that the lawyers try to select jurors whose past experiences and associations do not in any discernible way come into play when the facts of the case and the identification of the defendant and plaintiff are made known. A less rigorous standard is acceptable in the health professional and patient relationship: All that is needed when initiating a relationship with a patient is to be aware that transference and countertransference take place and try to be aware of how they might affect the interaction, although it may not be possible always to identify the person whom the patient is "seeing" in you or you are "seeing" in the patient.[8]

RECOGNIZE THE DIFFERENCE: FROM CASUALNESS TO PROFESSIONAL CARING

When health professionals foster a casual atmosphere, sometimes patients do not know how to interpret it. If it is misinterpreted, a patient may withdraw, become hostile, or show other signs of distrust.

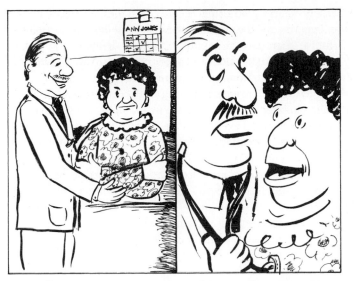

"Hello, Mrs. Jones. I'm Dr. Howard. May I call you Nancy?"
"Sure, Howie!"

Some of the most common actions subject to misinterpretation take place when a health professional engages in the following: (1) shares a secret or engages in private jokes with the patient, to the exclusion of others in the area; (2) quickly encourages the patient to establish a first-name-basis relationship; (3) tries to attract attention to himself or herself by little acts such as reading something funny or by bringing small presents to the patient; or (4) regularly spends extra time socializing with the patient and does little favors for the person in contrast to his or her treatment of other patients.

Some patients tolerate these and similar kinds of informal behavior very well. Others, however, realize that they are being treated differently from other patients or from how they think they are supposed to be treated and are unable to understand it. Rather than being pleased by this extra attention, they may grow distrustful.

The confident professional person can—but knows it is often wiser not to—rely solely on casual mannerisms. The patient readily discerns that these methods are being substituted for a deeper caring that only a more confident person dares to express.

Genuine caring is the subject of much consideration in the health professions today. Sometimes it is used to distinguish *treatment* (i.e., the technical aspects) from the other, more human dimensions of a health professional's role. We find this distinction misleading in some cases, because goals of care may best be achieved by sophisticated technological means such as a patient-administered morphine drip for the self-control of severe cancer pain.

In a recent article addressing the need to define "care" in one health profession (pharmacy), the author reviews several definitions currently in use and concludes, "Care and caring are ultimately defined as acts or behaviors which are a response to the values and needs of the individual, with professional care specifically intended to improve or maintain a person's health."[9]

Reich suggests that care means "paying attention"—it is not the warm fuzzy sentimentality so often expressed on the inside of greeting cards. True caring may become a challenge or even a burden. A person's life is composed largely of what he or she gives attention to or, put another way, cares about.[10] This is precisely what distinguishes care from sentimentality: sentimentality stresses the awareness that a person has an emotion, whereas caring always requires involved concern about the person's well-being. The association of this deeper understanding of care with the idea of respect is highlighted by the Latin root word for respect, *respicere,* which means "to look at."

New insights into society's understanding about the basic function of care are emerging. For instance, Carol Gilligan's classic study of moral development in children showed that girls and women tend to place their relationships at the center of their assumptions about the requirements for leading a good life. Therefore, finding the proper moral dimensions of caring within relationships becomes the central task of moral development.[11] Although boys sought independence, girls in her study continued to search for identity within the context of a relationship. This does not mean that girls could not build a strong sense of self or be independent in the sense that Erikson talked about as the task of intimacy and individuation, but rather that an understanding of humans as essentially relational beings informed their thinking. Additional studies have suggested that these themes are not gender specific. Placing care at the center of a relationship becomes crucial when human suffering is involved because caring is a salve to human suffering. As such, caring has been accepted as a virtue that should be expressed and valued in health professional and patient relationships.[12]

Caring as Attitude *and* Behavior

Although care has been treated as an attitude or, in the moral sense, a virtue that describes the kind of person a health professional *is,* more and more attention is being devoted to behaviors that can be identified as caring behaviors.[13] Part of the impetus for identifying such conduct is the emphasis on measurable outcomes in health care interventions.

You can see that the language and activity of caring might create a difficulty for health professionals, too. We live in a sexist society in which traits associated with women often are devalued. For instance, nurses and other professionals often are treated as second-class citizens because their professional roles explicitly entail and embrace conduct associated with caring. Caring and the persons giving and receiving care may become devalued in the eyes of others, and persons needing care may feel embarrassed or reticent to ask for and accept it.[14] Despite these difficulties, the weight of evidence continues to support the idea that caring, in all of its dimensions, adds to the effectiveness of the health professional–patient relationship in a time when all too often efficiency is substituted for the caring attitudes and behaviors patients equate with compassion or involvement in their situation.[15]

In short, there is a striking distinction between casual "you-are-special" gestures and deeper caring that results in benefit to the other person. Their complementary function is unmistakable, but to *substitute* the former for the latter is disastrous to the building of mutual respect in the relationship.

Caring—from the Patient's Perspective

One important insight is that a patient's perception of the difficulty he or she is experiencing often is different from that of the health professional. Earlier in this chapter we introduced the problem of thinging and how it undermines patients' trust. Patients are concerned primarily with what the problem signifies in terms of their daily lives, loves, and activities. Hardly ever is the technical aspect of what is wrong the governing factor. Health professionals are taught to look for the abstractive meaning of a condition: the chest sound, laboratory findings, x-ray films, the sight of the skin or tone of the muscle, and so forth. Contrary to this, the patient assigns a deeper *personal* meaning to the condition based on his or her understanding of the broader experience and effects of the illness. Chapter 9 shows that the patient's story (or stories) is the narrative he or she brings to the relationship as a clue to what this deeper personal meaning might be.

In John Updike's short story "From the Journal of a Leper," the young man begins his journal as follows:

> Oct. 31. I have long been a potter, a bachelor, and a leper. Leprosy is not exactly what I have, but what in the Bible is called leprosy (see Leviticus 13, Exodus 4:6, Luke 5:12B13) was probably this thing, which has a twisty Greek name it pains me to write. The form of the disease is as follows: spots, plaques, and avalanches of excess skin, manufactured by the dermis through some trifling but persistent error in its metabolic instructions, expand and slowly migrate across the body like lichen on a tombstone. I am silvery, scaly. Puddles of flakes form wherever I rest my flesh. Each morning, I vacuum my bed. My torture is skin deep: there is no pain, not even itching; we lepers live a long time, and are ironically healthy in other respects. Lusty, though we are loathsome to love. Keen-sighted, though we hate to look upon ourselves. The name of the disease, spiritually speaking, is Humiliation.[16]

What meaning does this person assign to his condition (Hansen's disease, commonly known as "leprosy")? What might you, as health professional, do to begin to address this profound suffering? Professional caring would require, in this case, that the patient's feeling of humiliation be a guide to how you respond to him, not only the distressing physical symptoms he describes. His example is just one powerful reminder that in lived experience, a patient takes the medical condition and places it into the larger context of meaning for his or her life. Your job is to address the medical condition, but always with an understanding of the bigger picture.

IT (ALMOST) ALL DEPENDS ON DEPENDENCE

People who seek your services to remain well or who become ill or injured share the experience of being in a new, unique relationship. Although, as discussed earlier in this chapter, there are several models of the health professional and patient interaction, the relationship is primarily one of authority–dependence, with the health professional being the person in authority in this regard. You, the health professional, are sought out explicitly to provide insight about staying healthy, evoke healing forces, apply appropriate technology, be a mentor, clarify values, be a role model, and mediate between the sufferer and society. Patients will have different responses to your authority depending on their own needs and on the way in which they have learned to respond to other authority figures in their lives (recall the possibility of transference discussed in an earlier section). Therefore, their interaction with you and your colleagues can be either a comforting, enabling interaction or a further source of suffering and challenge.

A patient probably does not fully understand his or her feelings toward the health professional; they may be expressed as awe or deference, as vague admiration, as infatuation, or even as intense hostility. To some extent, you can alter the patient's attitude if it seems to be interfering with the goal of the encounter.

Types of Dependence

Two types of dependence can be differentiated: detrimental (i.e., *over*dependence) and constructive dependence. These types of dependence are referred to many times in the rest of this book, so they should be noted carefully.

TABLE 11–2. Comparison of Detrimental and Constructive Dependence

	Detrimental Dependence	Constructive Dependence
Basis	Lack of sense of self	Mutual respect, feeling of self-worth
Stimulus	Overwhelming need	Genuine concern
Behavior	Blame the other for failures	Acceptance of responsibility for oneself and for the direction the relationship takes

Detrimental Dependence. Detrimental dependence in any relationship usually is based on an intense sense of self-depreciation and the desire to find personal identity in relation to someone else. It develops when one person has a neurotic need to cling to another who either does not know how to control the amount of involvement between them or needs the possessive aspect of the relationship or both. They consequently become intimately entangled in each other's problems to the point that they are no longer helpful to each other, but they are unable to terminate the relationship gracefully.

One classic example of this relationship is that of wives who lose themselves in their husbands' work or vice versa. They claim no greatness for themselves and may feel they do not even *exist* apart from who they are in relation to their spouses. Concomitantly, the spouse is made to feel entirely responsible for the other's well-being. The dependent person takes no responsibility for what happens. Although one may despise the other or there may be mutual distrust between them, they continue to control each other's lives. This dependence handcuffs both people to the relationship while each blames the other for their mutual imprisonment. They cannot express what they really feel about each other because the fate worse than their present imprisonment is rejection by the other person. The result is continuing mutual overdependence.

When a patient or health professional is seeking such dependence, that person may have a neurotic need to clutch the gains he or she believes lie in the relationship. A health professional may desperately need to be liked, either to prove his or her competence or simply to wield control over another person. Detrimental dependence may result if only one party exhibits the behavior, but it will undoubtedly result if both of them exhibit the behavior. This dynamic is especially devastating in a long-term health professional–patient relationship. Once the health professional and patient become overly dependent on each other, they will hesitate to discontinue treatment or evaluation procedures, even after it becomes apparent that the patient no longer needs the professional services of the health professional. They may arrange to see each other outside the clinical setting. If the patient does not improve, he or she may begin to blame the health professional; by the same token, the health professional may accuse the patient of not wanting to improve. Such is the double bind of detrimental dependence. To illustrate, consider the story of Arthur Cranston.

> At first, everyone thought Arthur Cranston was a delightful person. He was never late for his appointments, with you or others, cooperated thoroughly, and maintained a cheerful attitude in spite of his functionally debilitating symptoms. He began to telephone you between treatments, usually to ask a question in regard to his treatment regimen, but also to chat.
>
> Naturally, everyone was concerned when, after several treatments, he received no relief from his symptoms. A meeting of the health care team was called, and the members tried to outline another approach with the

hope that he might find some relief. You learned at the meeting that he also had begun calling the other members of the team, exhibiting the same behavior. Furthermore, you learned that he had been bringing small gifts to the others. You recall the time he brought in some donuts for you and your staff, a gesture that you appreciated and thought nothing more about at the time.

Now, after a few more weeks, his calls have become more frequent. He has also begun calling you at home, and you learned that the others have been receiving similar calls.

Yesterday he telephoned while you were with another patient. You asked the secretary to tell him you would call him back. The secretary did so. Later the secretary said, "Mr. Cranston said to tell you that he knows you are lying and just don't want to talk to him. He says he is coming over this afternoon and will wait in our receiving area until you have a few minutes. I told him you were pretty tied up this afternoon and asked if it was urgent. He swore at me and said, 'Of course it is.' " When you returned his call you realized that there was no urgency.

What might you be able to do to wean Arthur Cranston from his dependence on you and the other health professionals? A patient who enters the health care world with a need for total dependence on someone else becomes a problem for everyone. Health professionals find that the feeling of dependence is easily transferred from one person to another. It is the health professional's *role* that engenders the initial dependence; the individual health professional at any given time can only increase or diminish it.

Constructive Dependence. Constructive dependence is based on mutual respect. At some level, the patient acknowledges that he or she has a need and that fulfillment of the need means establishing some dependence on the health professional. It is, however, not a neurotic desire to cling to the other person. It does not entail loss of one's own identity in a relationship with another person. Both come together genuinely concerned, become personally (although not intimately) involved, and are able to terminate their relationship when it ceases to be mutually beneficial. This sense of trust and involvement can be established at their first meeting, benefiting both if it is their only encounter. If they continue to interact, mutual trust continues to grow.

Constructive dependence enhances each individual's potential and is characterized by each accepting responsibility for his or her own "progress" in the relationship. Because the limits of the relationship are understood by both, there is no fear of rejection. However, at the core of constructive dependence is a paradox. The two people who trust and respect each other find that in their closeness they are able to allow each other freedom.

Constructive dependence as it applies to the health professional–patient relationship occurs when people come together because of mutual need; the health professional needs to find satisfaction in applying professional skills, and the patient needs the services of the skilled professional. Both exhibit normal needs rather than the neurotic desires that lead to detrimental dependence. Their involvement is personal and not merely a business transaction; they express to each other those feelings and opinions that can be shared within the limited professional setting. When the patient no longer requires the services of the health professional, there will be no regret about ending their relationship because each one has benefited from it, whether it lasted for 10 minutes or 10 months. To illustrate, consider the story of Hilda Minier.

> Mrs. Minier is a retired schoolteacher who severely burned her face and arms when a camp stove exploded during a camping trip with her husband. She was treated on the burn unit for 3 months and now returns three times a week as an ambulatory care patient.
>
> She gets discouraged at times but has an overall optimistic disposition despite the obvious physical discomfort and the cosmetic difficulties she experiences as a result of her accident.
>
> On several occasions she has telephoned you to confirm that she is carrying out the home treatment procedures correctly. She speaks to the point and does not linger or make small talk. Sometimes you have asked to call her back because you are with another patient. She does not mind waiting. You think she deserves the reassurance and is reasonable in her extra demands on your time, though you know that she is quite capable of carrying out the home procedures accurately.
>
> On your birthday she sent you a birthday card at your home. Once she and her husband sent a fruit basket to the department, and you learned that a basket has been sent to other departments as well.

What are the differences between this interaction and the one involving you and Arthur Cranston? The key to understanding the difference lies in grasping the notion of dependence as it is expressed in the health professional and patient interaction.

RESPECT AS EMPOWERMENT

At the same time that the patient must successfully carry his or her share of responsibility for developing a constructive type of dependence, the health professional must join in the process by encouraging the patient to exercise the authority and autonomy that he or she still has available. For example, a patient who is institutionalized and has lost control over much of his or her life may still be able to command small details such as what to wear that day or when to eat. Sometimes the loss of independence signals to both patient and health professional that the patient really should be treated like a baby, having everything done for him. This is just plain nonsense. After a severe

back injury, one of the authors received the following note during a
bedridden period:

> NOBODY HAS EVER SAID THE
> UNIVERSE CANNOT BE EXPLORED
> FROM A RECUMBENT POSITION.

A patient who has confidence in his or her own dignity and potential seldom will
experience a feeling of total lack of control. The health professional can serve
as a constant source of encouragement and guidance in this process of
reempowerment.

Empowerment is realized partially through the patient's agency as a moral
decision-maker. One basic aspect of the contract is informed consent. As you
probably recall from your reading of Chapter 2, informed consent acknowledges a difference in power between you, the health professional, and the patient
and places the onus of responsibility on you to make the playing field more level.
In other words, it is your responsibility to inform the patient about what is going
to happen and to do so in such a way that he or she really understands what is
being agreed to. There is much to commend this approach.

At the same time, serious questions have been raised about this characterization of the relationship. For example, many have followed the concept of
"covenant" as a basis for the health professional and patient relationship. May
believes that the idea of a covenant includes the contract elements of mutual
expectations and agreement but goes further. Covenants, as they have been used
within theological contexts, place people in a situation in which they not only
provide goods but acknowledge being recipients of goods too. This approach
requires the professional to acknowledge all the benefits derived from health
care practice and from the opportunity to be with patients, clients, and their
families. Therefore, an element of professional gratitude enters the relationship,
empowering patients to do their best and possibly encouraging professionals to
go beyond the bare minimum of duty that would be agreed upon in a strict
contract approach.[17]

This covenantal characterization of the relationship deserves your considered attention as you find yourself engaged with the vast array of different kinds
of people whom we call "patients."

SUMMARY

The test of all of the ideas presented in this chapter is the extent to which any of
them support genuine respect toward patients, their families, and the ideals of
the health professions. Professional relatedness builds on basic human relational characteristics such as trust (and how reassurance fosters it), sensitivity to
the effects of transference and countertransference, attitudes and behaviors that
engender the feeling that one is cared for and deserving of attention, an
understanding of how dependence operates in a relationship, and the health

professional's commitment to empowering the other person. Practical as they are, they provide foundation blocks for building truly respect-based professional relationships.

REFERENCES

1. Sarton, M.: *A Reckoning.* New York, Norton, 1978, p. 204.
2. Erikson, E.: *Childhood and Society.* New York, Norton, 1950.
3. Secundy, M.G., and Jackson, R.L.: Engendering trust in a pluralistic society. In Thomasma, D.C., and Kissell, J.L. (eds.): *The Health Care Professional as Friend and Healer.* Washington, DC, Georgetown University Press, 2000, p. 66.
4. Veatch, R.M.: Models for medicine in a revolutionary age. *Hastings Cent. Rep.* 2:5–7, 1972.
5. Smith, S.: Three models of the nurse-patient relationship. In Spicker, S., and Gadow, S. (eds.): *Nursing Images and Ideals.* New York, Springer-Verlag, 1980, pp. 176–188.
6. Emanuel, E.J., and Emanuel, L.L.: Four models of the physician patient relationship. *JAMA* 267(16):2221–2226, 1992.
7. Freud, S.: *The Ego and the Mechanisms of Defense.* New York, International Universities Press, 1966.
8. Northouse, P.G., and Northouse, L.L.: *Health Communication: Strategies for Health Professionals.* 3rd ed. Norwalk, CT, Appleton & Lange, 1998.
9. Galt, K.A.: The need to define "care" in pharmaceutical care: an examination across research, practice, and education. *Am. J. Pharm. Ed.* 64: 223–233, 2000.
10. Reich, W.: Care. In *Encyclopedia of Bioethics.* 2nd ed. New York, Macmillan, 1995, pp. 331–336.
11. Gilligan, C.: *In a Different Voice.* Cambridge, MA, Harvard University Press, 1982.
12. Allmark, P.: Is caring a virtue? *J. Adv. Nurs.* 28:662–667, 1998.
13. Purtilo, R.: Health professional and patient relationship: ethical aspects. In *Encyclopedia of Bioethics.* 2nd ed. New York, Macmillan, 1995, pp. 2094–2103.
14. Mahowald, M.B.: Care and its pitfalls. In Haddad, A.M., and Beurki, R.A. (eds.): *Ethical Dimensions of Pharmaceutical Care.* Binghamton, NY, The Hawthorne Press, 1996, pp. 85–102.
15. Benner, P.: When health care becomes a community: the need for compassionate strangers. In Kilner, J.F., Orr, R.D., and Shelly, J.A. (eds.): *The Changing Face of Health Care.* Grand Rapids, MI, William B. Eerdmans, 1998, pp. 119–135.
16. Updike, J.: From the journal of a leper. *The New Yorker,* July 19, 1976, pp. 28-32.
17. May, W.F.: Code and covenant or philanthropy and contract? *Hastings Cent. Rep.* 5:29–35, 1975.

CHAPTER 12

Professional Boundaries Guided by Respect

CHAPTER OBJECTIVES

The student will be able to

- Describe how the idea of professional boundaries is relevant to respect
- Distinguish a respectful professional approach from one based on objectivity and efficiency alone
- Identify and discuss appropriate physical boundaries in relation to unconsented touching, sexual touching, and sexual contact after a professional and patient relationship has ended
- Describe three situations in which maintaining emotional boundaries is crucial to showing respect for patients
- Define "enmeshment"
- Identify some clues that may alert the health professional that his or her sympathy is becoming pity
- Define "overidentification"
- Describe what it means to "care too much"
- List five practical ways that professional boundaries can be better maintained

I remember the wintry day she called from a phone booth not too far from the office, barely hanging on. I got somebody to take me out to find her and bring her back to the office. I remember the moment when I realized that the absurd choice before me was to do grief work or find insulin. After a frustrating morning on the phone trying to find some public or private source of help—a struggle she was in no shape at the moment to handle—I took her to a drug store and bought the insulin myself.

I was feeling a bit of shame. There's an emphasis in our field now on maintaining proper boundaries, with the implication that those who do not are overfunctioning, co-dependent, and other compound words even more dreadful. Emotional disengagement was expected. Technically—

though no one forbade it—it was not part of my job to go find people in phone booths or pay for their medicine. I was aware of stretching the limits of what I usually do.

B. Jessing[1]

The health professional in the above quote is struggling with the appropriate limits of her "professional" involvement with her homeless client. She, like all health professionals, has been taught that we can overstep and in so doing may do more harm than good in the long run. Still, almost everyone can sympathize with her attempt to be respectful of her client's desperate situation. A good general rule is that the physical and emotional boundaries between you, the health professional, and patients must always be guided by the goal of facilitating a patient's well-being and maintaining profound respect in the interaction. However, as is the case with almost everything covered in this book, knowing the general rule does not necessarily help one with the complex human stories that face you in the line of work you have chosen. Therefore, this chapter attempts to provide some more details and examples of what it means to maintain professional boundaries.

WHAT IS A PROFESSIONAL BOUNDARY?

A "professional boundary" is the usual way of talking about physical and emotional limits that are appropriate to maintain while in the health professional and patient relationship. You have probably read accounts of health professionals losing their licenses or in other ways being sanctioned for engaging in sexual intercourse with patients or clients. The idea of sexual harassment includes conduct that falls short of having sexual intercourse but would be identified as ethically and legally unacceptable. We will briefly discuss these in a section that more broadly describes physical boundaries. Guidelines regarding emotional boundaries are designed to prevent psychological dynamics that are harmful to the patient or to you during the relationship. Most of these dynamics fall broadly into the category of detrimental dependence introduced in Chapter 11. We will discuss these, too. While studying this chapter bear in mind that some boundaries come from external sources (e.g., the time health professionals have to spend in the encounter) while others are internal (i.e., characteristics both health professional and patient bring to the encounter).

The guidelines for physical and emotional boundaries are derived from several sources. Some are from professional ethics codes; others are from laws. These in turn have grown out of the experience of health professionals and patients in the past. Sometimes the guidelines change based on insights from psychology regarding tensions that may arise from human needs for privacy, intimacy, and acceptance. Today studies of power within institutions and relationships add an additional component of understanding.

An apt place to begin your exploration is an examination of the self you bring to the challenge of maintaining appropriate limits of familiarity and intimacy with patients, clients, or their families. One way the wisdom of maintaining boundaries has been dramatized in the past is in the erroneous idea that being "professional" requires one to be aloof, objective, and efficient *at the price of good old personal warmth and affectionate conduct.* Sometimes this idea is suggested by the educational process, in which the need to acquire competence and clinical judgment appears to be all that professionalism requires. Although the authors warn against substituting casualness for genuine caring attitudes and behaviors (see Chapter 11), the intent is not to convey the impression that any step over the line into a friendly and relaxed demeanor may be unprofessional.

Where did this notion of a dichotomy between strictly personal and so-called professional qualities originate? There may be many sources. Some ancient philosophical and religious conceptions of healing are based on the idea that healing requires the intervention of a mysterious, impersonal power. For instance, in ancient Greek legend, life and death are in the hands of the gods who have some human traits but also have powerful superhuman potential to defy tragedy and death at times. The ancient God of the Israelites both smote and healed, but this healer's face was never seen. Unfortunately these ancient sources do not instruct us well in how to behave today. Most health professionals do not receive much instruction in how to construct and maintain boundaries.

The authors of this book are including this dichotomy, recognizing the extremely high personal price one would have to pay if becoming a "professional" required *separation* of the professional from the personal qualities that have helped you to develop friendships, business relationships, and relationships with loved ones. In fact, it would require becoming a split personality, as shown in Table 12–1.

Recognizing how important for your personal well-being it is to have an integrated set of qualities and to visualize yourself as a whole person creates a baseline from which you can design your professional approach. In other words,

TABLE 12–1. Professionalism Misconceived

Professional Self	Personal Self
Is efficient	Cares; is concerned about efficiency
Is competent administrator	Is warm, enthusiastic human being
Avoids getting involved in conversations about patient's personal life	Asks patients questions concerning his or her personal life
Demands respect from patient	Encourages openness and honesty in patient
Places premium solely on sound application of technical skills	Places premium on social interaction with person
Protects self by maintaining distance	Risks self by encouraging closeness

---

TABLE 12–2. Professionalism Rightly Conceived: Personal-Professional Self

Incorporates actions that communicate caring into the patient–health professional interaction; recognizes efficiency as a trait that can express caring when it does not impose rigid limits on the interaction

Combines a pleasant approach with competence

Shows interest in the patient as a person with values, needs, and beliefs but does not encourage a relationship that will lead to overdependence (detrimental dependence)

Is respected by the patient, who recognized the professional's integrity; acknowledges that complete, open, mutual sharing with each other is not necessary to the functioning of a public-sector relationship

Maintains a balance between providing sound health care services and fostering friendly interaction

---

the *integration* of your professional and personal qualities, as shown in Table 12–2, allows you to proceed from a sound foundation of wholeness in your attempt to construct workable boundaries. We turn now to that topic more specifically.

RECOGNIZING WHAT A MEANINGFUL DISTANCE IS

In human interaction, psychological and physical distance takes on deep meaning, determined by the degree of intimacy it represents for both parties. At one pole, there may be a complete sense of separateness, and at the other there is the realm of togetherness that is highly personal, informal, and familiar (i.e., intimate). At any point along this continuum, certain behaviors are put into play, whereas others remain in the background. In health professional and patient interactions the degree of intimacy must be guided by the propriety and character of this particular relationship. A key is that the health professional must meet the reasonable expectations of the patient while not overstepping into too familiar ground, not remaining too aloof, and not abandoning the patient. The degree of distance must take its reference point of meaning, then, from the appropriate contours of this particular relationship. One important caveat is that the health professional dare not place too great an expectation on the patient or his family for emotional support. When this happens, the professional's dependence is becoming detrimental to the patient (see Chapter 11). You will probably think of some "test cases" of this generalization in which more intimate communication would be appropriate. However, to illustrate our caution further we turn to some specific limits on physical contact and emotional attachment that have resulted in guidelines, policies, and laws based on society's notions of meaningful distances in this relationship.

PHYSICAL BOUNDARIES

As a general rule we are a society that does not condone very much touching, especially among strangers. You may find a clerk in a store who physically touches the palm of your hand in returning change. You may be jostled in a crowd. Strangers may impulsively hug the man or woman next to them in the midst of an important sports event. However, the occasions when touching among strangers is socially sanctioned can probably be counted on the fingers of one hand. At the same time, many health professionals' tasks require them to be in physical contact with people who are their patients, and to do so respectfully. In addition, displays of affection expressed by a pat on the shoulder or a gentle hug or signs of support occasioned by holding the patient's hand are all behaviors you may be comfortable engaging in as a part of your interaction.

Because touching often is not socially condoned, but can be a very effective means of establishing rapport or showing reassurance—and may be required to effect a diagnostic or treatment regimen—the acceptable contours of physical contact between health professional and patient deserve your attention.

Unconsented Touching

The legal foundations of informed consent are some of the most basic societal acknowledgments that professional contact departs dramatically from accepted social norms of physical contact. The legal concept of battery is based on society's deep prohibition against unconsented touching. By giving informed consent the patient is saying, in effect, I give you—and others involved in my care—consent to stroke, rub, poke, or even puncture or cut me, depending on what you are licensed by society to do as a part of your professional procedures. If the person on the street attempted such activity with a stranger he or she would end up in jail. Cartoonist Gary Larson pokes fun at this type of license and points to the potential for abuse of this privilege in the cartoon in Chapter 2.

Obviously the permission to make physical contact already puts the health professional and patient relationship into a special category where usual, socially acceptable distances are breached on a regular basis. This helps you to understand one important reason why we addressed informed consent in Part One, identifying it as the contractual basis of the health professional–patient relationship.

This right to make physical contact does not give you permission to automatically impose on a patient's sensitivities or dislikes regarding physical contact. Many cultural, social, and personal factors will come together to create a patient's comfort zone regarding physical contact and you should be guided by a sensitivity to individual differences.

Sexual Touching. Some types of physical contact are deemed unacceptable in the health professional and patient relationship under any conditions, even with the consent of the patient or client. Under law you cannot make contact with a patient with an intent to harm him or her physically or psychologically. If you do, you will be charged with sexual or other physical abuse.

The type of touching that has received the most attention is physical contact delivered with an intent to excite or arouse the patient sexually. Although sexual intercourse is the most *verboten,* the prohibitions are not limited to it. For example, the American Medical Association's 1997 *Code of Medical Ethics: Current Opinions with Annotations* addresses the broader notion of *sexual misconduct.*[2] Why should it be forbidden if a competent, adult patient consents to or even seems to invite sexual contact? The strongest argument against this type of contact is that it betrays the reasonable expectations built into the essence of the health professional and patient relationship. Patients have a right to receive the best care possible without having to satisfy the professional's needs.

However, what about the idea that sexual activity between professional and patient may be taking place between two consenting adults? An objection to this argument is that sexual activity never is free from other types of claims on the other person, so that both patient and health professional may begin to recreate the conditions of the relationship in light of the power of its sexual dimensions rather than the conditions under which a patient gave informed consent in the first place. In short, it is never considered fair that the patient would have to meet your need for sexual pleasure, sexual intimacy, sexual fulfillment, dominance in a relationship, or any other gain, no matter what the patient might believe will be gained.

Sexual Harassment. The importance of the idea that sexual distance must be maintained in public settings is being aired today in the notion of "sexual harassment." The U.S. Equal Employment Opportunity Commission (EEOC) defines harassment as unwelcome sexual advances, requests for sexual favors, and other verbal or physical conduct and includes activity that creates a hostile or unwelcome work environment for the person who feels "harassed."[3] Most state licensing acts have provisions prohibiting such behavior by professionals, and many institutions include prohibitions in their policies. You will have ample opportunity to learn more about the particulars of the legal issues involved in this evolving area of the law. An important aspect of the issue of sexual harassment that has not been explored deeply enough is the harassment or other sexual behaviors that may issue from patients, clients, or their family members toward professionals. For example, one study of physical therapists reported that 63% of respondents had experienced some form of sexual harassment perpetrated by patients or clients.[4] At the heart of the discussion is the degree of distance and quality of exchanges that must be maintained for respect to be expressed and for human dignity to flourish for everyone involved.

What About Dual Relationships?

In the past the typical belief has been that once a health professional and patient relationship formally has ended, two consenting, competent adults ought to be free to do whatever they please. This makes good intuitive sense on the face of it. We call your attention, however, to literature on the dynamics of "dual relationships" and some caveats that are being posed. In their article entitled "Dual Relationships and Professional Boundaries," Kagle and Giebelhausen define dual relationships as those in which "[a] professional . . . assumes a second role with a client, becoming . . . friend, employer, teacher, business associate, family member, or sex partner. The dual relationship may begin before, during, or after the [professional] relationship."[5] Their review of the literature on dual relationships in the professions lead them to conclude that for the most part:

> Professionals who enter into dual relationships often rationalize their behavior, arguing that the situation is unique. . . . However, dual relationships are potentially exploitive, crossing the boundaries of ethical practice, satisfying the practitioner's needs and impairing his or her judgment.[5]

They provide evidence and one case example of how even a friendship initiated after the termination of the professional relationship became injurious to the former client. They are especially cautious about the opportunity for abuse in sexual relationships. On the other hand, a woman who felt betrayed by her psychotherapist's unwillingness to continue a relationship beyond the physical-emotional boundaries of the professional and client relationship, especially after the formal relationship had ended, has written a book entitled *When Boundaries Betray Us*. Beyond all else her painful experience is a call for thoughtful health professionals everywhere not to become too legally obligated to the boundaries that preclude possibilities for dual relationships, especially once the health professional and patient relationship has ended.[6]

More research in this general area is needed. You can see that the present thinking about dual relationships is not conclusive. Not even all major health professions prohibit it. The American Medical Association's opinion on sexual misconduct addresses only current patient relationships, noting that a subsequent sexual or romantic relationship is acceptable if it does not permit the physician to "exploit trust, knowledge, emotions or influence derived from previous professional relationships,"[7] and many professions remain silent on the issue. To take seriously the potential for harm to a patient or former patient is to err on the side of better judgment. Although an exception may present itself, a good rule is to honor physical and emotional boundaries with great thoughtfulness and care.

We turn, then, to three types of experiences in which emotional boundaries become tools for maintaining respect in the health professional–patient relationship.

PSYCHOLOGICAL-EMOTIONAL BOUNDARIES

You have already examined the idea of detrimental dependence (Chapter 11). We turn now to a more in-depth examination of some specific ways the emotional responses and psychological attachments of the health professional or patient can interfere with respect for the patient. The term "enmeshment" summarizes these situations aptly:

> In interaction with the client, the nurse who has become enmeshed often develops an emotional connection with or an emotional availability to the client that may be impossible to maintain over the life span of the client. This can ultimately lead to client feelings of anger or emotional pain and to a sense of abandonment. The process of enmeshment may also complicate provision of adequate care at a later time. This can occur if the patient sees the other care team members as not caring sufficiently or as providing inadequate care, in comparison with the nurse who is enmeshed.[8]

In these situations a self-conscious distance zone should be created to enable each person to gain or regain perspective on the appropriate nature of this public-sector relationship and the expectations each can reasonably have of it.

Pity

Emotional boundaries may have to clearly be set to maintain full respect for the patient if, in your attempt to respond well to her or him, you become so entangled in the apparent futility of the patient's plight that it becomes an occasion for pity and therefore impossible to think about the patient or act in a way that really serves the patient's best interests.

Most health professionals can name at least one type of illness or injury that profoundly affects them emotionally. Sometimes their feelings are so strong that they cannot bear to treat patients with that particular condition. For instance, you can probably think of a condition that would be so horrendous for you to have yourself that you would feel sorry to the point of pity for a person who has that condition. You might name cancer, severe burns, aphasia, or psychosis. Younger health professionals may have difficulty treating persons suffering from illnesses that affect young people, one factor described in the phenomenon of "AIDS burnout" in the late 1980s.[9]

It is not at all unnatural for you to become periodically so involved in patients' dilemmas that you take these problems home with you. Almost any health professional can recall the time he or she had trouble falling asleep or was moved to tears or laughter by a sudden tragic or joyful announcement touching a patient's life. There is, however, a significant difference between this depth of professional caring, which stimulates a purely human response, and fruitless or destructive enmeshment. The difference can be illustrated with the following story:

Michael Anderson was admitted to the psychiatric ward of City Hospital after the police brought him there from the streets. The police found him unconscious in a doorway of a downtown office building. Michael is a 29-year-old alcoholic. His mother died when he was 12 years old, and he left home to live on the streets shortly after that. He recently learned that his father died of a heart attack shortly after he ran away from home.

Craig Hopkins, a health professional student in clinical education, is also 29 years old. His similarity to Michael Anderson, however, ends there. Craig Hopkins grew up in an upper-middle-class home and served as an officer in the Marines. He has never had close contact with an addict before, but he finds Michael very warm and human during his initial interactions. Michael is admitted to the detoxification unit where he will spend the next week or so. They both chat when Craig has a few minutes, and, over the next few days, Craig arrives at the conclusion that Michael has had more than his share of misfortune.

The next day, when Craig goes into Michael's room, he finds Michael doubled up, writhing in agony. With a trembling voice, Michael tells him that the doctor has not given him anything to take the edge off his withdrawal from alcohol. To Craig's surprise, Michael grabs him by the wrist and pleads, "Please, please, I can't stand this agony. If you will just get me something to drink, just enough to make it over the hump, I swear I'll never touch another drop. If I can't get a little relief, I will kill myself. The doctor is a sadist."

Craig Hopkins tears himself away and leaves the room. That night, however, he cannot sleep. He is haunted by the picture of an asthenic man who has survived the death of his parents but has succumbed to the bottle; he sees clearly the beads of sweat that clung to Michael's face as he spoke; he thinks that Michael is clearly all alone in the world; he is angry at Michael's physician for not making detox a little easier for Michael.

The next day, when Craig goes toward Michael's room, a nurse stops him, saying that Michael is in a restless sleep and experiencing some visual hallucinations. The nurse says, "You've got to watch these alcoholics. They're all liars. They'll do anything to manipulate the staff to give them more of the stuff."

Craig remembers Michael's pleading eyes the day before and is overcome with a desire to make a sharp retort to the nurse's statements. He goes instead to Michael's room and deftly slips a half pint of whiskey into the drawer of the bedside stand and makes enough noise so that

Michael stirs from his tortured sleep and sees what he is doing. He is not sure why he does this, but he knows it is important to quickly turn and leave.

What do you think about Craig's conduct? He has reached the point where he is responding impulsively rather than with genuine caring because the situation is so painful to him. Such a feeling exceeds sympathy and is more closely related to pity. Because pity distorts the objective perspective necessary to resolve the real problem, he ceases to be of help. In fact, he may include himself among the patient's many problems.

Pity can be communicated to the patient in one meeting as well as over a period of time. Facial expression can instantly convey one's feelings. Quick nervous movements, coupled with a sudden departure, are sometimes correctly interpreted as expressions of pity. The desire not to talk about the patient's problem, and trite comments such as, "It'll be *fine*, I'm sure," can also be interpreted to mean, "Poor, poor you."

You cannot solve this type of problem arising from pity simply by enmeshing yourself more deeply into the patient's personal life. Of course, your pity is in response to a real need of a patient. What is called for is sympathetic acknowledgment of the person's dilemma, but clarity that your professional role sets boundaries on what you will be able to do to intervene constructively in his or her plight.

Overidentification

The second situation in which emotional boundaries and psychological distance must be maintained to assure mutual respect arises when you, the health professional, have trouble seeing the patient as a unique individual. The patient may so perfectly embody a stereotype that in your eyes he or she becomes the stereotype. The patient may so remind you of someone else that he or she becomes that person (see the discussion of countertransference, Chapter 11), or you may have had an experience so similar to the patient's that you believe your experiences to be identical. In all three instances such a reaction is called overidentification and is another variety of enmeshment. Because elsewhere we have discussed dynamics present in stereotyping and countertransference, we concentrate our discussion on the third type of situation.

At first it seems a mistaken idea that having had similar experiences may actually hinder the effectiveness of health professional and patient interaction at times. But everyone has had the experience of beginning to relate a traumatic (or exciting) event only to have the other person interrupt with, "Oh! I know *exactly* what you mean!" and then go on to describe his or her own story. One feels cheated at such times, thinking, "No, that's not what I meant, but you are more interested in telling me about yourself than in listening to me!" The way such overidentification works within the health professions can be illustrated in another story:

> Mrs. Garcia, an elementary school teacher, became interested in teaching language skills to hearing-impaired children after her third child, Lucia, who was born deaf, successfully learned to communicate by attending special classes for those with hearing impairment. Mrs. Garcia enrolled in a health professions course directed toward training teachers of hearing-impaired persons.
>
> During her clinical education, she was surprised and alarmed that some of the mothers requested that she not be assigned to their children. Finally, she approached one of the mothers whose child she had been working with and with whom she felt comfortable. "What's wrong?" she asked. "Do they think I'm incompetent because I am an older student? Is it my personality? I want so much to help these children, and I can't understand what I'm doing wrong." The embarrassed mother replied, "Well, since you asked, I'll give you a direct answer. *I* don't feel this way, but some of the mothers think that you don't understand their children's difficulties because every time they start to tell you something about *their* children, you immediately interrupt with an experience that *your* child had."

In your opinion, how might this situation have been handled to avoid Mrs. Garcia's natural tendency to overidentify on the basis of her own intense situation? A first step would be for her to recognize that the tendency will be there. It will also be helpful to remind herself periodically that attempts to relate to the patient by pointing out superficial similarities between her own experience may be interpreted by the patient as her desire to talk about her own problem. Her basic task is not to be falsely led to believe that a closeness has been established. Rather, she must learn to maintain greater distance until the uniqueness of the other person emerges.

Caring Too Much

The final situation we discuss in this chapter is the most complex. It addresses the awkwardness that ensues when a relationship that began with appropriate boundaries has still led to circumstances signaling to you that a new set of boundaries must be established. This type of situation often is precipitated by the true affection that many people in health professional and patient relationships learn to feel for each other. The affection may spill over to, or be primarily directed to, the patient's family or other loved ones, too. One study suggests that professionals who have been brought up to view themselves as "caregivers" in the family may be more susceptible to overstepping this boundary than others because they become sensitively drawn into the other's life situation more.[10] We identify some signs that affection, a positive component of the relationship, has spilled over into enmeshment and make some general suggestions about what can be done to rectify the situation.

Obviously, affection is more likely to develop in health care settings where longer term professional relationships exist. One example of how a problematic dynamic can arise is illustrated in the following story.

> Jack Simms has been an ambulatory patient at University Rehabilitation for 6 months. His affable, optimistic spirit has made him very popular with the staff. At 23 years of age, he was involved in a car accident in which his fiancée was killed, and he suffered a traumatic brain injury. Some health professionals have long suspected that Jack's optimism is a veneer for the deep sorrow and frustration resulting from this sudden, dramatic change in his life. However, attempts to encourage him to visit with the staff psychiatrist have been largely unsuccessful, a problem exacerbated by the fact that his insurance plan covers only 6 hours of psychiatric evaluation and treatment anyway. One day he tearfully tells Karen Morgan, a health professions student who has been treating him, that he is depressed and desperately lonely. Up to this point, their interaction has been full of banter and they have felt quite comfortable with each other. Karen does not divulge to the rest of the staff Jack's expression of depression and loneliness, but that night on the way home, she stops by a local pub where he has invited her to "come and have a drink" following work.
>
> In the following weeks, she begins to visit him more often. She finds him attractive, they share common interests, and he is obviously happy in her company. During this time, however, Karen also leads her own private life, going on dates and interacting with a world of other people. However, Jack hangs around the clinic before and after treatments, and he counts the minutes until she arrives at the pub.
>
> During her Christmas vacation Karen visits friends in a distant city and has a marvelous time. When she returns, bursting with enthusiasm and eager to share her stories, she finds Jack sullen and angry at her for staying away from him for so long. He has arranged for her to receive a present from him, which he plops angrily on the clinic desk. He says, "That's for you. Take it if you want." Then he wheels himself out of the clinic angrily.

Jack's reaction indicates that he feels Karen has betrayed their relationship and abandoned him. He has now reached the point where someone he thought was a friend has "rejected" him. Karen, who acted in good faith on her feelings of warmth and affection for Jack, has thus unwittingly fostered detrimental, rather than constructive, dependence. Her subsequent attempts to explain her sudden withdrawal may have profound, lasting negative effects on Jack. Instead of being a friend and confidante—maybe eventually a lover—as he had hoped, she will become just another of a long line of rejections he has experienced. He has relied on her more than she had intended or was able to manage.

There are no sure and fast rules about how to proceed when genuine affection and enjoyment of the other is prodding the relationship along. Many of the warning signs of detrimental dependence discussed in Chapter 11 can be useful. In fact, the most powerful antidote to enmeshment is the health professional's strong personal identity and the presence of a satisfying personal life.[11] Periodic reexamination of your own motives and conduct or others' assessment of your relationship can help, too. Although it is important to maintain appropriate professional distance, you will best be served by showing genuine warmth and affection but always tempering that with awareness that the other person's needs and wishes may exceed or differ from your own. Periodic reflection on the conduct you are observing is wise.

MAINTAINING BOUNDARIES FOR GOOD

One key to maintaining boundaries in a way that will serve everyone's good is to be ever mindful that you can express genuine care for a patient by maintaining distance in some situations. We have made a few suggestions and conclude this chapter by going through each case once more to make more specific comments for your consideration and reflection.

In the case report in the preceding section, Craig Hopkins responded to Michael Anderson because he pitied him. However, patients abhor pity, even if it serves some small immediate purpose. Pity is destructive and belittling to the patient, who eventually will recoil from it.

Many patients who become objects of pity are suffering and do not know how or when to limit personal revelations when they find a professional person with a sympathetic ear. You can monitor the extent to which patients reveal confidences by simply asking if they really want to tell so much. Health professionals in general are in no position to solve most of the patient's personal problems unless they are trained to work in a psychiatric setting. A guideline is that if you are not professionally prepared for work in a psychiatric setting, you should readily refer the patient to someone—a chaplain, a psychologist, or a social worker—who is professionally skilled in providing this kind of assistance. The referral capacity is one of the strengths of a team approach to genuine care.[12] The health professional makes a mistake by responding with a display of overwhelming emotion—pity, in this case—while failing to put the person in contact with other means of support.

Finally, in such situations, checking one's feelings with other professionals can be helpful. The incident between Craig Hopkins and the nurse is a case in point. She told him that Michael Anderson was simply manipulating the hospital staff, to which accusation Craig responded antagonistically. The nurse made a generalized statement that is often correct of such patients but could have been questionable in this particular circumstance.

However, if Craig had listened to what she said, he might have gained a clearer insight into this patient or into others like him. Rather, he became defensive and was unable to listen objectively. In addition, he did nothing that might have helped the nurse attain a better understanding of Michael's situation.

In the case of Mrs. Garcia, troubling personal feelings or biases stemming from stereotyping, countertransference, and overidentification surfaced in the patient and health professional relationship. Coworkers can be valuable here. In a situation in which the health professional's close relationship with the patient prevents him or her from seeing the patient objectively, another professional person working with the patient may view the situation from a different perspective and thus provide some insight into the health professional's troubling responses. When the health professional refers a patient to someone else or shares disturbing feelings with coworkers, he or she is maintaining a healthy, respectful distance from the patient by bringing other people into the relationship.

Mrs. Garcia's effectiveness as a teacher was hindered by her own previous experiences, which led to overidentification. Overidentification, once it becomes a part of the health professional's thinking, cannot be easily erased. However, an important step toward adequate interaction is to keep a distance from one's own experience, only occasionally and thoughtfully sharing stories of similar experiences with the patient and his or her family. Respectful interaction is achieved when the health professional first stresses the uniqueness of the patient's experience and only then allows comparisons with the health professional's own experience. This behavior gives the patient an opportunity to describe fully his or her unique experience and express the feelings attached to it before the health professional superimposes any similarities on it. Then, as the health professional shares his or her own ideas and judgments, the patient will begin to realize that the health professional's own account reveals concern about and insight into the patient's problem.

In the final case report, the problem involved the health professional (Karen Morgan) who paid too much attention to the patient (Jack Simms). In such a case, it is always wise for the health professional to refrain from visiting the patient outside the treatment or testing situation until he or she is absolutely certain that the patient's feelings and life situation are such that an injury to the patient's feelings and dignity will not result.

Another way to maintain constructive physical and emotional boundaries is to remind the patient of the real situation between them. A young man, for instance, should know that the health professional he adores is engaged to someone else. By discreetly sharing with the patient personal incidents from everyday life, the health professional will be better able to maintain a "reality factor" in their relationship that will be helpful to both. It is the health professional's responsibility to give and receive pertinent personal information in such a way that workable limits are maintained in the relationship.

SUMMARY

This chapter promotes respectful interaction through your awareness of, reflection upon, and willingly and intentionally acting on constraints within the relationship. We have shown that the maintenance of professional boundaries is not achieved by employing a cold or impersonal approach. Indeed, such an approach may only increase the person's conviction that he or she is not understood by you, the health professional. You are faced with the challenge of carefully structuring the individual situation so that the dignity of both you and the patient is respected. The next chapter emphasizes situations in which the complementary and exciting challenge is one of creating a comfortable, appropriate closeness.

REFERENCES

1. Jessing, B.: Back to square one. In Haddad, A., and Brown, K. (eds.): *The Arduous Touch: Women's Voices in Health Care.* West Lafayette, IN, Purdue University Press, 1999, pp. 29–30.
2. American Medical Association: *150th Anniversary Edition of Code of Medical Ethics: Current Opinions with Annotations.* Chicago, American Medical Association, 1997, Section 8.14.
3. EEOC-FS/E4: Facts about Sexual Harassment; EEOC Guidelines on Sexual Harassment 29 CFR 1604 11a. 93, January 1992.
4. deMayo, R.A.: Patient sexual behaviors and sexual harassment: a national survey of physical therapists. *Phys. Ther.* 77:739–744, 1997.
5. Kagle, J.D., and Giebelhausen, K.B.: Dual relationships and professional boundaries. *Social Work.* 39(2):213–220, 1994.
6. Heyward, C.: *When Boundaries Betray Us: Beyond Illusions of What Is Ethical in Therapy and Life.* Cleveland, Pilgrim Press, 1999.
7. American Medical Association, Section 8.14 op. cit.
8. Rich, R.A., and Hecht, M.K.: Staffing considerations. In Haddad, A. (ed.): *High Tech Home Care: A Practical Guide.* Rockville, Aspen, 1987, pp. 117–127.
9. Wachter, R.M., Cooke, M., Hopewell, P.C., and Luce, J.M.: Attitudes of medical residents regarding intensive care patients with AIDS. *Arch. Intern. Med.* 148:149–152, 1988.
10. Farber, N.J., Novack, D.H., and O'Brien, M.K.: Love, boundaries and the patient-physician relationship. *Arch. Intern. Med.* 157: 2291–2294, 1997.
11. Davis, C.: *Patient Practitioner-Interaction. An Experiential Manual for Developing the Art of Health Care.* Thorofare, NJ, Slack, Inc., 1998, pp. 3–11.
12. Cassel, C., and Purtilo, R.: Ethical and social issues in contemporary medicine. *Sci. Am. Med.* Fall 1999, pp. 34–42.

CHAPTER 13

Professional Closeness: Respect at Its Best

CHAPTER OBJECTIVES

The student will be able to

- Identify the optimal mode of respectful interaction between patient and health professional and two key components of this "professional closeness"

- Discuss how integrity conveys respect for others' values thereby fostering professional closeness between patient and health professional

- Describe six guidelines for helping the health professional make maximum use of the time spent with a patient

- List several types of "attention to detail" that make patients know the health professional respects them as individuals

- Identify five levels of intimacy and their appropriateness for a health professional and patient relationship characterized by respect-in-action

Most of the many words that have been written about "doctor-patient communication" have come from doctors; there are textbooks devoted to the subject, and communication "competencies" are now taught in a number of medical schools. It would be difficult for me to come up with a list of competencies I look for in a doctor, but I know when I have met one I will trust. Mark Kris, who heads the thoracic-oncology service at Memorial, was this kind of doctor. The first thing Mark did, after looking at my medical records and having me carefully retell the story of what had happened to me over the past few months, was to give me a thorough examination. This was the first physical I'd had since this drama began; everyone else had just looked at the X-rays and scans. After he finished, he asked me how I felt. It was the only time in these months that anyone had asked me that question. . . .

A. Trillin[1]

223

This quote expresses one patient's brief reflection on her relationship with a health professional. It holds some clues you will recognize as professional closeness by the time you finish this chapter. Not every encounter will attain this level of refinement, but a committed and skilled health professional will always strive for it.

Professional closeness is the ideal (and attainable) form of interaction between a health professional and patient. The patient (or, if the patient is unable to participate actively, the family) contributes trust and a willingness to partner with the health professionals in reaching mutually agreed-upon goals. In turn, many health professionals adopt a robust commitment of faithfulness to the patient. It is rooted in the moral urgency of standing by people when they are the most vulnerable. Two essential elements that such health professionals bring to a relationship are integrity and individualized care.

INTEGRITY IN WORDS AND CONDUCT

Integrity comes from the root *integritas,* meaning "wholeness." Adjusting one's attitude and approach so that a patient and family can experience a sense of wholeness between what you say and what you do, a fittingness between their needs and your demeanor and actions, gives the security needed for their trust in you.[2] Patients will look to you from the start for reassurance that the relationship is going to benefit them. Such reassurance often is offered through words. For example, in the novel *I Never Promised You a Rose Garden,* the ward administrator tells Deborah, "It [the cold pack] doesn't hurt—don't worry." Those words sound like words meant to generate trust, comfort, and Deborah's willingness to cooperate with the health professional's plan.

However, Deborah, who is undergoing treatments in a psychiatric hospital and is very frightened of what has already been done to her in the name of treatment, has exactly the opposite response. She thinks, "Watch out for those words . . . they are the same words. What comes after that is deceit."[3] Her situation illustrates the fact that words meant to be reassuring may not have the intended effect of engendering a feeling of security at all if consistent conduct does not follow them.

Our encouragement to be self-reflective about integrity is designed to help you achieve it even when interaction is brief. In fact, meeting the challenge of creating professional closeness in a single meeting or during a short period of time may be more important today than ever before. The rapid social change that the health care system is experiencing as societies move to more and more complex networks of caregivers in large health plans is causing many to ponder the question: How will this rapid transition in human relationships affect people? Some professionals are very pessimistic, prophesying a dramatic breakdown in trust and effectiveness between health professionals and patients.[4] However, others' outlooks are less bleak, suggesting that many behaviors appropriate for longer term relationships will be able to be adapted to the new situation.

PAYING CLOSE ATTENTION TO THIS PERSON

We suggested at the outset of this chapter that professional closeness involves not only integrity but individualized care. Individualized care amounts to paying close attention to this person and acting accordingly. You have already learned some differences between casual contact and genuine caring in the professional and patient relationship (see Chapter 11). Caring is so essential to exhibiting respect for patients that we now take the idea of caring a step further.

What does it mean to "see the patient as a unique person"? Recall from previous chapters in Part V that first it means you must not treat a person as a thing. One version of this phenomenon is thinking of the patient primarily as the condition that brought her or him into contact with you. However, the challenge presents itself in your more general professional activity as well. Persons always should be treated as ends in themselves. Any attitude, action, practice, or policy that allows the patient's well-being to take second place to some other end is a threat to the potential for professional closeness. When you are paying close attention to the person, you are willing and able to honor even the smallest detail to convey your awareness that this patient is not only special but also is a person unique from all others. An often overlooked but extremely important expression of your care is the way you handle this patient's scheduled time with you. It is surprisingly easy to manipulate a patient's schedule for the sake of your own (or your institution's) efficient functioning—to mask your dislike of or favoritism toward a patient, to allow yourself a longer lunch hour with a friend, or for a thousand other reasons. In fact, we live in a society that

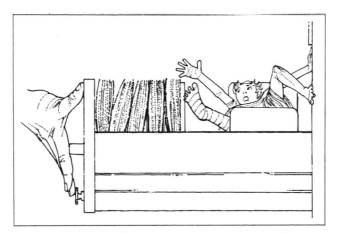

The health professional who manipulates objects in everyday life is in danger of manipulating the patient in the same impersonal manner.

makes it commonplace to manipulate people, but it is inconsistent with respectful interaction.

Almost everyone struggles with effective management of time, and health professionals are no exception. We elevate this challenge to the level of suggesting that poor time management will convey to patients that you do not care about them even if you think you do, thereby creating a barrier to professional closeness.

At the same time, expending the energy to manage your work time with the goal of professional excellence means that you are fine-tuning your caring behaviors. Consequently, sometimes your vigilance to the clock will be compromised for higher goals. Several guidelines can help you know when exceptions are in order.

The first is to commit yourself to never cutting corners with a patient unless it is absolutely necessary. The patient deserves your full professional commitment to his or her well-being. Owing to shortages of personnel, your like or dislike of some patients, and other reasons, it is easier in some situations than others to cut corners. If professional closeness is your goal, that conduct is not a prerogative for you. When you must take shortcuts, patients are likely to feel more cared for if you explain to them why they are getting short shrift.

The second rule is to allow the professional situation to guide you rather than the clock. Every health professional knows that on some days a particular patient needs some extra time to work through a problem, which can wreak havoc on a schedule. Then there are patients who for good (or poor) reasons are late or need to linger and make small talk, diverting your time and energy from other patients. Time management becomes a major challenge, but to set it against a backdrop of trying to be as caring as possible will help to mitigate the damage that will be done. Although some patients you have kept waiting may become impatient, your focused attention on doing all that you are able to do for them when their turn comes will create the conditions for professional closeness more readily than if you rigidly let the clock determine your day.

Finally, managing time with the goal of providing genuine care also can mean remembering certain clues about how to act with the patient during the time you actually are together. Here are some hints:

1. Remove the person from the usual office or clinic traffic or other areas where distractions are likely to occur.

2. Sit down when talking to the person to give the impression that he or she is the only person in the world who needs care.

3. Refrain from calling attention to how busy you are, or you will seem to be paying even less attention to the patient than you actually are. If there was an unavoidable delay in getting to the patient, explain why; if you cannot hide your distraction, explain that, too.

4. Approach the person slowly and graciously, even though you may have had to run to be on time for your appointment.

5. Look the person in the eye when conversing instead of glancing all around the room. A lack of eye contact communicates lack of interest and further increases his or her feeling that time with you is being wasted.

6. Protect the time that you have with the person by telling other people in the area that you are busy and will be happy to talk with them later. The patient who is scheduled to spend 15 minutes alone with you, but shares this time with 10 intruders or telephone calls, will feel more cheated than the one who enjoys 5 uninterrupted minutes.

Time will be a challenge and perhaps an enigma for you, partly because of your curiosity and interest in so many wonderful things and partly because of the many external pressures competing for your energies. This sign should be posted in every professional's workplace:

PUT WHAT IS IMPORTANT BEFORE WHAT IS URGENT

Establishing work habits that are guided by the patient's well-being as your highest priority will help you keep the important values in appropriate focus. One personal outcome will be that because patients will feel cared for, your commitment to this element of professional closeness will allow you to realize the satisfaction that comes from doing your job well.

LITTLE THINGS MEAN A LOT

An important way to enhance a person's self-worth or dignity, thereby enhancing the conditions conducive to professional closeness, is to acknowledge little personal details, which too often go unnoticed. One of the authors recalls a student's astonishment when just before graduation he was reflecting on his own developing way of being with patients.

> "This might surprise you," John said, "but do you know what I'd say is the most important thing I've learned in the last several weeks of my experiences in the clinics? I'd call it learning that little things mean a lot! Do you think that's ridiculous? For instance, I have learned the importance of pouring a glass of water for a thirsty patient, listening to the 9th inning of a baseball game between parts of a treatment, laughing at something the patient says, wiping a nose. Perhaps these things sound silly to you." I reassured him that they all counted as expressions of deep respect for who the person is as a unique individual.

John had learned that attention to personal details, however mundane, that are important to the patient is an effective way of showing a patient that he or she matters. It is fertile soil upon which professional closeness can take root and grow. These little details take many shapes, but we remind you of a few common ones here.

Personal-Hygiene Detail

When a patient has a hygienic need, attention to it before any other activity or exchange will make him or her very grateful. This is not to suggest that you need to wait on the patient with toothbrush, deodorant, and nail clippers in hand or that hygienic activity should in any way compromise time that should be spent utilizing professional skills. However, sometimes a simple act, such as providing a tissue when the patient needs one, makes the difference between an embarrassed person and an attentive person.

Personal-Comfort Detail

A person sometimes experiences a certain amount of physical discomfort in a treatment, diagnostic, or testing situation. It is easy to forget how often we shift posture, scratch, blink, swipe, or shrug just to get comfortable; yet there are conditions or techniques that prevent persons from performing these basic comfort functions. An extreme but instructive example is offered by Jean Dominique Bauby, the former editor of the magazine *Elle,* who suffered a stroke to his brainstem. This injury prevented him from any bodily movement whatsoever except to blink, but it left intact all of his sensations. This severe condition is called "locked-in syndrome." Mr. Bauby leaves an incredible memoir of his experience, achieved by blinking words with his left eye. Imagine his situation:

> This morning, with first light barely bathing Room 119, evil spirits descended on my world. For half an hour, the alarm on the machine that regulates my feeding tube has been beeping out into the void. I cannot imagine anything so inane or nerve-racking as this piercing beep beep beep pecking away at my brain. As a bonus, my sweat has unglued the tape that keeps my right eyelid closed and the stuck-together lashes are tickling my pupil unbearably. And to crown it all, the end of my urinary catheter has become detached and I am drenched. Awaiting rescue, I hum an old song by Henri Salvador: "Don't you fret, baby, it'll be all right."[5]

There are many ways a patient, even one with severe physical limitations such as Mr. Bauby, can be made more comfortable; they may involve straightening or cleaning the patient's glasses, wiping away sweat, supporting the person's arm while drawing blood, or running for an extra towel.

Many times patients are not asked simple questions such as whether the room temperature is OK, and if not what can be done to make the person warmer (or cooler).

Have you been stuck in a situation where you could not make yourself comfortable? You can remember that situation as a starting point of your own imagination when you are with patients. Asking "Are you comfortable?" or "Is there anything else I can do for you while I am with you to make you more comfortable?" will always be appreciated.

Personal-Interest Detail

Almost everyone has some area of interest, whether it be a hobby, job, family, or other focus. Showing interest in the person does not require probing unduly deeply into his or her personal life, something we warned against in Chapter 7. Some patients will want to chat about life outside of the moment and others will not. At the same time, asking an inpatient about the noon menu, listening to the ninth inning of a ball game, commenting to the ambulatory patient about something he or she is wearing, reminding a teenager that her favorite rap artist has a special show on TV that night, and spelling Mr. Schydlowski's name correctly on his appointment slip all count as appreciated attempts to personalize care. Birthdays and holidays are important occasions to recognize a person. On Mr. Arnold's birthday, write "HAPPY BIRTHDAY, DICK ARNOLD" in bold letters on the schedule board or let other staff know so that they can acknowledge it, too. You will think of other expressions of this type of respect to put into everyday action.

Expanding-Awareness Detail

If you have been confined to a home, hospital, or bed, you know how quickly one loses track of time and becomes out of touch with the rest of the world. By sharing an incident observed on the way to work, by reviewing a play seen the evening before, or by taking the patient to a window to see a child and dog playing together, you can extend the patient's environment beyond the immediate area, bringing him or her into contact with the outside world. One of the authors once brought apple blossoms into a four-bed room in an extended care facility only to have two of the patients burst into tears, saying they missed the smells of spring more than anything since being forced to make this their permanent residence. This opened the door to a discussion about springtime memories.

The one danger of paying attention to any or all of the types of details discussed above is that they may be substituted for actual professional services. It is possible to lose sight of the proper priorities. The professional person who would rather fluff pillows than proceed with a treatment or who would rather chat than work cheats the patient. He or she may be like a "friend" to the patient, but the regular substitution of personal detail for professional skills denies the patient the one thing he or she needs most from you.

REALITY TESTING AS A FORM OF RESPECT

Professional closeness also is fostered by your willingness to help patients "test" how they should act in the face of change occasioned by illness or injury or even of frustration caused by temporary alterations in their social or work patterns. This type of testing is more common among persons who suffer from severe or long-term conditions, but almost everyone who becomes a patient must undergo some kind of adjustment that can lead to the need to "try out the new self." Patients, many of whom may feel more confident with you than with others during this period, may say or do things that are designed to see what kind of response certain statements or behaviors will invoke. This is called "reality testing." One simple, forthright way to respond is for you to let a patient know which behaviors are *unacceptable* in your professional relationship (for example, jokes that are crude or have derogatory ethnic or sexual overtones). When a patient tries to divulge personal details that you judge inappropriate, you should let that person know that those things are better left unsaid.

Confronting patients about their unacceptable behavior may embarrass and upset them initially, but it will prevent conduct that may hinder their success in society. Just as importantly, it models the fact that your respect for them must be met by what you consider their respectful behavior toward you. However, it is equally crucial that you express delight and approval when you are happy about something the patient does. If the patient compliments you, you should accept the compliment graciously. Small, appropriate gifts also can be accepted graciously from patients, although you must be careful not to allow the patient to use a gift as a means of trying to unduly ingratiate himself or herself.[6]

What does it mean to "unduly ingratiate"? The idea of "gratuities"—the accepting of gifts from patients or families—long has been discussed in professional ethics codes, oaths, and other thoughtful writings in the health professions because sometimes patients do want to express genuine gratitude for the help you have given them. Refusing such gifts can be a sign of disrespect toward the patient or family if they have a need to say a heartfelt "thank you." However, gifts also can be used to influence you to give disproportionate time or attention to the patient or in other ways to upset the finely tuned attitudes and behaviors that allow you to show equal respect to everyone. The rule of proportionality—letting the gift fit the occasion—is a general guideline to follow. If you feel uncomfortable with the size, nature, or timing of the gift you should follow your instincts in graciously refusing it, acknowledging to the giver that you appreciate the thought that went into it. One approach that may help is to suggest a small token of appreciation (e.g., a box of candy) that can be shared with your colleagues, thereby diffusing a more highly personal focus of the gift on you.

In summary, by making a patient aware of unacceptable and acceptable behaviors you can help her or him gain some realistic idea of how that person may be received back into the larger social situations that await him or her. Your respect for the person is expressed by maintaining an honest and consistent response to the patient's many tentative actions. The respect you show through these actions, when carried out in a spirit of genuine caring, will generate a relationship of professional closeness.

FINDING A COMFORTABLE LEVEL OF INTIMACY

At the core of professional closeness is the challenge of finding a comfortable level of intimacy with an individual and testing that against the opportunities, tasks, and constraints of the health professional and patient encounter. Several years ago the authors found a capsule summary of intimacy levels expressed through conversation that still seems relevant and helpful for your consideration of the health professional–patient relationship. Therefore, we present these levels here along a continuum from the least intimate type of interaction (where there is a solid sense of separateness) to the most intimate type of interaction (where there is togetherness as characterized by informality, a sense of private lives together, and familiarity).[7]

Level 5: Cliché Conversation. No genuine human sharing takes place at this most superficial level. "How are you?", "It's good to see you," and "Have a good day" are said without thought, and standard answers are expected. The person who responds to "How are you?" with a detailed description of how he or she really feels is frowned on or, more likely, left to talk to himself or herself. This level protects people from each other and minimizes the likelihood of any further involvement. With rare exception, any physical contact during this exchange of "niceties" is seen as putting an unwanted claim on the listener or may be perceived as hostile.

Level 4: Reporting Facts. Although this goes beyond cliché politeness, almost nothing personal is revealed at this level either. Some sharing does take place, but only information about general subjects such as baseball scores, fashion, or a book.

Level 3: Personal Ideas and Judgment. People venture to give some information about themselves at this level. This may be done by expressing an idea, judgment, or decision, which is usually guarded and is monitored by the listener's response. If the listener looks disapproving, bored, or confused, the person probably will hesitate to share more at this level. Sometimes this type of exchange takes place on a plane or an extended wait in a queue. A person may venture a conversation with someone he has seen many times at his usual hangout. Although cultural norms of touching will vary and some individuals are more physically demonstrative, there will probably be very little physical contact during this level of interaction.

Level 2: Feelings and Emotions. Only people who trust each other reveal themselves at this level. Understanding between friends or people with whom one works cannot grow unless there is a mutual sharing at this level, commonly known as gut-level communication. A person will not want to share at this level if he or she believes the other person is judging the emotions themselves as good or bad. The individual wants the other person to understand that the emotion being expressed is genuine. There may be more freedom to accompany the communication with some degree of friendly touching or comfort.

Level 1: Peak Communication. Profound mutual trust and honesty are shared at this, the deepest level. There is almost perfect mutual understanding. Obviously, not many human interactions take place at this level. It is an all-encompassing intimacy experienced rarely by most people and never by some. Although not always the case, physical contact may be acceptable, welcomed, or even central to this degree of intimacy.

These five levels of intimacy in conversation are valuable touchstones because they describe accompanying behaviors and emotions appropriate to different types of situations. What levels do you think are appropriate in the health professional and patient relationship? We believe that seldom does this relationship include level 1 communication because this degree of intimacy usually requires physical or emotional involvement that is not conducive to maintaining respect for the patient. Given that health professionals and patients basically are strangers involved in a public-sector relationship, the deep involvement of level 1 is more likely to become detrimental dependence, which trespasses boundaries, or lead to a dual relationship (discussed in Chapters 11 and 12, respectively) instead of a healthy intimacy. At the same time, the shared trust in level 2 can support sharing happiness, sadness, and other emotions when the patient's or family's situation merits such response.

Some health professionals routinely discourage such emotional expression because it is uncomfortable for them to watch an adult break down and sob or grow furious. Without saying a word, the health professional can prevent the patient from expressing his or her fears; a "don't-tell-me" smile, an "I'm-too-busy" shrug, a "you're-above-that-kind-of-thing" wink, or a pleading "I-won't-know-what-to-do-if-you-cry" look will deter the most distressed patient or family member but does not foster professional closeness.

However, if professional closeness issues from deep caring of one human being for another, then the patient and family should have the option of revealing themselves through sharing their fears and other emotions with you. Furthermore, you should be prepared to be understanding when a patient is emotionally distraught; when this happens, several guidelines can be followed.

First, identify that the patient or family member has an emotional or feeling-level problem. This is not always easy to do because he or she, often afraid and embarrassed, may have clever means of disguising true emotions. What does he or she really feel? Is it anger, hurt, or fear?

Second, verbalize to the person the emotion he or she appears to be expressing by saying the following: "Mr. Lee, you seem sad today," or "Mrs. Cerosi, I think you must be angry about something. Am I right?" The patient may readily admit to the emotion. If your guess is wrong, the patient may blurt out what he or she is really feeling. However, in some cases, the person will, at least initially, deny that anything is the matter.

Third, allow the person to express his or her true emotion. This, of course, does not mean that the patient should be allowed to take advantage of you, to begin throwing objects across the room, or to engage in a free-for-all. As in any such relationship, an underlying foundation of mutual respect must be maintained and honored.

In short, patients and families often are in a situation in which they may need to reveal some deep-seated feelings without fear of rejection or ridicule. In some instances, then, a patient will reveal himself or herself simply by telling you about personal matters. In other instances, more emotionally charged information will erupt. Your thoughtful and heartfelt response helps to assure the patient that he or she is fully respected as a human being, and professional closeness is more likely to occur.

SUMMARY

Professional closeness is respect-in-action at its best. It is achieved when all the appropriate factors that should characterize a respect-based health professional and patient relationship are realized to their fullest. Previous chapters have detailed the importance of self-knowledge and patient knowledge geared toward earning a patient's trust and have shown ways to gain that trust. This chapter has highlighted the fact that the patient's (and also his or her family's) feeling of security and partnering with you is enhanced by your integrity and your ability to individualize care through sensitive attention to detail regarding this patient. Ultimately, you are in a position to help the person engage in reality testing about how he or she will be accepted by others. Your willingness to explore the appropriate depth and form of intimacy ideal for this relationship exemplifies your motivation to achieve professional closeness.

REFERENCES

1. Trillin, A.: Personal history. Betting your life. *The New Yorker.* Jan. 29, 2001, pp. 38–42, quote p. 41.
2. Beauchamp, H., and Childress, J.: *Principles of Biomedical Ethics.* 4th ed. New York, Oxford University Press, 1999, p. 471.
3. Greene, H.: *I Never Promised You a Rose Garden.* New York, Holt, Rinehart & Winston, 1964, p. 56.
4. Eisenberg, L.: Good technical outcome, poor service experience. A verdict on contemporary medical care? *JAMA* 285:2639–2641, 2001.
5. Bauby, J.D.: *The Diving Bell and the Butterfly.* [translated by Jeremy Lagatt], New York, Alfred A. Knopf, 1997, p. 57.
6. Purtilo, R.: *Ethical Dimensions in the Health Professions.* 3rd ed. Philadelphia, W. B. Saunders, 1999, p. 113.
7. Powell, J.S.: *Why Am I Afraid to Tell You Who I Am?* Chicago, Argus Communications, 1969, pp. 54–62.

PART FIVE

Questions for Thought and Discussion

1. Mr. Zbigrewski has been treated for several weeks by Ms. Montgomery, a young intern at the local ambulatory care clinic. On her birthday, he slips her an envelope as he goes out the door. When she opens it, she finds a birthday card and a check for $50.
   a. What questions would you have to answer to interpret the significance of this gift?
   b. What problems may arise in the patient and health professional relationship if she returns the money?
   c. What problems may arise if she keeps the money?
   d. How, if at all, would your thinking change about this situation if the check had been for $25,000?

2. Mrs. Lo comes to your department for a test. Within the first 5 minutes that you are with her, she tells you that she is a friend of your coworker and thinks you should know that your coworker uses marijuana and cocaine. According to Mrs. Lo, your coworker has also been a "pusher" and has served time in jail in another city. Your coworker is pleasant and well liked by patients and colleagues and, as far as you can discern, is professionally competent. She does take all of her sick time, but so do a lot of the others.
   a. What should you say to Mrs. Lo when she offers you this information?
   b. Should you tell your coworker what Mrs. Lo has told you? If you do, are you breaking a confidence with Mrs. Lo? Can you now develop professional closeness with Mrs. Lo?
   c. What, if any, difference will this information make in your attitude toward your coworker?

3. Jack Q. is a homosexual who has AIDS. He is extremely depressed, and much of his bitterness is directed toward his family members, who have refused to visit him. He has other challenges as well. Several of the health professionals do not want to treat Jack in spite of universal precautions and an ethical duty to do so. Jane A., a nurse, refuses on the basis that she is pregnant and does not want to endanger her fetus. Ardoni Y., a social worker, demurs on the basis that he believes that homosexuality is a sin and it is against his religion to interfere with God's talking to Jack in this way. Rita P. tells her supervisor that she has had more than her share of AIDS patients during the past 2 months and wants someone else to take Jack. Finally, Karen N., a physical therapist, asks to be excused on the basis that she has an immune system defect.

Discuss the actions of these health professionals on the basis of what is required for professional respect toward Jack. Are any of their excuses for not wanting to treat Jack legitimate? Why or why not?

4. Name three virtues you think are the most important for ensuring respectful interaction between a health professional and patient. Why do you choose these as more important than others?

5. M.K. is a patient you initially found very enjoyable to be around. However, recently this patient has been taking every opportunity to touch you. Today it was a pat on the rear end. You are starting to feel extremely uncomfortable around M.K. What steps should you take to bring this unacceptable behavior to a halt?

PART SIX

Respectful Interaction: Working with Patients Effectively

Having studied the basic foundational pieces of respectful interaction, you now have an opportunity to apply your learning to several types of patients you will see in the course of your professional career. We have chosen to address them by age group, over the lifespan, being mindful that individual differences often outweigh the similarities we are emphasizing in these different age cohorts.

Part Six begins with Chapter 14, highlighting the challenges and joys of working with newborns, infants, and toddlers. Understandably, the family is a key element of consideration for these age groups. Chapter 15 moves the focus of your attention to school age children and adolescents.

In Chapter 16 we discuss your interaction with people who become patients during young adulthood and the "middle years." Only in recent times have these life periods been given more than a cursory glance, and we share some of the insights that researchers and others are finding.

Chapter 17 examines key issues related to working with the older population. Of all age groups this one is increasing more in diversity and size worldwide than any other group. No matter what your chosen field, you will have occasion to work with persons who have lived a long time.

Throughout the lifespan, the person who becomes a patient is faced with many of the challenges we have been discussing so far. You have a substantial role in respectfully helping them to meet those challenges.

CHAPTER 14

Respectful Interaction: Working with Newborns, Infants, and Toddlers

CHAPTER OBJECTIVES

The student will be able to

- Discuss how families serve as bridges to respectful interaction with newborns, infants, and toddlers
- Identify five processes of the family health system that can lend insight into family and patient dynamics
- Make several suggestions that will help support healthy functioning of the family during a child's illness
- Distinguish some key differences that need to be considered in one's approach to newborns, infants, and toddlers
- Discuss in general terms Erikson's sequential view of the psychological development of infants and toddlers
- List some everyday needs of the infant that may help explain an infant's response to the health professional
- Describe the steps showing how consistency of approach usually builds trust in an interaction with infant patients
- Describe five types of play, and show how each can facilitate respectful interaction with a pediatric patient
- Describe how the toddler's developing need for autonomy enters into the health professional and patient relationship

I mean, this is not, you know, a piece of machinery that . . . we want to make work. It's, it's a child and he, you've got all those dynamics of mom and dad, and grandma, and brothers and sisters. And, and you know, all of those things need to be, are, are just as important, just as important as whether that kid is breathing or not. . . . Part of the recovery of the child depends on, and their future depends on, dealing with these issues too. Because of the attachment that the family has for that child.[1]

All health professionals will interact with newborn, infant, and toddler patients at some time, although most health professionals do not work solely or even primarily with these groups. These patients must be treated with the respect they deserve as unique individuals like everyone else. Furthermore, the opportunity they are given to experience human dignity and support in their time of illness, injury, or other adversity can become a resource to help them manage future difficulties.

Most of us take for granted that a newborn will live into his or her 7th or 8th decade of life. This has not always been so. At the start of the twentieth century in the United States, more than half of reported deaths involved persons 14 years of age or younger. Today, the infant mortality rate is 7.2 infant deaths per 1,000 live births.[2] However, the decline in infant mortality rate overall is not shared equally by all groups. Mortality is still higher for infants and children in poor families with poor living conditions. In 1998, the mortality rate for black infants was more than twice that for white infants. Better opportunities for good initial health care and overall longevity in white groups point to deep, internal, society-wide problems, the health consequences of which must be reckoned with. Furthermore, in the United States, the leading cause of death for children ages 1 through 14 (and even into adolescence and early adulthood) is accidents.[3] Demographic observations such as these suggest the types of health problems you will most commonly encounter in very young patients. Both health professionals and patients will benefit from a skillful and knowledgeable approach to interaction with patients in young age groups.

This is the first of several chapters that will examine your interaction with patients across the lifespan. It begins with the family as a focus of care and then moves to working with new parents and newborns, infants, and toddlers. The section on growth and development includes information that applies across childhood and adolescence as well, although working with each age group has its own challenges. Provided here is a wide range of relevant topics concerning interaction with young patients that should provide a basis for more in-depth exploration in your other coursework during your professional program.

HUMAN DEVELOPMENT AND FAMILY

In the past in mainstream health care in the United States, treatment focused exclusively on the patient as a solitary individual. It was not commonplace to attend to families as the focus of care. Today we see how important it is to care for patients, especially children, in the context of their families: the family is implicitly and explicitly recognized as a critical social unit surrounding and influencing its members and, in turn, being influenced by its members. We will begin by discussing the evolving concept of "family" in contemporary society. If we are to work with families as collaborators in maintaining the health of children and in the care of ill, injured, or disabled family members, then we must understand how families define themselves, how they function, and how best to interact with them.

Family: An Evolving Concept

The term "family" has been defined in a variety of ways. How would you define family? It is safe to say that your notion of what constitutes a family is influenced by your values, culture, and professional perspective. For example, a sociologist may define a family in terms of its socioeconomic status, or a psychologist may focus on the interpersonal dynamics of individuals who claim family ties. The most common type of familial bond is through spousal and blood relationships. However, none of these definitions is sufficient to describe the types of relationships and arrangements that make up the modern family. Current statistics suggest that family size and the number of two-parent families is decreasing while the number of single-parent families is increasing. Families may comprise several generations of blood kin, a mix of stepparents and children, or a combination of friends who share in household responsibilities and childrearing. Technological advances such as artificial reproduction also challenge traditional stereotypes about what constitutes a family. For example, motherhood and the family unit can be determined by genetic, gestational, or social relationships.[4] Society is being forced by scientific and social advances to redefine what is meant by "family."

Thus, an inclusive definition of family is needed, one that allows the members of a family to define themselves as a family unit and acknowledges the variety of cultural styles, values, and alternative structures that are part of contemporary family life. In fact, families define a unique culture; that is, a unique behavioral complex that is socially created, readily transmitted to family members, and potentially maintained through generations.[5]

To work with families, you must understand how families function. Family theories describe families, how they operate, and how they respond to events both internal and external. There are numerous family theories, and each makes assumptions about the family. Most health professionals use a combination of family theories in their work with children and their families, but all have in common the fact that they move the focus of health care from the individual member who is ill, injured, or disabled to the family as a unit of care. We will focus on a particular method of viewing the family, the family health system, developed by Anderson and Tomlinson.[6] According to this method, care is directed toward five processes: (1) interactive, (2) developmental, (3) coping, (4) integrity, and (5) health. The story of Ian will help you by showing how the family health system model applies to a particular child and his family.

> Ian was a low-birth-weight infant with short bowel syndrome. Short bowel syndrome is characterized by maldigestion, malabsorption, dehydration, electrolyte abnormalities, and both macronutrient and micronutrient deficiencies. Owing to new medical and surgical treatments, the

survival rate ranges from 80% to 94%.[7] Ian will require long-term parenteral nutrition; that is, he will not be able to take food orally and will be dependent on intravenous solutions to provide the bulk of his nutritional needs. Ian is the first child of Dylan and Adrianna Chapel, both in their early twenties. After a stay in the neonatal intensive care unit, Ian was sent home with his parents, who have provided care since that time with the help of a home care agency and a nutritional support company. The Chapels do not have their own parents or other relatives nearby. The majority of Ian's care falls on them.

Ian is now an active 2-year-old. Mrs. Chapel is the primary caregiver during the day and most evenings. Mr. Chapel works as a paralegal in a law firm and attends law school at night. The Chapel's insurance coverage is through a group plan at the law firm where Mr. Chapel works.

Assume you are assigned to work with the Chapel family during an on-site educational experience with the home care agency providing primary care. The goal of your interaction with Ian and his family is to help promote family adaptation to his chronic condition (short bowel syndrome) and to empower the Chapels to develop and maintain healthy lifestyles. By reviewing the five processes listed earlier, you can get a picture of the family's functioning and possible areas for intervention.

First, the *interactive* process of the family is composed of communication, family relationship, and social supports.[8] In your assessment of the interactive process of the Chapel family you will explore the types of communication patterns they use; the effect of Ian's illness on the communication of the family both internally and externally; the types of relationships within the family; and the quality, timing, amount, and nature of social support they receive. Open communication should be encouraged. One aspect of care could be to assist the Chapels in mobilizing the informational and emotional support they need to cope with Ian's illness. Because the Chapels do not have family support in the immediate community, they may have to rely on informal support systems such as friends and coworkers and formal support systems such as respite care agencies to assist them in the care of their child. Perhaps there are other children who have short bowel syndrome or who have to rely on parenteral nutrition in the community. The caregivers of such children may have or could form a support group to help troubleshoot common problems and offer advice.

Second, assessment of the *developmental* process includes the family developmental stage and individual developmental stages. The Chapels, as a family, are in the second stage of family development as described by Duvall in his classic work.[9] Stage II of the family life cycle involves integrating an infant into the family unit, accommodating to new parenting roles, and maintaining the marital bond. Ian is moving from infancy to becoming a toddler. You will be introduced to basic development needs of toddlers later in this chapter, but briefly Ian will be interested in his environment and want to explore it. Ian will become increasingly mobile and develop language during this stage. All of this is influenced by the presence of his chronic condition. Therefore, it would be appropriate for you to assess how well these developmental tasks are being achieved. You could instruct the Chapels about the developmental milestones Ian should achieve and the tasks involved. For example, Ian needs freedom of mobility to learn to walk, so his nutritional solution could be placed in a backpack to allow him to move freely. Children with short bowel syndrome may also require frequent visits to the bathroom throughout the day when the time comes for toilet training. To decrease the Chapels's frustrations, you could plan ahead for this next developmental milestone and work with them to plan a structured routine that is consistently implemented and results in success for all involved, especially the child.

There is some evidence that about 10% to 15% of children with short bowel syndrome will experience neurological or developmental defects such as a delay in physical development or visual-spatial defects.[10] Thus, you would also want to watch for possible developmental delays to plan for early therapeutic interventions.

The process of *coping* has been identified as problem solving, adaptation to stress and crisis, and management of resources.[11] In your work with the Chapels, you should assess their ability to handle stress and the impact that Ian's illness has on everyday activities. Has Ian's illness caused a change in the family's life plans? For example, did Mrs. Chapel plan on returning to work outside the home after the birth of her son? If so, can the family adapt to the loss of income or are support services available to allow Ian to be cared for during the day so that Mrs. Chapel can work? Were the Chapels intending to have several children? Have Ian's care needs changed this? Overall, you would want to assess how the family deals with crises in general.

You can support the Chapel's coping processes by offering advice on the progression of the illness, discussing the normal feelings of frustration and guilt that accompany the care of a chronically ill or disabled family member, and offering resources to help the family cope more effectively, such as respite care and other support groups. Can you think of others?

The Chapels will also have to cope with financial difficulties. Even with the best health insurance, there are lifetime limits on coverage; in addition, there are many out-of-pocket expenses related to the care of a child with this diagnosis. Although most children experience small bowel adaptation over time and can be weaned from parenteral nutrition, some children cannot be weaned and require surgery or even an intestinal transplantation.[12] Thus, the Chapels may be facing years of out-of-pocket expenses and expensive hospital stays, procedures, and medications. This kind of financial pressure can be very stressful for any family.

The *integrity* process of family life involves family values, rituals, history, and identity.[13] These aspects of the family process greatly affect its behavior. Family rituals, one facet of the integrity process, provide a useful framework for assessing threats to a family's integrity. Family rituals include celebrations and traditions such as activities surrounding birthdays or bedtime routines for children. Suggestions for evaluating family rituals include assessment of the following[14]:

- Does the family underutilize rituals? Families who do not celebrate or mark family changes such as birthdays, deaths, anniversaries, and so forth may be left without some of the benefits that accompany rituals such as bringing the family together or marking changes in life and family roles.
- Does the family follow rigid patterns of ritual? In families who are rigid, things are always done the same way, at the same time, and with the same people. Families who are rigid do not respond well to necessary changes that disrupt routines and rituals occasioned by illness and injury.
- Are family rituals skewed? A family with skewed rituals tends to emphasize only one aspect of family life (e.g., religion) and ignore others. For example, a family might spend all of its time celebrating with the father's side of the family on religious holidays and ignore the different rituals cherished by the mother's relations.
- Has the ritual process been interrupted? For example, the birth of a disabled or chronically ill child may threaten family identity and permanently disrupt family rituals. In the case of the Chapels, they have elected to stay home for traditional family holidays because almost all holidays involve a focus on food. For the foreseeable future, Ian cannot tolerate most food orally, so the Chapels will have to consider what this interruption in ritual means to their life together and may have to develop other rituals at holiday time that do not focus so prominently on food.
- Are the rituals hollow? Rituals that are performed just for the sake of performing them have lost their life and may be stressful for the family rather than a source of joy and strength.

In addition to changes in ritual that occur over time in families, many role changes also occur, particularly when chronic illness is involved. For example, Mrs. Chapel has become the primary caregiver. She may or may not have expected to take on this role. Essential interventions include helping the Chapels redefine major family roles and maintain their new responsibilities.

The final process of family experience is related to *health*. This process includes health status, health beliefs and practices, and lifestyle practices.[15] You would want to assess the family's definition of health and how they define the health of the individual members. Besides the responsibilities involved in caring for a child who requires parenteral feedings, what do the Chapels do to maintain their own health? How do the Chapels deal with health problems? To whom do they turn? Interventions in the area of health process include education, encouragement, and counseling regarding the short- and long-term aspects of Ian's care.

In summary, Ian and his parents' situation illustrates the family health system as one useful approach to the care of families and children. The family health system applies to all families whatever the composition and stage of familial development. You are encouraged to explore other models of working with a family and their effectiveness in achieving optimal family health. Regardless of the model you choose, it is clear that family relationships are an important consideration in understanding the conduct of any patient and for developing an effective mode for respectful interaction with that patient. Care can best be accomplished if it is considered a collaborative venture between the family and the health care team. The elements of family-centered care in Table 14–1 provide a context for recognizing the family's central role.

Legally, the parents or another formally appointed guardian are the voice of the young child except in rare instances in which the state intervenes to protect the child from caregivers who, the state judges, are not acting in the child's best interest. The most grievous situation results when there is growing suspicion or knowledge that the patient is a victim of child abuse or neglect. In the case of a dysfunctional family in which abuse is suspected, however much you may empathize with the family's suffering, you must turn your attention to the protection of the victimized child. The Child Abuse Prevention and Treatment Act (CAPTA), originally passed in 1974, has been amended several times. The most recent amendment, called the Child Abuse Prevention Treatment and Adoption Act Amendments, was adopted on October 3, 1996. CAPTA mandates

---

TABLE 14–1. Elements of Family-Centered Care

1. Recognizing that the family is the constant in a child's life, while the service systems and personnel within those systems fluctuate
2. Facilitating parent-professional collaboration at all levels of health care
   Care of an individual child
   Program development, implementation, and evaluation
   Policy formation
3. Honoring racial, ethnic, cultural, and socioeconomic diversity of families
4. Recognizing family strengths and individuality and respecting different methods of coping
5. Sharing with parents on a continuing basis and in a supportive manner complete and unbiased information
6. Encouraging and facilitating family-to-family support and networking
7. Understanding and incorporating the developmental needs of infants, children, and adolescents and their families into health care systems
8. Implementing comprehensive policies and programs that provide emotional and financial support to meet the needs of families
9. Designing accessible health care systems that are flexible, culturally competent, and responsive to family-centered needs

---

From the National Center for Family-Centered Care of the Association for the Care of Children's Health, Bethesda, Md.

reporting of child abuse and neglect in all 50 states.[16] A good general rule is that you should be suspicious of maltreatment when reports of the history of the child's injuries do not coincide with physical findings. Furthermore, you must become acquainted with appropriate reporting procedures, which vary from state to state. Of course, caregivers, parents, and others who engage in maltreatment of children are also deeply troubled. Your support of policies and practices that treat the issue as a family affair will help solve bigger family problems.

In summary, the family is usually a sound and reliable bridge to building better understanding of the needs of infants, toddlers, and young children. We now turn our attention to the growth and development of the child, another important factor in working with pediatric patients.

Useful Principles of Human Growth and Development

Development occurs in numerous ways—physical, emotional, and intellectual—and all aspects of development affect one another. Although professionals often talk about growth and development simultaneously, growth can be thought of as quantitative and development can be thought of as qualitative. We will address growth first. Human growth proceeds in accordance with a number of general principles that are helpful in understanding what occurs in the growth process, when, and why. These general growth principles are (1) orderliness, (2) discontinuity, (3) differentiation, (4) cephalocaudal, and (5) proximodistal and bilateral.

Orderliness. Growth and changes in behavior usually occur in an orderly fashion and in the same sequence. Thus, all fetuses can turn their heads before they can extend their hands. Almost every child sits before he or she stands, stands before walking, and draws a circle before drawing a square. All babies babble before talking and pronounce certain sounds before others. Likewise, certain cognitive abilities precede the next. All children can categorize objects or put them into a series before they can think logically.

Discontinuity. Although growth is orderly, it is not always smooth and gradual. There are periods of very rapid growth—growth spurts—and increases in psychological abilities. Parents sometimes speak of the summer that a child grew 2 inches. Many adolescents experience a sudden growth spurt after years of being the ones with the smallest stature in their class.

Differentiation. Development proceeds from simple to complex and from general to specific. An example of differentiation in the infant is seen in an infant's ability to wave his or her arms first and later develop purposeful use of his or her fingers. Motor responses are diffuse and undifferentiated at birth and become more specific and controlled as the child grows. Beginning motor activity in the toddler involves haphazard and unsystematic actions, progressing to goal-directed actions and specific outcomes.[17]

Cephalocaudal. Cephalocaudal means that the upper end of the organism develops sooner than the lower end. Increases in neuromuscular size and maturation of function begin in the head and proceed to the hands and feet. After birth, an infant will be able to hold its head erect before being able to sit or walk.

Proximodistal and Bilateral. Proximodistal means that growth progresses from the central axis of the body toward the periphery or extremities. Thus, the central nervous system develops before the peripheral nervous system. Bilateral means that the capacity for growth and development of the child is symmetrical—growth that occurs on one side of the body occurs on the other side of the body simultaneously. These principles apply throughout the lifespan, from infancy to old age.

Theories of Human Development to Guide You

Development can be discussed from a cognitive, identity, sexual, or psychosocial basis. We focus primarily on cognitive development because it entails how a person perceives, thinks, and communicates thoughts and feelings. Some time is spent on psychosocial development because of the profound impact this has on the professional's interactions with patients. Although this chapter focuses on the cognitive and psychosocial development of the infant and toddler, the same theories are applicable to the school-age child and adolescent discussed in Chapter 15.

The manner in which a child learns to think, reason, and use language is vital to the child's overall growth and development.[18] Traditionally, health professionals have based their interventions with children on the stages of cognitive development described by Jean Piaget (1896–1980).[19] Piaget's theory is a logical, deductive explanation of how children think from infancy through adolescence. Piaget described the earliest stage of cognitive development as sensorimotor. At this stage, infants take in a great deal of information through their senses. Tactile and verbal stimulation and auditory and visual cues can have positive, long-range results. The early beginnings of cognitive development can be stimulated by talking to the infant and by face-to-face interactions.

Piaget labeled the cognitive abilities of toddlers as preoperational. Toddlers learn to think and understand by building each new experience upon previous experiences. Miller summarized Piaget's depiction of the cognitive stage of toddlers in terms of egocentrism (seeing the world from a "me-only" viewpoint), rigidity of thought ("Mom is always right"), and semilogical reasoning ("my dog died because I was a bad boy").[20] Children in this stage are confused about cause and effect, even when it is explained to them, and think in terms of magic (i.e., wishing makes it so). However, more current researchers refute Piaget's beliefs and claim that he may have underestimated the cognitive abilities of toddlers. These researchers suggest that children have far more potential to understand complex illness concepts than they have previously been given credit for.[21] Thus, some toddlers may be capable of appreciating the perspective of another and adapting their behavior accordingly. For example, a hospitalized 3-year-old from a multilingual family knew which language to speak to the nurses and which to speak to his grandmother.[22] Others propose that, rather than viewing the toddler as incapable of thinking a certain way, one should view him as a novice. Children have much less life experience than adults. Thus when children gain experience through chronic illness, for example, or perform tasks involving their own expertise, they can demonstrate adultlike performance and more sophisticated thinking and reasoning.[23] The debate in the area of cognitive development is ongoing. For example, evolutionary developmental psychology, which takes into account genetic and ecological mechanisms that affect development as well as the effect of cultural contexts, has recently added voices in the discussion regarding variability in development.[24,25] The various ideas of developmental theorists are important to explore because they have direct implications for how best to work with young children.

As with cognitive development, there are numerous stage/phase theories about the psychological and social dynamics of child development. Development, seen this way, is a process or movement. "Movement from potentiality to actuality occurs over time and in the direction of growth and progress. It is not surprising, then, that most conceptualizations of development incorporate the notion of improvement—of 'better' more integrated ways of functioning."[26] Almost all stress the importance of bonding or forming attachments as the primary developmental task. No one has done more to promote this idea than Erik Erikson, a psychologist who, in the 1950s and 1960s, proposed eight stages of psychosocial development.[27]

According to his theory, the development of trust, shown in Chapter 12 to be fundamental to the effective patient and health professional relationship is one of the tasks facing the child in all relationships. He or she is engaged in a process that will affect his or her ability to engage in respectful interaction with everyone. During infancy, the child is introduced to trust and begins to experience (or to not experience) its power.

The psychosocial development of the toddler involves acquiring a clearer sense of himself or herself that is separate from that of the primary caregiver, becoming involved in wider social relationships, gaining self control and mastery over motor and verbal skills, and developing independence and a self-concept. Later in this chapter, we spend time considering specific examples of how you can effectively interact with infants and toddlers by anticipating the developmental tasks specific to their age group. A caveat is warranted at this juncture about developmental stages. All stage models are just that—models—

and it is difficult to place a child in a specific stage merely by chronological age. Stages are only a way to describe an ongoing process.

FROM NEWBORN TO INFANT

The anticipation of the birth of a child is fraught with emotions ranging from joy to fear. The birth process has largely moved from the home to the hospital. Many hospitals attempt to duplicate the comforts and familiarities of home by designing birthing suites complete with a videotape recorder and rocking chair. With the move to shorter lengths of stay for a normal delivery, it is unlikely that you will have much opportunity to work with these tiniest of patients unless you choose to work in labor and delivery or neonatology.

The Normal Newborn

The normal newborn is highly vulnerable but also amazingly adaptable to the new environment outside the womb as noted in this classic article on the mind of the newborn.

> A baby enters the world prepared to attend to change in physical stimulation. Contrasts in light, motion, sound, smell, touch, and taste attract his attention. When objects in his field of vision differ in the amount of black-white contrast, for example, the infant looks at the place of greatest contrast. Infants also respond to differences in wavelength, as though they perceive green, blue, yellow, and red exactly the way adults do. In short, a baby is prepared to discover the dimensions of the external world and does not have to learn how to locate the information.[20]

The newborn period ends at the first month of life. After that, newborns are called infants. Newborns have many needs, especially when health problems are present at birth. They also are human beings worthy of full respect. The field of neonatology, especially the intensive care of newborns, deserves consideration because it stretches our concept of what a "newborn" is.

Life-Threatening Circumstances

New technology is always changing the possibility for survival in the neonatal intensive care unit (NICU). Smaller and smaller neonates who have had shorter gestations in the womb are seen in NICUs. So many variables enter into survival for these tiny patients. Sometimes a neonate who weighs more than the fragile neonate in the next isolette is the one who does not survive. Each year tens of thousands of babies are born too early and too small and end up in an NICU. In each case, parents and physicians share a common goal—to make each baby healthy. New medical technologies are saving babies who until only recently would have died. Unfortunately, the costs can be staggering, and the result may be a baby whose future is limited by debilitating health conditions. With little or no preparation, parents are being asked to decide when the technology is doing more harm than good. It is interesting to note that in retrospect, parents do not identify involvement in decision making. In Pinch's longitudinal study of parents' experiences in the NICU, "families remembered their general acceptance of all proffered treatments. Parental knowledge increased substantially after discharge, and the dominant perception was that they were not informed sufficiently in the NICU."[29] Thus, respectful interaction with parents and these fragile newborns requires that you take extra care to inform them about the progress and status of their children.

Moving into Infancy

A newborn very quickly grows into early infancy. When working with an infant, you will be in a position to make independent clinical judgments about his or her best interests and to observe the interaction between parents and their new baby. Happily, the parents almost always provide the primary supportive bridge between you and the infant patient, interpreting the baby's expressions, babbles, and postures and providing insight into how continuity of approach to the infant can be maximized. During this time, parents have to learn cues from their infants, and sometimes you can teach the parents as well as learn from the parents' comments and behavior.

The needs of infants sometimes are difficult to determine because these patients lack substantial verbal skills to express their wants and needs. (Even adults sometimes have great difficulty asking for what they need.) Professionals who rely on a patient's ability to ask for what he or she needs take a narrow view of needs assessment.

INFANT NEEDS: RESPECT AND CONSISTENCY

There are two contexts by which to view the infant's needs. The first focuses on the stage of psychosocial development that we have already discussed and the second on immediate concrete needs such as the need for a drink of water, food, pain relief, or a diaper change. You have an opportunity to demonstrate respect for the infant by responding effectively to each type of need. Remember that parents often have explicit ways of doing things for their infant that can help too. For example, parents may hold the infant in a certain way, play a favorite game such as pretending to sneeze or rubbing the baby's back that will, at a minimum, help calm the infant while you look for other reasons for the infant's distress.

A primary approach is characterized by the three "C's": consistency in approach, constancy of presence, and continuity of treatment. Consistency is especially important because it builds trust (infant self-confidence) through the following steps:

1. An infant's need exists.
2. The infant exhibits generalized behavior.
3. The caregiver responds.

4. The need is satisfied.
5. The need recurs.
6. The infant predicts the caregiver's response.
7. The infant repeats previous behavior.
8. The caregiver responds in a consistent manner.
9. The need is satisfied.
10. The infant's trust toward the caregiver develops.
11. The need recurs.
12. The infant is confident that the caregiver will respond appropriately.[30]

Of course, infants do have different temperaments, which create differences in responses to the health professional. These individual differences are welcomed by the health professional because they support the belief that humans are unique, each deserving of unique respect.

Everyday Needs of Infants

By now you should have discovered in this book that the "solutions" to challenges during interaction with patients sometimes are concrete and mundane and dictated by common sense. Fussy, irritable, crying infants are in the position of becoming the least liked (and probably least cared for) patients on the pediatrics unit. Crying is one way infants try to communicate distress. More likely than not, because of the infant's age and stage of development, this distress is related to a concrete, immediate need. Respectful interaction with infants in distress requires careful attention to several types of detail.

Comfort Detail. Small children most often become irritable when they experience physical discomfort. Careful attention to comfort is a key to their sense of well-being. This becomes all the more reason to check for factors that could lead to discomfort whenever possible. It is too easy to assume that a baby's crying or other belligerence is because he or she is a fussy or cranky baby. Examine the bed shirt, diaper, and crib sheets. Are they wet from urine, sweat, or a spilled medication? Are they wrinkled and creating pressure spots? Does the baby have abrasions, punctures, or other bodily tenderness that cause contact pain? Is tape pinching the baby or has an intravenous line infiltrated? Check the ears, nostrils, and throat. Is there something lodged in one of them? Are the throat and mouth dry? Check the medical record. What did the baby eat and when? Is he or she taking fluids? Is he or she hungry or thirsty, perhaps? Is he or she having some predictable side effect from a medication?

Health Professional Detail. Discomfort can also be caused by something the health professional is wearing or doing. Is your outfit scratching the baby? Is the color or design too complex? Do you have on jewelry that scratches, scrapes, or pinches? Are your hands clammy and cold? Are you bony? Your conduct is like a mirror to the young child. If you are anxious or uncomfortable with caring for an infant, the infant will sense it.

In addition to the immediate discomfort the health professional may cause any infant by inattention to these details, a more persistent negative response could be a sign of deeper discomfort. A good general rule is to remain consistent, approaching the infant similarly in each interaction in hopes that the familiarity itself will be a comfort. Also, watch how the infant interacts with others, especially those who appear to be successful in calming him or her. Try altering your approach to match those that seem to help the infant.

Environmental Detail. Like all of us, infants have various comfort zones, which include temperature, space, and other environmental factors. Is the room quite warm? Do other children seem to be more irritable today? Is the infant sweaty or clammy? Are there new noises in the area from nearby construction, an open window, or a newly placed monitor? Are there different smells in the air because of painting in the hallway or a new disinfectant used by the cleaning staff? Where is the crib placed? Try placing it in another position or placing the infant in a different position in the crib. Is he or she exposed to open spaces on both sides of the crib or is one side against the wall? Try alternatives to this arrangement. Are there sounds in the wall from steam heat or water pipes?

In short, you should be attentive to the behavior of the young patient and to the people who are associated with her care. Responsiveness to infant needs is generally best met during this developmental phase through predictable interaction. Infants, like all humans, are unique beings with various temperaments and their own histories and responses to environmental input. It is critical that you pay careful attention to detail when you assess a disturbed infant's needs.

THE TODDLER: BECOMING A "SELF"

Much of the material related to respectful interaction with the infant patient and his or her family can be applied to the child past the stage of infancy into other stages of childhood and adolescence. As a child grows, however, some new challenges confront both parents and health care providers. This is especially true of the toddler, a difficult and challenging stage of development for all involved.

A review of Erikson's stages shows that the young patient's psychosocial tasks in moving from infancy to becoming a toddler and then an older child focus on becoming one's own "self," separate from others.

Respect for a toddler can be enhanced when the child actually asks for what he or she wants. Of course, sometimes the toddler will have difficulty making himself or herself understood and may be embarrassed by his or her own awkward attempts to act grown up. Especially important to the child is the need to succeed at "adult" tasks (which include anything new from the early tasks of learning how to walk and to feed oneself no matter how long it takes).

Play is an important vehicle through which a toddler patient's sense of worth can be fostered. According to developmental psychologists, play may be the child's richest opportunity for physical, cognitive, language, and emotional development. Freiberg states that there are several types of play, any of which can be encouraged as part of treatment or other aspects of interaction with the child. These include (1) symbolic play, which is used by children to make something stand for something else; for example, when the young patient "becomes" the more powerful health professional by wearing the health professional's clothes or stethoscope; (2) onlooker play, which involves watching others, such as when the health professional entertains the child or when the child observes others at play but does not participate; (3) parallel play, which is side-by-side play characterized by activity that is interactive only by virtue of another's presence (the participation by observation and side-by-side types of play may help to decrease a young patient's loneliness, even though he or she cannot fully interact with others); (4) associative play, which involves shared activity and communication; and (5) cooperative play, in which rules are followed and goals are achieved. Associative play and cooperative play are generally beyond the capabilities of the toddler.[31]

TODDLER NEEDS: RESPECT AND SECURITY

Attention to personal detail outlined in the section on infants applies to interaction with the toddler as well. Fortunately, in most cases toddlers can verbalize their basic needs ("Me hungry," "Me go?" "More," or "No") and express their curiosity by pointing to something and asking, "Dis?" Their illness, the intimidating surroundings, or their shyness, however, may make young children even more reticent than most patients to make their needs known in this direct manner. They often show their feelings of insecurity about what is happening to them by being cranky or acting overly fearful and demanding.

Children, like all patients, tend to regress when they become ill. Having so recently moved out of infancy, toddlers sometimes return to infantlike behavior. You need to be aware that this is a normal tendency and that you should not condemn young patients who do not "act their age." In the following story, a nurse tells of a toddler with Burkitt's lymphoma, a particularly fast-growing cancer, who was not doing well and was essentially silent.

> . . . . I don't know how I knew this, but something said to me that he needed to be held right then. I asked him if he would like to rock in the rocking chair, and of course he didn't answer but he did not resist when I picked him up. We sat in that rocking chair for an hour and a half, and I could feel him settling in. I had on this knit sweater with a print, and when he finally sat up I laughed and said, "Jason, you've got waffles on your face!" He said, "I know, I've got them on my knees too." That was the first time he spoke, and after that we couldn't shut him up.[32]

A combination of gentle support for age-appropriate behaviors and tender care, such as holding and rocking, can encourage the toddler to feel more secure.

SUMMARY

This chapter has presented an overview of a variety of theories that seek to explain how human beings develop biologically, psychologically, and socially over the lifespan. The progression from infancy to early childhood is shaped by many influences, the most important of which is the family. As an infant becomes a toddler, he or she starts taking steps, literally and figuratively, toward a lifelong journey that is unique to each child. Recognizing the uniqueness of the child as an individual as well as the product of a developmental phase will help you to better understand the many dimensions in which respect can be conveyed, and the success of the your interactions will be maximized.

REFERENCES

1. Pinch, W.J.E., and Spielman, M.L.: Ethics in the neonatal intensive care unit: parental perceptions at four years postdischarge. *Adv. Nurs. Sci.* 19(1):72–85, 1996, quote p. 77.
2. Centers for Disease Control and Prevention, U.S. Department of Health and Human Services. Deaths: final data for 1998. *National Vital Statistics Rep.* 48(11):1, 2000.
3. Ibid, p. 2.
4. Rae, S.B.: Whose child is this? Defining the mother in surrogate motherhood arrangements. *J. Women's Health* 3(1): 51–64, 1994.
5. Sparling, J.W.: The cultural definition of family. *Phys. Occup. Ther. Pediatr.* 11(4):17–28, 1991.
6. Anderson, K.H., and Tomlinson, P. S.: The family health system as an emerging paradigmatic view for nursing. *Image J. Nurs. Scholarship* 24(1):57–63, 1992.
7. Sigalet, D.L.: Short bowel syndrome in infants and children: An overview. *Semin. Pediatr. Surg.* 10(2):49–55, 2001.
8. Anderson and Tomlinson, 1992.
9. Duvall, E.M.: *Family Development.* 5th ed. Philadelphia, Lippincott, 1977.
10. Beers, S.R., Yaworski, J.A., Stilley, C., Ewing, L., and Barksdale, E.M., Jr.: Cognitive deficits in school-age children with severe short bowel syndrome. *J. Pediatr. Surg.* 35(6):860–865, 2000.
11. Anderson and Tomlinson, 1992.
12. Vernon, A.H., and Georgeson, K.E.: Surgical options for short bowel syndrome. *Semin. Pediatr. Surg.* 10(2): 91–98, 2001.
13. Anderson and Tomlinson, 1992.
14. Imber-Black, E., Roberts, J., and Whiting, R.: *Rituals in Families and Family Therapy.* New York, Norton, 1988.
15. Anderson and Tomlinson, 1992.
16. Child Abuse Prevention Treatment and Adoption Act Amendments (P.L. 104-235), 1996.

17. Puskar, K.R., and D'Antonio, I.J.: Tots and teens: similarities in behavior and interventions for pediatric and psychiatric nurses. *J. Child. Adolesc. Psychiatr. Ment. Health Nurs.* 6(2):18–28, 1993.
18. Mott, S., James, S., and Sperhac, A.: *Nursing Care of Children and Families.* 2nd ed. Reading, MA, Addison-Wesley, 1990.
19. Piaget, J.: *Six Psychological Studies.* New York, Vintage, 1964.
20. Miller, S.A.: *Developmental Research Methods.* Englewood Cliffs, NJ, Prentice Hall, 1987.
21. Rushforth, H.: Practitioner review: communicating with hospitalized children: review and application of research pertaining to children's understanding of illness. *J. Child Psychol. Psychiatry Allied Disciplines* 40(5):683–691, 1999.
22. Menig-Peterson, C.L.: The modification of communicative behavior in preschool-aged children as a function of the listener's perspective. *Child Dev.* 46:1015–1018, 1975.
23. Yoos, H.L.: Children's illness concepts: old and new paradigms. *Pediatr. Nurs.* 20(2):134–140, 145, 1994.
24. Geary, D.C., and Bjorklund, D.F.: Evolutionary developmental psychology. *Child Dev.* 71(1):57–65; 2000.
25. Suizzo, M.A.: The social emotional and cultural contexts of cognitive development: neo-Piagetian perspectives. *Child Dev.* 71(4):846–849, 2000.
26. Clark, M.C., and Caffarella, R.S. (eds.): *An Update on Adult Development Theory: New Ways of Thinking About the Life Course. New Directions for Adult and Continuing Education.* San Francisco, Jossey-Bass, 1999, p. 20.
27. Erikson, E.H.: *Identity and the Life Cycle.* New York, W.W. Norton. 1959
28. Kagan, J.: The baby's elastic mind. *Hum. Nature.* 1(1):72, 1978.
29. Pinch, W.J.E., and Spielman, M.L.: Ethics in the neonatal intensive care unit: parental perceptions at four years postdischarge. *Adv. Nurs. Sci.* 19(1):72–85, 1996, quote p. 77.
30. Schuster, C.S., and Ashburn, S.S.: *The Process of Human Development.* Boston, Little Brown and Company, 1986, p. 180.
31. Freiberg, K.L.: *Human Development, a Life Span Approach.* 3rd ed. Boston, Jones and Bartlett, 1987, pp. 229–230.
32. Montgomery, C.L.: *Healing Through Communication.* Newbury Park, CA, Sage, 1993, p. 78.

CHAPTER 15

Respectful Interaction: Working with the Child and Adolescent

CHAPTER OBJECTIVES

The student will be able to

- Distinguish some key differences that need to be considered in one's approach to children beyond the toddler stage and to adolescents
- Discuss in general terms the key developmental tasks of children and adolescents
- Describe how the five types of play introduced in Chapter 14 are relevant—or not relevant—to respectful interaction with older children
- Identify several aspects of the child's existence that may be creating problems for the child
- Describe how a child's developing need for successful relatedness enters into the health professional and patient relationship
- Make several suggestions that will help minimize the disequilibrium of the family during a child's illness
- List some compelling reasons for giving respectful attention to an adolescent's desire to exercise authority in regard to health care decisions and describe legitimate limits on that authority
- Discuss four sequential coping phases of adolescent patients

When I was seven, my father who played the violin on Sundays with a nicely tortured flair which we considered artistic, led me by the hand down a long, unlit corridor in St. Luke's School basement, a sort of tunnel that ended in a room full of pianos. There, many little girls and a single sad boy were playing truly tortured scales and arpeggios in a mash of troubled sound. My father gave me over to Sister Olive Marie, who did look remarkably like an olive.

P. Hampl[1]

Much of the material related to respectful interaction with the infant or toddler and his or her family can be applied to older children. As a child grows, however, some new challenges confront the child, parents, and health care providers. Therefore, in this chapter we add some dimensions to the groundwork we laid in Chapter 14 to highlight some of the most important differences as well as focus on the situation of adolescent patients.

THE CHILDHOOD SELF

A young child's psychosocial tasks in moving from infancy to childhood focus on the need to recognize that one has a "self," separate from others, but that ultimately many aspects of that self must survive and thrive in relationships with others. Therefore, much activity and energy are focused on being different from others at the same time that much is invested in learning how to be accepted by others and having some say in relationships. As we address later in this chapter, these tasks become paramount during the adolescent years, but the fundamental building blocks begin much earlier.

NEEDS: RESPECT AND RELATING

Writer Annie Dillard poetically describes the first part of the child's developmental task, that of becoming a "self" different from others. She recalls it this way in her autobiography, *An American Childhood:*

> I woke up in bits like all children, piecemeal over the years. I discovered myself and the world, and forgot them, and discovered them again. . . . I noticed this process of awaking and predicted with terrifying logic that one of these years not far away I would be awake continuously and never slip back and never be free of myself again.[2]

Children, in general, want to make it alone and have learned not to accept the full dependence of infancy and the toddler years, but yet are not really independent either. When they become patients, like most people they regress. The dependence side of the scales tips heavy and the good fit of selfhood that the child is slipping into suddenly escapes. In this confusing never-never land of being neither infant nor fully child nor adult, children must try to reestablish some sense of equanimity and self-identity during their time of being a patient in addition to making their need for success in a relationship known.

Most children beyond the toddler years have learned to communicate verbally and have many more experiences upon which to rely compared with an infant or a toddler. Thus, their resources for effective relating are greater than those in their earlier years. School-aged children are capable of leaving the security of their families and the familiar setting of home to enter new worlds such as the piano class described in the opening to this chapter. Sister Olive Marie is one of many authority figures, such as teachers, coaches, and other role models, with whom the child will interact. However, for the most part health professionals present types of authority that are often unfamiliar to the child. Family and school authority figures usually do little to prepare him or her for the health professions setting and its unique challenges and choices.

Play and Toys

Play appropriate to the child's age and social development can be an important vehicle to help ease the tension he or she is feeling about being able to relate to the people in the health care setting. In Chapter 14 we introduced five types of play and suggested that at the toddler stage and immediately beyond it children are comfortable with symbolic, onlooker, and parallel play. However, as the child grows, associative play, which involves shared activity and communication, and cooperative play, in which rules are followed and goals are achieved, become the norm. Some older children who become patients will regress to an earlier stage, but many will be able to assume roles at the higher levels of play, which will allow them to act out their predicament of being in such a new situation. For example, at level 4 they may play hospital with a professional or family member, assuming the powerful role of the nurse or someone else in charge, thereby revealing their own anxieties and how they perceive their situation. Clues to how they think their tension could be eased may be revealed in their attempts to minister to the play partner who has now become the patient. At level 5 they may succeed admirably at table games, card games, or sports, using their participation and mastery as an effective way of relating.

Young patients often play with toys, too, so that a truck, doll, puzzle, or other object may be an effective means of helping to establish a relationship. At the same time, children can be very sensitive about being "too old" for certain types of toys, so that health professionals and others must think carefully about which toys to select.

School Issues

When children of school age become patients, health professionals are faced with additional challenges. Even a short illness or injury may mean a disruption in school attendance and may not only put the child behind in schoolwork but also can have devastating consequences socially. During the school years children organize most of their relational activity around family and school; therefore, they are at risk of being "out of the action" in every way when removed from the educational environment. At the very least you should be aware of this loss and show interest in his or her school-related activity if, indeed, any is being carried on at the moment.

Most children with chronic illnesses or long-term disabilities will receive special attention regarding education through the school system itself. Disability can be defined as a long-term reduction in ability to conduct social role activities, such as school or play, because of a physical or mental condition. A significant portion of children, estimated to be 6.5% of those younger than 18 years, have experienced some degree of disability.[3] The Americans with Disabilities Act prohibits discrimination on the basis of disability in employment, state and local government services, public accommodations, commercial facilities, transportation, and telecommunications.[4] You can find out about the different components of ADA at http://www.usdoj.gov/crt/ada/adahom1.htm. The Individuals with Disabilities Education Act (IDEA) (formerly called P.L. 94-142 or the Education for all Handicapped Children Act of 1975) requires public schools to make available to all eligible children with disabilities a free appropriate public education in the least restrictive environment appropriate to their individual needs (20 U.S.C. 1400 et seq.). However laudatory this is, the law does little to address the accompanying problems that sometimes arise: able-bodied children may be cruel toward peers who have medical conditions, parents may believe that their child is not getting as good care as they would like or disagree with the "individualized education program" that has been developed for their child, teachers may feel that they do not have enough time to devote to the needs of all the children in their classrooms, and children with serious but not permanent conditions may not qualify.[5] When you come into contact with families who are trying to work through some of these issues, you can often encourage them as well as direct them to the appropriate resources when problems arise. For example, if parents disagree with the individualized education program, they can request a due process hearing and a review from the state educational agency if applicable in their state.

In short, during the school-aged years a child's feelings of self-worth and experiences of relatedness usually are tied to school. Any means by which you can convey sympathy for the child's predicament and respect for his or her capacities will enhance the child's fragile identity and self-esteem and help ensure success in the relationship.

Family—A Bridge to Respectful Interaction

All of the family dynamics described in Chapter 14 apply as the child grows older. The growing child, however, does present some additional challenges to the family and health professional working with the family.

It has been noted that the child's desire to become more independent is one of the major developmental tasks of this growth period while at the same time he or she may feel extremely lonely and insecure when illness strikes. The family often is torn between wanting to support the child as an independent "big girl" or "big boy" while being attentive to his or her needs. They may also be dismayed by the child's obvious regression or respond to their own feelings of guilt for the child's illness with overprotectiveness. Your awareness of their struggles and needs is essential if you are to be successful.

Respect for the child's input, especially when his or her opinions seem to differ from those of parents, is essential, too. Many policies now acknowledge the importance of listening to children, even if their opinions do not govern legally. For example, the prevailing feeling is that children usually know when they are seriously ill and can handle difficult information about their health and future prospects as long as they have the support of their families. In an era when health professionals and patients are trying to find better ways of setting humane limits on treatment, children's insights into appropriate limits some-times are overlooked, even though they know when they have reached the place where they cannot tolerate any more interventions. Children often are aware of their parent's anxiety, opposition, or denial, and they try to act as referees among family members or between health professionals and family. Additionally, brothers and sisters of the ill child are also affected by the stress such illness creates in the family. In a study of the siblings of hospitalized children, the brothers and sisters noted stress that included feelings of loneliness, resentment and fear, and positive feelings of resilience such as lessons learned and independence.[6] You can help siblings cope by providing support and informa-tion. Anything the health professional can do to keep the supportive context for siblings alive is well worth the effort. You can also help by trying to keep family disequilibrium at a minimum while acting primarily as an advocate for the child.

This balancing act sometimes is easier said than accomplished. The following story from one of the authors' experiences highlights how such a dilemma can arise. As you read this story, think about your reasons for wanting to share the information about this child's condition with him or wanting to withhold it.

> When John was 7, he fell from a swing, had some joint pain of the lower left extremity, and was unable to fully extend the knee. Numerous radiographic studies were completed, and results were largely normal. However, John could still not fully extend his knee and continued to complain of tenderness. Finally, a magnetic resonance image revealed a lesion that turned out to be non-Hodgkin's lymphoma (NHL). John received combination chemotherapy and appeared to be in remission for several years. As John has gotten older the physician who has followed John and his family has grown somewhat concerned about his mother's overprotectiveness. Although it was less noticeable when he was younger it has been the topic of conversation among the professionals when he and his mother have come to the clinic. For instance, she mentioned that she still dresses John and accompanies him almost everywhere.
>
> John is now 10 and during a follow-up visit to the oncologist, it was discovered that he had a recurrence of NHL. Although the prognosis for children with NHL has improved, the outcome for children with recurrent NHL remains bleak.[7]
>
> John had always asked many questions about his condition, and so it seemed odd to the nurses and others that he was uncharacteristically

silent on the matter of his illness now, even though his condition continued to worsen. His mother visited for a minimum of 6 hours every day and warned everyone that John was not to be told that he had a recurrence of cancer.

During the last week, John has had several serious episodes. Last night he had a cardiac arrest and was resuscitated. The resident physicians and nurses would like to put him on a "no code" status so that if his heart stops again he will be able to die peacefully. They also would like him to know the seriousness of his illness and that he has cancer, because they think he has a right to know he is going to die.

Today the physician approached John's mother about whether John could be told about his illness. She flew into a rage and threatened to move John to another hospital immediately if they did not promise to never tell him under any circumstances. Although the health professionals know she has a legal right to remove him from the hospital, few of them think she actually will. Their opinions on whether he should be told are now divided.

Several suggestions may help you to decide what to do when you are faced with dilemmas concerning how much information to share with child patients:

1. *Make your own position clear* to yourself and to the patient's parents. Do you believe the child is able to handle information about his or her condition? Why or why not? Under what conditions would you feel morally bound to disclose relevant health information to this child? Under what conditions would you withhold such information even if you believed that doing so could increase the child's distrust in you?

2. *Explore the resources available in your health care setting* to support families as they work out their anxieties and difficulties. As one author notes, "The purpose is . . . to support, not supplant, the family. An atmosphere of acceptance and assurance allows each family to manage their own lives and to arrive at a solution most adequate for them.[8]

In summary, children bring to the health care interaction hopes, fears, and dreams that reflect their need to establish autonomy and initiative as a "self" while maintaining the security of relationships with family, friends, and others. The delicate balance between being an individual and being part of relationships that is difficult under the best of circumstances is further challenged by illness or other incapacity. The efforts of health professionals and family alike are required for successful adaptation or recovery. The benefit is that within a context of respect for the child as a unique individual, health professional and patient will be able to work together to meet the patient's best interests.

THE ADOLESCENT SELF

The word "adolescent" means literally "to grow into maturity or adulthood." During the later stages of child development, all children are thrust into the difficult position of having to show industry and individuality in the larger world, to assert who they are, to command authority in some areas, and to explore the mysteries of developing sexuality. In short, they must complete the work of establishing an identity. This period is accompanied by dramatic physiological, anatomical, and psychological changes.

Early and Late Adolescence

Most psychologists and others writing about adolescence divide it into two stages, early and late, each with developmental tasks. Early adolescence lasts for about 2 years and is characterized by growth spurts, maturing of reproductive functions and sex organs, increased weight, and changes in body proportions. These profound changes understandably may have profound psychological results.

Anyone who is around early teens knows that their self-images govern everything they do. The teen years are a time of intensely seeking one's "self." In its extreme form the self is the way the body looks and nothing more. However, for many teens the absorption with the self goes beyond bodily appearance alone. Adolescents are generally concerned with fitting in with their peers. They will try various roles in an attempt to integrate their developing social skills with goals and dreams.

This early period of adolescence is so unsettling that psychologists and others have termed it a period of adolescent turmoil. However, other researchers indicate that adolescence may not be as fraught with emotional issues as has been previously thought. In an ethnographic study of early adolescent girls, both popular and not so popular, the findings revealed a close relationship with parents and certainly not the trauma and stress suggested by common discourses (or myths) about adolescence. Teachers, parents, and health care professionals may expect trouble from adolescents due to or attributed to "raging hormones," but in this study the trauma did not materialize.[9] At a minimum, there is clearly asynchrony between physical development and psychosocial maturation that may be the source of some conflict and also in part offers an explanation for the number of teen pregnancies and instances of sexually transmitted diseases.

After this period of rapid and profound change, the young person moves into late adolescence. Here self-identify fully emerges (if the person has successfully completed the life tasks leading up to this moment), with all of its attendant self-regulation and self-discipline. Some adolescents do not move on to this stage of development because they literally do not survive. For the black population, homicide is the leading cause of death for those aged 15 to 24.[10]

During the postpubertal years, most persons also become more self-conscious of a philosophy of life and a value system:

Many factors first influence the development of an ideology—parents, peers, significant others, religious training, and cultural and social background. Some theorists speculate that from the time of adolescence the person is dealing with the "child of the past," that each early experience in the child's social life and culture directly and indirectly affect his or her development of a philosophy of life. . . .[11]

The impact of a peer's behavior on an adolescent is significant. In a study of 527 adolescents in grades 9 through 12, substance use (cigarette, marijuana and alcohol use), violence (weapons and physical fighting), and suicidal behavior (suicidal ideation and attempts) were related to their friends' substance use, deviance, and suicidal behaviors, respectfully. On the positive side, the more prosocial behavior of friends had a negative correlation with violence and substance abuse.[12] Other factors, such as family function, depression, and social acceptance, influenced adolescents' health-risk behavior as well.

NEEDS: RESPECT, AUTONOMY, AND RELATING

Autonomous decision-making raises some delicate questions for health professionals who are working with an adolescent patient because this person often wants to aggressively assert his or her authority in decisions. It is not always clear whether the adolescent is capable of making wise authoritative decisions. Only in recent years has there been an attempt to address the legal rights of adolescents. The most prominent view, referred to as the Mature Minors Doctrine, allows for parents or the state to speak on behalf of a minor's interests only as long as the minor is unable to represent himself or herself. Thus, the level of the young person's development emerges as a decisive factor. In keeping with the legality of the Mature Minors Doctrine, you can try to assess the maturity of an adolescent patient in regard to his or her ability to cope effectively with illness or injury. The question whether an adolescent is a "mature minor" must be decided by health care professionals independent of parental judgment.[13]

There are some compelling reasons to give decision-making authority to mature adolescents. Some adolescents would never consult a health care provider with a problem if they knew it would require parental consent before treatment. Also, in their developing autonomy, they would never share delicate information with the provider if they thought confidentiality would be violated. Coupled with the reluctance of adolescents to speak about risky behavior or other health issues, they often do not receive recommended and preventive counseling or screening services appropriate to their age group.[14] Health professionals need to encourage discussion of risky behaviors such as smoking and alcohol consumption as well as diet, weight, exercise, and topics related to sexual activity.

One important study showed that, for the adolescent, the process of sustaining himself or herself during a serious illness is made up of four sequential phases[15]:

> *Cognitive discomfort* describes the extent to which the patient experiences mental uneasiness and a desire to be relieved of it. Two strategies used by patients in response to cognitive discomfort are (1) thought stopping, that is, breaking down negative or disheartening thought processes, and (2) thought reflection, or giving careful, deliberate consideration to negative thoughts.
>
> In the *distraction* phase, activities are used to replace disturbing thoughts with more acceptable ones. Nine strategies are used in this phase: (1) doing something to keep busy; (2) reasoning that "It could always be worse"; (3) thinking "I made it this far"; (4) looking ahead to when it will be over; (5) using cognitive clutter; (6) thinking "God will take care of me"; (7) looking back at how bad it was; (8) thinking about survivors; and (9) thinking about others who have been patients.
>
> The phase of *cognitive comfort* brings on a period of solace and uplifted spirits for the patient.
>
> Finally, in the *personal competence* phase, a feeling of hopefulness occurs plus perception of the self as resilient, resourceful, and adaptable in the face of threat.

An adolescent engaged in the process of these phases is likely to be able to make some authoritative judgments about his or her illness and treatment. A problem is that, because this sequence takes time, the patterns of your interaction with the patient often are set before the adolescent can prove himself or herself capable of authoritative decision-making. At the very least, you should be aware of the adolescent's attempts to take command of the situation and to respond thoughtfully to an extremely difficult challenge. Failure to respect his or her efforts is a failure to show respect for the patient generally.

Family and Peers—Bridges to Respectful Interaction

Families and friends should not be excluded from the health care interaction process for patients in this age group either. The aforementioned emphasis on the importance of the adolescent's autonomy and authority should in no way be seen as undermining the importance of treating the patient as a part of a family unit when one exists.

Most adolescents like to argue about adult rules, even those they accept. Listening to family exchanges about rules that the adolescent disagrees with often will provide insight into the conduct of the adolescent toward you, too. Also, the health professional should not assume that the adolescent's attitude toward parents means there is not a deep dependence on them or heartfelt caring from the family. Further assessment is needed to ascertain whether family disequilibrium is creating a breach in that support system.

Health professionals often benefit from including an adolescent patient's close friends and peers in interactions. Peer group activity is essential for identity formation, and all illnesses or injuries are jolts to the adolescent's identity. Getting to know the person's friends by name, seeking their support, and trying to understand their feelings about the patient's condition can be helpful to all.

SUMMARY

In this brief overview of children and adolescents the theme of respect revolves around at least two ideas, patient autonomy and effective relatedness. There are numerous ways in which the young patient will try to exert autonomy and find a way of relating with you effectively. By showing imagination—and at times, patience—you will have an opportunity to build a close and rewarding relationship.

One of the greatest challenges for you as a health professional is to think of the development of people from birth to adulthood as a continuum, with some moving along it faster than others. We have provided some guidelines that will help you think generally about people as they pause—then continue to pass through—older childhood and adolescence. The individual patient will present himself or herself as a unique individual still in the process of forming and refining an identity. You have a responsibility to be sure that, in the midst of activities such patients may engage you in, their health care needs are met. Having said that, we move ahead to the next chapter and the unique challenges associated with treating people in the adult years.

REFERENCES

1. Hampl, P.: *I Could Tell You Stories: Sojourns in the Land of Memory,* W.W. Norton Company, London, 1999, p. 21.
2. Dillard, A.: *An American Childhood.* New York, Harper & Row, 1988, p. 11.
3. Newacheck, P.W., and Halfon, N.: Prevalence and impact of disabling chronic conditions in childhood. *Am. J. Public Health* 88(4): 610–617, 1998.
4. Americans with Disabilities Act of 1990, 42 U.S.C. 12101 et seq.
5. Sullivan, P.M., and Knutson, J.F.: Maltreatment and disabilities: a population-based epidemiological study. *Child Abuse Negl.* 24(10):1257–1273, 2000.
6. Fleitas, J.: When Jack fell down. . . Jill came tumbling after. Siblings in the web of illness and disability. *MCN Am. J. Matern. Child Nurs.* 25(5):267–273, 2000.
7. Kobrinsky, N.L., Sposto, R., Shah, N.R., et al.: Outcomes of treatment of children and adolescents with recurrent non-Hodgkin's lymphoma and Hodgkin's disease with dexamethasone, etoposide, cisplatin, cytarabine, and L-asparaginase, maintenance chemotherapy, and transplantation: Children's Cancer Study Group CCG–5912. *J. Clin. Oncol.* 19(9):2390–2396, 2001.

8. Fleming, S. J.: Children's grief: individual and family dynamics. In Corr, C. A., and Corr, D. M. (eds.): *Hospice Approaches to Pediatric Care*. New York, Springer, 1985, p. 211.

9. Finders, M.J.: *Just Girls: The Hidden Literacies and Life in Junior High*. New York, Teachers College Press, 1996.

10. Centers for Disease Control and Prevention, U.S. Department of Health and Human Services. Deaths: final data for 1998. *National Vital Statistics Rep.* 48(11):2, 2000.

11. Daub, M.M.: Prenatal development through mid-adulthood. In Hopkins, H.L. and Smith, H.D. (eds.): *Willard and Spackman's Occupational Therapy*. 7th ed. New York, Lippincott, 1988, p. 68.

12. Prinstein, M.J., Boergers, J., and Spirito, A.: Adolescents' and their friends' health-risk behavior: factors that alter or add to peer influence. *J. Pediatr. Psychol.* 26(5):287–298, 2001.

13. Cook, R., and Dickens, B.M.: Recognizing adolescents' 'evolving capacities' to exercise choice in reproductive healthcare. *Int. J. Gynecol. Obstet.* 70(1):13–21, 2000.

14. Bethell, C., Klein, J., and Peck, C.: Assessing health system provision of adolescent preventive services: the Young Adult Health Care Survey. *Med. Care* 39(5):478–490, 2001.

15. Hinds, P.S., and Martin, J.: Hopefulness and the self-sustaining process in adolescents with cancer. *Nurs. Res.* 37:336–339, 1988.

CHAPTER 16

Respectful Interaction: Working with the Adult

CHAPTER OBJECTIVES

The student will be able to

- Compare some of the unique challenges of development in the middle years with those of childhood and adolescence
- Discuss the meaning of work for adults
- Discuss "responsibility" as it applies to the middle years of life and how it may affect the response to health professionals working with an adult patient
- Describe some social roles that characterize life for most middle-aged persons and consider ways in which showing respect for a patient requires attention to those roles
- Discuss how stress enters into attempts to carry out the responsibilities of each of the aforementioned roles and some health-related consequences of great stress
- List some basic challenges facing health professionals who are working with a middle-aged person going through a midlife crisis

"Here are some guidelines on how to be an adult," said the consulting editor at a magazine where I worked several years ago. "I wrote them in honor of your twenty-first birthday, which if I'm not mistaken is today." The man handed me a sheet of paper. The list began, "Adults always speak in a calm quiet voice. When angry an adult says, 'I think I must tell you that I am angry.' " The list ended, "Adults are very careful about the drains, and often have trouble walking on beaches: sometimes they cannot synchronize their legs properly to adjust for the sand."

A. Lamott[1]

WHO IS THE ADULT?

It may be true that of all the life periods, adulthood has been the least understood and least studied. It follows that health professionals will probably be least adept at interacting respectfully with persons in this age group. The relative ease with which health professionals generally approach adult patients does not ensure that the needs of a person of middle years will then automatically be better met. Although ease of initial interaction is an important ingredient in effectiveness, it is not in itself sufficient. If only there were an accurate list of what it means to be an adult. In fact, adulthood is far more complicated than youth.

A stereotype about adult life is that it is only a waiting period or holding place made up of work, establishing a family, or dealing with menopause on the way to retirement and old age. In reality, there is a wide variation in the type and timing of transitions and activities in adult life that is far richer than this stereotype suggests. For these reasons, it is important to examine some vital issues concerning life as an adult in this society.

Adulthood can be legally defined by chronological age or at the time a person begins to assume responsibility for himself or herself and others.[2] It can also be defined by achievement of certain developmental tasks such as being independent; establishing a personal identify in a reflective way; finding a meaningful occupation; establishing long-term relationships; contributing to the welfare of others or making a contribution to family, faith community, or society at large; and gaining recognition for one's accomplishments on a community basis. Finally, adulthood can be defined in psychological terms, that is, the level of maturity exhibited by a person. Mature persons are able to take responsibility, make logical decisions, appreciate the position of others, control emotional outbursts, and accept social roles. The opening quote pokes fun at the adult attribute of accepting minor frustrations with the seldom heard phrase, "I think I must tell you that I am angry," as if all adults remain calm and composed when they are angry. What it means to be an "adult" is a combination of many factors, the most important of which you will be introduced to in these pages.

NEEDS: RESPECT, IDENTITY, AND INTIMACY

"One of the striking things about adult development as a field [of study] is its age. It is entirely a twentieth-century phenomenon, in no small part because the concept of adulthood has crystallized only in this century."[3] Adult development is not marked by definitive physical and motor changes such as those seen in toddlers (e.g., learning how to walk), but it is full of challenging and largely unpredictable experiences. Adult life is marked by concepts such as midlife crisis, generativity, and the empty nest, but not every adult has these experiences. We would be better able to predict the response of a 5-year-old to a major illness than we would that of a 30-year-old. Additionally, there may be differences between the way middle age is experienced by men and women. Also, the specific point in history that a person enters adulthood may have profound implications for adult life. For example, many women who entered adulthood during the women's movement of the 1960s and 1970s had more opportunities regarding work and sexual freedom than the previous generation of women. Finally, development may also differ because of sexual orientation, race and ethnicity, class, and education, to name a few. Thus, no single theory is adequate to explain adult development. Even if we hold several variables constant (e.g., age and sex), it is still difficult to predict how two middle-aged patients would react to the same diagnosis. Consider the example of Ms. McLean and Ms. Jeon, both of who have just learned that they have in situ cancer of the cervix.

> Sara McLean, age 34, has a family history positive for cervical cancer. Her maternal aunt and older sister both died of cervical cancer. Ms. McLean has recently become engaged and plans to be married in 6 months. She put off committing to a permanent relationship and starting a family until she completed graduate work in clinical psychology. With the support of her husband-to-be, she had planned on balancing a career as a private therapist with raising a family. She is devastated when the oncologist presents information about the treatment of choice for her condition—a total hysterectomy.
>
> Eunice Jeon, age 33, also has in situ cancer of the cervix. She has no family history of cancer and has always prided herself on her "hearty" family stock. All of her grandparents are alive and well. Ms. Jeon married her high school sweetheart the weekend after graduation. The Jeons have four children aged 5, 8, 10, and 12. Mr. Jeon is an emergency medical technician and plans someday to enroll in medical school after he finishes his bachelor degree. Ms. Jeon works as a secretary/receptionist at the Catholic grade school her children attend. She is troubled by the diagnosis, but when presented with treatment options merely asks, "When can we schedule the surgery? I want to get this taken care of as soon as possible."

Both of these women's feelings and reactions are the result of their life experiences to this point, which in turn, are determined by their roles. In Ms. McLean's case, her response to the diagnosis is influenced by her roles as daughter, sister, niece, fiancé, and psychologist. Ms. Jeon's response is influenced by her roles as mother, wife, daughter, granddaughter, and receptionist. These life roles are only a few that we can ascertain based on the information presented in the brief cases. It is highly probable that both women have many more roles. Ms. McLean planned her life around finishing her education. Ms. Jeon's has revolved largely around her family. In short, just looking at their ages, it would be impossible to predict how Ms. McLean and Ms. Jeon will interpret this crisis.

Adult patients are generally more capable of entering into a professional relationship as an equal partner than younger people. Even though adult patients are better able to protect their own interests and make their wishes known, they are still worthy of the respect that we accord to younger, generally more vulnerable, patients. Respect continues to be one of the hallmarks of effective interaction as we work our way through the lifespan.

A developmental task unique to the adult is the development of a self-definition or identity. Identity has its roots in self-perceptions in relation to specific social settings. For example, after completing an educational program, a person may refer to himself or herself as "an engineer" or "a physical therapist." The professional role has become part of the person's identity. Identity provides continuity over time and across problems and changes that arise in life. Illness and injury invariably result in changes in the patient's identity as was previously mentioned in Chapters 7 and 8. So there is a sense of maintenance of self through identity and yet room for change to accommodate the vicissitudes of life.

Intimacy is another developmental task of the adult. According to Erikson, adult development is marked by the ability to experience open, supportive, and loving relationships with others without the fear of losing one's own identity in the process of growing close to another. Intimacy is experienced in a variety of relationships with family members, lovers, and friends. This stage of adult development is sometimes referred to as love—the balance of intimacy and isolation. The major developmental facets of adult life are referred to repeatedly as we explore the social roles, meaning of work, and challenges of midlife.

Psychosocial Development and Needs

Maturity requires the acceptance of responsibility and empathy for others. The concept of achievement central to adult life can be defined in a number of ways. Some "midlife crises" discussed later in this chapter seem to stem from a person's having adequately assumed responsibility and realized his or her achievement potential, whereas others arise when the individual has failed to do so.

A profile of a person in the middle years of life will necessarily involve a consideration of his or her sense of "responsibility." When we ask if someone is willing to "assume responsibility," we are concerned with acts that the person can do and has voluntarily agreed to do. Given these conditions of ability and agreement, we want to know whether the person can be trusted to carry out the acts, regardless of whether the agreement was explicit (i.e., a promise to abide by the terms of a contract) or implicit (i.e., a promise to provide for one's own children or parents). Underlying the idea of acting responsibly is an assumption that the individual *is* a free agent, i.e., one who is willing and able to act autonomously. Thus, a person coerced into performing an act is not considered to have accepted responsibility for it.

During the middle years, there is another aspect to acting responsibly: it involves having a high regard for the welfare of others. In this second stage of adult development, the adult must find a way to support the next generation by redirecting attention from self to others. Successful mastery of this stage results in "care."[4] This involves empathy for the predicaments that befall others in life. The acts may flow from a free will, but the will must operate in accordance with reasonable claims and justifiable expectations of other people. The claims of society on a person peak during the middle years, so "acting responsibly" must be interpreted in terms of how completely the person fulfills the conditions of those claims. For instance, in Hindu culture, one stage of acting out a karma involves active engagement in the affairs of family and business. Only when an individual has successfully completed these tasks does he or she move on to higher, more contemplative levels of existence.

One way to view the matter in our culture is to recall the discussion of values in Chapter 1. The basic value of self-respect is discussed at some length and shown to be among the most essential ingredients of "the good life." During the middle years, most people perceive self-respect as vulnerable to the judgments of others: one's self-respect at least partially depends on the extent to which he or she commands the respect of employer, family, and friends. This idea is related to our concept of "reputation," and one commands respect by giving due consideration to society's claims. Hiltner notes, correctly we believe, that, to a large extent, even the personal values of the middle years must include a regard for others. For most, it is a highly social period when interdependencies are complex and pervasive.[5]

One factor distinguishing the contemporary person of middle years from like persons in other periods of history is that today some of the psychological components of adolescence are extended to a much later age than during other historical periods. Thus, a 25-year-old individual who feels some of the weight of the societal claims placed on people of middle years may still be financially dependent on his or her parents (or spouse), may still be in school, may be living in the family home, and may still be actively exploring sexual preferences and lifestyles. Individuals who do not work on the identity versus role confusion stage during late adolescence or early adulthood will find themselves years later going back, so to speak, to try to resolve the issues that were not addressed. For example, in a study of gay males in middle adulthood, the researcher found that "these men were facing issues befitting their chronological age (non-gay issues which had been worked on while leading a double-life) as well as unresolved identity issues from the past."[6] The key point of this study is that these men were initially working through the earlier stage of development rather than reworking earlier developmental issues that can occur throughout adult development.

Parents might believe that they have moved through a developmental task of the family, that of raising children, only to find that adult children return to their parents' home after a divorce or unemployment. Therefore, a parent or parents who might have been rejoicing in an empty nest and time for each other may experience the stress of having adult children under their roofs once again and with grandchildren in tow. Furthermore, a significant number of women have delayed pregnancy until midlife and find themselves attempting to integrate child rearing, marriage, and recreational and work roles in their late 30s and early 40s. Thus, the delayed acquisition of independence, earlier physical maturation characteristic of modern cultures, pressures on young people to grow up fast, return of adult children to their parents' home, and delayed childbearing all complicate the traditional views held about progression through adulthood. At best, one can conclude that the lines between adolescent and middle-year life periods and the beginning and ending of parenting responsibilities are by no means distinct!

Social Roles in the Middle Years

There are several social roles that most fully characterize this period.

Primary Relationships. It is almost always during the middle years that a person decides with whom lasting relationships will be developed. Fortunately, an increasing number of older people are also developing new relationships, but they are usually people who were able to sustain deep and lasting relationships in the middle years as well.

The primary relationship takes priority over all others, the most common type being the relationship with a spouse. Choosing a spouse or other permanent companion and becoming better acquainted (i.e., learning to know the person, discovering potentials and limits, similarities and differences, and compatibilities and incompatibilities) are processes interwoven with the more basic activities of eating, sleeping, acquiring possessions, working, worshiping, relaxing, and playing together.

Those who do not enter into a marriage relationship sometimes develop a deep and lasting involvement with a friend or sibling. One of your first tasks, especially in ongoing interaction with a patient of middle years, is to find out if there is a key person in his or her life and, if so, who that person is. This can be accomplished without unnecessary probing into the person's private life. Particularly in times of crisis the patient looks to that key person for comfort, sustenance, and guidance. However, sometimes the person you assume would be the most supportive is not. Consider the story of Mary Ogden and Pam Carlisle:

> Mary Ogden, age 61, is a retired, single teacher who is hospitalized for treatment related to severe diabetes. The entire small community where she has resided and taught for 35 years adores her. Through the years she has received numerous awards for community service. She is a cooperative, cheerful person, who, in spite of her illness, continues to be an inspiration to everyone. She is especially fond of Pam Carlisle, the head nurse on the unit where Mary is being treated.
>
> On the afternoon before Mary's planned hospital discharge, an unscheduled visitor comes to the nursing desk insisting to speak to Pam about a highly personal matter. The visitor is Agnes Ogden, an elderly lady

who informs Pam that she is the sister (and only living relative) of Mary. The visitor seems sincere and asks that Pam provide details of her sister's condition so that she might be better prepared to aid her with both her physical illness and personal affairs. Pam complies with her request, actually feeling relieved that there is someone to share this burden with her. The following morning Pam visits Mary's room and finds her profoundly irate for the first time. She informs Pam that she has not been on speaking terms with her sister for many years, that she considers her sister to be untrustworthy, and that she thoroughly resents her sister's having the knowledge of her personal affairs and illness. Mary develops a distrust of Pam and becomes depressed, agitated, and uncooperative.

What could Pam have done differently to foster Mary's trust rather than to destroy it? What would you have done when Agnes came to you requesting information? How might you rebuild the trust that once existed between you and the patient should such a breakdown occur?

Parenting. Caring for children often is a part of adult life. The sex role stereotypes traditionally assigned to mothering and fathering are breaking down in many families so that both parents share the whole range of parenting skills. The concept of parenting is being expanded, too: there is the "single parent," who provides the full care usually shared with another; same sex couples are parenting; and, finally, a small but growing number of people are attempting to live within extended family situations in which parenting is shared by several persons.

Whatever the challenges of each model, all of these people share the awareness that our society believes the child's welfare depends on the quality of parenting. The age-old recognition that a child's physical well-being depends on adult care is now buttressed by more recent assertions that the child's potential for fulfillment and satisfaction in later years is also determined by the parent. Such beliefs can create overwhelming guilt in some parents when their children do not follow the path that these parents believe is the most beneficial.

The least that can be said of parenting relationships is that they are among the most enduring and complex of human interactions. The health professional who fails to consider them in an ongoing relationship with a patient neglects an integral part of the patient's identity.

Care of Older Family Members.   Not only do many adults care for children as a part of their daily responsibilities, but they also care for their parents, parents-in-law, and other older friends and relatives. It has been successfully argued by Brody in her landmark work that parent care has become a normative but stressful experience for individuals and families.[7] The decrease in premature death has resulted in a sharp increase in the natural lifespan. Thus, more people are living into older age. At the same time that the population of older people increased, the birth rate declined, resulting in a shortage of filial caregivers. It is estimated that 2.1 million people older than 65 years of age require assistance with two or more activities of daily living. Seventy-two percent of unpaid family caregivers are women, the majority of whom are mid-life daughters or daughters-in-law.[8] Parent care is not limited to one age period of the caregiver's life but may span across several age periods in adult life. The consequences of parental caregiving are not fully understood, but it clearly exerts an impact on adult life for an unpredictable amount of time, unlike child rearing, which has built-in time limits of dependence and a progressive move to greater independence from the parent. Additionally, we are just beginning to appreciate the cultural differences that play a part in caring for elderly family members. For example, in a study of Mexican-American families and elder care, it was found that there is a clear sense of responsibility to care for the elder members of one's family.[9] Thus, women in this culture may go about readjusting their work obligations in different ways than women in other cultures. The cultural lens is an important aspect of viewing this role of adult life.

Political and Other Social Activities. Involvement in political and social organizations has traditionally been at a peak during the middle years. Responsibilities stemming from membership in such organizations are often second only to those of work if measured in terms of energy consumption and personal commitment. A sense of identity in the middle years depends heavily on belonging to a particular political party, religious group, service organization, or honorary society. Not only are these organizations and public service activities a source of identity, but they are also a vehicle for contributing to one's profession or community. There are, of course, other sources of claims on adults, but those cited constitute some highly significant ones.

Work as Meaningful Activity

Work, like family and adulthood, is a concept that can be variably defined. Work as meaningful activity can occur in a variety of settings and assumes many patterns. Therefore, the meaning of work and the responsibilities it requires will depend, of course, on the person's value system, expectations, and aspirations as well as the specific environment, job title, and position within a hierarchy. For some, work is performed primarily in the home; for a great many others, it entails a significant amount of time away from home. Adults in the middle years are judged to spend about half of their waking hours engaged in work. The kind of work they do largely determines their income, lifestyle, social status, and place of residence. Because of the amount of time and energy expended, the type of factual information one acquires over a lifetime is often influenced by the working situation. Studies of professional socialization suggest that, at least for the white-collar and professional worker, the kind of work done also defines the worldview.

Work-related responsibilities still differ for men and women. You have undoubtedly observed what most women experience in their work roles: the reasonable expectations include not only doing a job in the labor force as well as men but also maintaining the quality and amount of work performed in the home.

Women respond to these various needs or demands by trying to balance their impulse to care and the level of personal support available.[10] When the limits of caregiving are reached, something else has to give. In many cases, women make changes and adjustments in their employment in order to continue in the caregiving role.[11] It is a clear indication of what role takes priority in women's lives.

Two types of responsibility are associated with the work role: (1) to do one's job well and (2) to fulfill the reasonable expectations of others (e.g. employer, peers, or family members). The professional relationship has the added dimension of helping: one is expected to help those who need professional services. Work relationships are different from simple friendships in a number of ways, although the former can be lasting, deep, and complex.

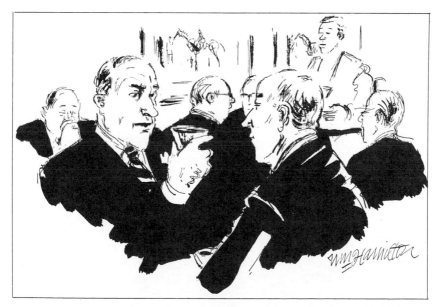

"I've learned a lot in sixty-three years. But, unfortunately, almost all of it is about aluminum."

From *The New Yorker,* November 11, 1977, p. 27. Drawing by William Hamilton; © 1977 The New Yorker Magazine, Inc. Used with permission.

The car pool phenomenon is an intriguing combination of the work and friendship roles; here people who are grouped together for the purpose of getting to and from work also usually engage in camaraderie over a considerable period of time and more regularly than with their own family members. We have known some car pool members who interact as friends or acquaintances during the commute, then assume their "proper" role with each other within a hierarchical working environment.

Your task is to assess how the patient views his or her work situation, particularly the relationships in it. Whether a patient's work involves providing quality child care, laboring on the section crew to replace railroad ties, or presiding over a meeting in the executive suite, the work entails responsibility both toward a job to be done and toward other human beings. Treatment goals must be tailored to help the patient either carry out these responsibilities or to accept the fact that it is no longer possible to do so.

Those who work with adult patients in the areas of occupational health are keenly aware of the relationship among health, injury, and illness and the worker's role. Consider the following case.

> Masie Baldwin has worked as a nursing home aide for the past 15 years. She is the sole provider for her three children, one of whom has just started college. Although Ms. Baldwin has attended the mandatory in-service sessions on proper body alignment and lifting of patients, she has not always followed the proper procedure. Ms. Baldwin stated to her fellow workers more than once, "I'm big and strong. I don't like waiting for help or lugging out the lift to get patients up. I can get them up and out of bed without help." Unfortunately, while getting Mr. Collins out of bed, Ms. Baldwin injured her lower back and neck. Ms. Baldwin has been on worker's compensation leave for the past month and is now involved in a "work-hardening" program to determine if she is capable of returning to work in the nursing home. The health professionals working with Ms. Baldwin observe that she is highly motivated to return to work, but frightened of reinjury. Her confidence in her strength and sense of invulnerability has been badly shaken. During a particularly trying day in the work-hardening program, she tells her therapist, "If I can't work in the nursing home, I don't know what I'll do. It's the only kind of work I've ever done. All my friends are there."

What "meanings" do you feel Ms. Baldwin gives to her work? How does her identity tie to her work roles? What are some of the challenges you might face in working with Ms. Baldwin?

It is important for you to return to the developmental identity and view it in light of the adult social roles and responsibilities we have discussed so far. We have emphasized responsibility in terms of relationships in the middle years and work roles and have suggested that self-respect during this period is largely determined by meeting the justifiable expectations of others. However, self-respect unquestionably also depends somewhat on believing in and being true to oneself. Thus the person of middle years who meets all of society's expectations can still be unfulfilled.[12] That, in fact, is precisely the plight of many people today who have not pursued personal interests and goals at all or very minimally. This situation can be viewed as an inability or unwillingness to assume responsibility toward oneself, and it leads to a form of the midlife crisis that is discussed in this chapter. Accepting the consequences of one's own behavior is vital; all of us share, to some extent, the problem expressed by the motto on President Truman's desk, "The buck stops here." The sense of "being somebody," such an integral part of adolescence, must become more fully defined in the middle years. In this period, individuals are expected to be able to show more clearly who they are and what they are able to contribute to the welfare of loved ones and to society.

Biological Development during the Adult Years

In human beings the lifespan is thought to be about 110 to 120 years. In Western nations the average life expectancy is said to be 76.1 years (71.5 years for men, 78.4 years for women), although this varies according to race and other variables.[12] The 15 leading causes of death for all age groups are listed in Table 16–1.[13]

Cause of death varies according to race and sex, too, but this table should give you a general idea of the types of illnesses you will encounter most often with adult patients.

From adolescence on, human beings continue to grow and mature. Aging can be defined as "the sum of all the changes that normally occur in an organism with the passage of time."[14] Aging, like adulthood itself, is complex and varies from one person to another. Aging also gives rise to feelings of anxiety in a way no other area of human development does. Failing intellectual or biological functions in the middle years can become a preoccupation for your patient. For example, during this period the pure joy of physical activity experienced in younger years may acquire a sober edge. One of us overheard a man who for years has enjoyed running just for the sport of it tell his friend, "Yeah, my running will probably guarantee that I live five years longer, but I will have spent that five years running!" Adults may also worry about changes in their mental capacities when they forget something or misplace the car keys. Suddenly, forgetfulness is no longer something to be taken lightly but could portend more serious problems generally associated with old age such as Alzheimer's disease.

Perhaps the anxiety that aging provokes is due to the close relationship between biological development and illness, decline, and death.[15] Rather than view aging in this way, gerontologists have proposed the concept of "compressed morbidity," which suggests that people may live longer, healthier lives and have shorter periods of disability at the end of their lives. The focus of health care

TABLE 16–1. Cause of Death

Rank	Percentage of Total Deaths
1. Diseases of the heart	31.0
2. Malignant neoplasms, including neoplasms of lymphatic and hematopoietic tissues	23.2
3. Cerebrovascular disease	6.8
4. Chronic obstructive pulmonary diseases and allied conditions	4.8
5. Accidents and adverse advents	
Motor vehicle accidents	1.9
All other accidents and adverse events	2.3
6. Pneumonia and influenza	3.9
7. Diabetes mellitus	2.8
8. Suicide	1.3
9. Nephritis, nephrotic syndrome, and nephrosis	1.1
10. Chronic liver disease and cirrhosis	1.1
11. Septicemia	1.0
12. Alzheimer's disease	1.0
13. Homicide and legal intervention	0.8
14. Atherosclerosis	0.7
15. Hypertension with or without renal disease	0.6
All other causes	15.8

Based on the Ninth Revision, International Classification of Diseases, 1975.

then becomes one of prevention, health improvement for chronic disease and postponement of disability or death rather than cure.[16] In Chapter 17, we will discuss different views of aging and their impact on your interactions with older patients.

Stresses and Challenges of Midlife

The more responsibilities a person assumes, the more vulnerable he or she becomes to the symptoms associated with stress. Stress is recognized as a threat to the well-being of the present generation and will increase if steps are not taken to deal with it. Major problems associated with stress in adult life finally are gaining the attention of investigators, health professionals, workplace counselors, and religious groups.

Chapter 4 addressed some aspects of stress in students, and Chapter 7 suggests types of patient challenges likely to produce stress at any age. Middle-years stress is similar in its most general form. The specific sources differ, but the means by which a young person has learned to deal with stress will be carried into adulthood. One significant difference is that, in the middle years, no clearly defined end to some sources of stress—no "gracious exit" from an impossible situation—may be in sight. The stress attending next week's exam can be more easily managed than that arising from the realization that one has a stressful lifestyle in general.

Some stresses result from personal life choices. The responsibilities assumed in marriage and other primary relationships (e.g., child rearing, parent care, and work) all create stress, as do unemployment and some factors in the social structure itself. Each is discussed separately.

Primary Relationships. Marriage relationships during the middle years have been studied more extensively than other types of primary relationships, but it is reasonable to believe that all such relationships produce stress situations. Common sources of stress in the marriage relationship include nonfulfillment of role obligations by a spouse, lack of reciprocity between marital partners, and a feeling of not being accepted by one's spouse. Illfeld maintains that sources of stress that are damaging to the marital relationship are those of an ongoing nature instead of those of a discrete event. He further proposes that these common, mundane stressors in everyday life take more of a toll in suffering than does the impact of a dramatic life crisis.[17] Couples with children often experience stress around the departure of their children, leaving both (and not only the woman, as is often thought) with the "empty nest syndrome." The empty nest has traditionally been a gendered approach to theorizing about changes in midlife. In addition to the empty nest, women's middle age is often discussed in terms of menopause and new opportunities for activity and self-expression. For many women who work outside the home, the empty nest is not an issue of concern. Also, menopause is not universally viewed as the critical event of middle age that many popular authors claim it to be.[18] A more violent expression of stress, the primary source of which may not arise from the relationship itself but is acted out within it, is the battered spouse syndrome. Some persons involved in situations of domestic violence are receiving attention from self-help groups and other organizations, but not all are. They may well be present among your patients or clients, exhibiting symptoms that deserve attention. For generations they have remained hidden and silent, victimized by the fear of stigmatization and having no place to go. Refuges, as they are called, are now springing up around the country, and an increasing number of health professionals are volunteering their services for the treatment and rehabilitation of these women and men and their abusers.

Parenting. The tremendous responsibility associated with parenting also leads to stress situations in the middle years. Child abuse and neglect, which are increasing (or, perhaps, are being reported more systematically), are other tragic examples of what can happen when stress is not controlled. Most stress related to child rearing leads to less deplorable results, but nonetheless it does take an immense toll on both parent and child.

Care of Elderly Family Members. As has been previously mentioned, the majority of the burden for parent care falls on adult women. Many quit their jobs to fulfill the responsibility of caring for one or more elderly family members. Women caregivers also report strains on their own health that are a result of the stresses of daily caregiving. The most common health consequence of caring for an older, sick relative is depression.[19] This often goes undetected and untreated. Add to this the other demands competing for these women's time and energy and you can see how stressful parent care can be. The stress is often borne with considerable grace as adult children often express the desire to care for their parents and the satisfaction and joy it brings them in concert with the burdens. Unfortunately, elder abuse, like spousal and child abuse, is on the rise. Much needs to be done in the way of effective social policy development to assist families in caring for their frail elderly relatives so that they do not reach the limits of their endurance.

Work. For many individuals in the middle years, stress related to work is their primary stress, manifesting itself in a wide range of disorders. The source of stress may be job dissatisfaction in general, coupled with the notion that there is nowhere else to go. It may be that the job is basically satisfactory but that some component is an ongoing source of stress, such as a coworker who is a continual "thorn in the flesh." Some jobs are in themselves highly stressful. One of the most studied high-stress jobs is a position in an intensive care unit. Another is work in an airport control tower. These studies demonstrate that a job with high responsibility where the consequences for a mistake are dire creates the highest stress. Boredom and repetition also create stress. Work-related stress can be a key factor in the development of serious health problems such as cardiovascular disease and alcoholism or other substance abuse problems.

Unemployment. A particular form of stress related to the work role is caused by the inability to hold a job. The increase in admissions to psychiatric hospitals in the last 10 years has been highest among men in their middle years who have lost their jobs and cannot find another. In a society that rewards its members for paid work, the stress of working can be less threatening to health and well-being than the stress of being unemployed.

Thus, it becomes evident that the middle years, in which a person is in many ways at his or her prime, are also years of responsibility and stress. The burdens, although each taken alone may be a small constraint, sometimes have the overall effect of making the middle-aged person feel exhausted and overwhelmed. Although these years are sometimes characterized as a plateau or holding pattern, they are much more varied than that: they are filled, instead, with alpine meadows, treacherous cliffs, cool blue pools, and swift undercurrents.

Doubt at the Crossroads and Midlife Crisis

The task of assuming responsibility and its attendant stresses, the great desire to achieve, or transitions in career, family life, and health condition may at some critical moment trigger an opportunity to take stock. The feeling accompanying the experience is most clearly expressed as doubt. It differs from the vacuous zero point of boredom and lacks the volcanic fervor of other types of stress. Doubt allows no rest; indeed, it is a relentless churning that nakedly reveals almost all the dimensions of one's life. The masks that have allowed the masquerade to go on, the clatter that has accompanied the parade, the walls that have kept fearful monsters from view, all suddenly evaporate and leave a pregnant silence. The self stands alone.

This midlife crisis has received more attention than have many other aspects of experience that people face during their middle years. Numerous theories have been set forth to explain what happens, most of them reflecting, as we have just done, that it is a period of expanding more fully into one's own life space. It is a head-on look in the mirror.

The experience itself, characterized by doubt about the headstrong course one has been on, has a paradox built into it. The paradox is aptly expressed by the German phrase *Torschlusspanik,* which means "the panic of the closing gates." Ostensibly, the state-owned apartments in parts of Germany are locked at 11 o'clock, and any hapless resident who fails to return home by then must find a park bench for the night. Thus, as 11 o'clock nears, those residents still on the outside muster tremendous energy to get everything done and still make it to the gates before it is too late. On the one hand, the challenge is terrific; on the other, the dread is overwhelming. Both the potential for completing or achieving the goal and the clearly defined limits of those goals are brought simultaneously into sharp focus.

The various transitions that are a part of adult life allow people to come to terms with new situations. Bridges conceptualizes a transition as a three-phase psychological process people go through: ending, neutral zone, and new beginning.[20] A transition begins with an ending. Something must be left behind to move to the next phase. A transition may be sought or thrust upon a person. For example, consider the case of Tanya Zorski who worked as a claims processor at an insurance company for the past 10 years. Recently, Tanya's employer merged with another company, resulting in "downsizing" or firing of many people in the claims department, including Tanya. Tanya's transition begins with the ending of her job. The next phase of transition is the neutral zone. After letting go, willingly or unwillingly, she must examine old habits that are no longer adaptive.[21] As Tanya begins to look for another position, she will discover that the computer skills that had been adequate at her old job, are not marketable. Employers want people with experience in leading-edge computer programs, and Tanya does not possess these skills. During the neutral zone phase, people start to look for new, better-adapted skills or habits. People may take this opportunity to pursue a long-held dream. The final phase is the new beginning. Tanya may move into a new beginning in her life by pursuing a degree in nursing. She may reason that if she is going to invest the energy, time, and financial resources in learning new skills, she might as well do it in a profession that she has wanted to join since she was young.

Although changes in midlife have often been labeled as a "crisis," perhaps the language is too strong. "Instead, perhaps, many individuals make modest 'corrections' in their life trajectories—literally, 'midcourse' corrections."[22] These corrections to one's life course are often the opportunity for growth. As is the case with Tanya Zorski, the more life-changing an event, the more likely it is to be associated with learning opportunities. "In fact, learning may be a coping response to significant life changes for many people."[23]

Regardless of whether a vision is being claimed or reclaimed, the task is to prepare for the adjustments and challenges still to come.

WORKING WITH THE PATIENT OF MIDDLE YEARS

This chapter deals almost exclusively with the psychosocial processes people face in their middle years. The fact is that life tasks associated with the middle years primarily are psychosocial ones.

Your patient in his or her middle years who arrives at the health facility may be working to maintain health or is experiencing a physical symptom. Because the middle years is not "supposed to be" characterized by painful or other troubling physical symptoms, those patients may feel especially angered or confused by this physical intrusion into the work of being a responsible person and pursuing goals! A woman of middle years who was being interviewed recently in a seminar reported that she had "bow-and-arrow" disease. The doctor had told her that she had multiple myeloma, a bone marrow disease, but the fact that she heard "bone marrow" as "bow-and-arrow" probably more accurately expresses how many adults experience their illnesses or injuries. The idea of being struck down in one's prime and that of the "untimely" accident or death are often applied to this age group. The denial, hostility, and depression that patients feel about being so attacked are factors to which you should give your attention, whether your interaction occurs only once or extends over a long period of time.

Because psychological and social well-being are preeminent for people of middle years, treatment must be attuned to both. Of all the challenges described in Chapter 7, the loss of independence most epitomizes the overall loss experienced by the adult patient. Of course, the person's former self-image is threatened, too, but this is almost a direct outgrowth of the loss of independence. A patient who can no longer go about meeting the responsibilities expected of him or her and pursuing the numerous life goals now established will usually feel trapped, vulnerable, and frustrated. The primacy of these concerns in middle life should help you to understand why a patient seems overly concerned about having to get a baby sitter for an hour or having to be home at a given time or why he or she is willing to forego treatment rather than to take time from work for a trip to the health facility.

Furthermore, an adult patient experiencing acute stress poses special problems and challenges. Each one must be treated according to the particular manifestations of the stress. Part of your duty is to assess how many of his or her physical or psychological symptoms arise from stress. This, of course, must often be done with a psychiatrist or psychologist, but not always. Indeed, listening to what is on a patient's mind may not only help to decrease his or her anxiety at the moment but may also enable you to make minor adjustments in schedule, routine, or approach that will further diminish it.

Many of the suggestions given throughout this book apply to all age groups. However, if you are alert to some of the central concerns and roles of middle life, you may well find that your success in achieving respectful interaction with the patient of middle years is heightened.

In the next chapter you have an opportunity to examine some changes that are faced by the person who has successfully lived through the middle years. As you will see, these changes involve some of life's greatest challenges, both positive and negative.

SUMMARY

Even though biological capacities begin to diminish in middle adulthood, adults generally have sufficient capacity for a personally satisfying and socially valuable life. The major life tasks for adults are to establish personal identity, develop intimate relationships, and feel and act on the desire to make a lasting contribution to the next generation. Although some people never resolve the issues that are brought into focus during the transitions of midlife, fortunately most do. Some emerge from the process with a new job, a new mate, and a new life view. The various aspects of adult development that were presented in this chapter are a sampling of the ways you can look at the complex process of how people grow and develop as adults, with an eye to how these observations can help to you to be respectful in your interactions with middle-life patients, clients, and families.

REFERENCES

1. Lamott, A.: *Hard Laughter.* New York, North Point Press, Farrar, Straus and Giroux, 1980, p. 50.
2. Bee, H.L.: *Journey of Adulthood.* 3rd ed. Upper Saddle River, NJ, Prentice Hall, 1996.

 3. Clark, M.C., and Caffarella, R.S.: Theorizing adult development. In Clark, M.C., and Caffarella, R.S. (eds.): *An Update on Adult Developmental Theory: New Ways of Thinking About the Life Course. New Directions of Adult and Continuing Education.* San Francisco, Jossey-Bass, 1999, p. 3.

 4. Reeves, P.M.: Psychological development: becoming a person. In Clark, M.C. and Caffarella, R.S. (eds.): *An Update on Adult Developmental Theory: New Ways of Thinking About the Life Course. New Directions of Adult and Continuing Education.* San Francisco, Jossey-Bass, 1999, pp. 19–28, quote p. 21.

 5. Hiltner, S.: Personal values in the middle years. In Ellis, E.O. (ed.): *The Middle Years.* Action, MA, Publishing Sciences Group, 1974, pp. 27–34.

 6. Peacock, J.R.: Gay male adult development: some stage issues of an older cohort. *J. Homosex.* 40(2):13–29, 2000, quote p. 22.

 7. Brody, E.M.: Parent care as a normative family stress. *Gerontologist* 25(1):19–29, 1985.

 8. Robinson, K.M.: Family caregiving: who provides the care, and at what cost? *Nurs. Econ.* 15(5):243–247, 1997.

 9. Clark, M., and Huttlinger, K.: Elder care among Mexican American families. *Clin. Nurs. Res.* 7(1):64–81, 1998.

10. McGrew, K.B.: Daughters' caregiving decisions: from an impulse to a balancing point of care. *J. Women Aging* 10(2):49–65, 1998.

11. Pohl, J.M., Collins, C.E., and Given, C.W.: Longitudinal employment decisions of daughters and daughters-in-law after assuming parent care. *J. Women Aging* 10(1):59–74, 1998.

12. Moos, R.H., and Billings, A.: Conceptualizing and measuring coping resources and processes. In Goldberger, L., and Breznitz, S. (eds.): *Handbook of Stress: Theoretical and Clinical Aspects.* New York, The Free Press, 1982, pp. 212–230.

13. Centers for Disease Control and Prevention, U.S. Department of Health and Human Services. Deaths: final data for 1998. *National Vital Statistics Rep.* 48(11):5, 2000.

14. Matteson, M.A.: In Matteson, E.S., McConnell, E.S., and Linton, A.D. (eds.): *Biological Theories of Aging in Gerontological Nursing: Concepts and Practice.* 2nd ed. Philadelphia, W.B. Saunders, 1996, pp. 159–171, quote p. 160.

15. Mott, V.W.: Our complex human body: Biological development explored. In Clark, M.C., and Caffarella, R.S. (eds.): *An Update on Adult Developmental Theory: New Ways of Thinking About the Life Course. New Directions of Adult and Continuing Education.* San Francisco, Jossey-Bass, 1999, pp. 9–18, quote p. 9.

16. *Healthy People 2000.* Washington, DC, U.S. Department of Health and Human Services, 1990.

17. Illfeld, F.W.: Marital stressors, coping styles and symptoms of depression. In Goldberger, L., and Breznitz, S. (eds.): *Handbook of Stress: Theoretical and Clinical Aspects.* New York, The Free Press, 1982, pp. 482–495.

18. Gergen, M.M.: Finished at 40: women's development within the patriarchy. *Psychol. Women Q.* 14:471–494, 1990.

19. Cohen, D.: Detection and treatment of depression of caregivers. *Home HealthCare Consultant* 5(6):32–36, 1998.

20. Bridges, W.: *Managing Transitions: Making the Most of Change.* Reading, MA, Addison-Wesley, 1991, p. 4.
21. Ibid, p. 6.
22. Stewart, A.J., and Ostrove, J.M.: Women's personality in middle age: gender, history, and midcourse corrections. *Am. Psychologist* 53(11):1185–1194, 1998, quote p. 1188.
23. Zemke, R., and Zemke, S.: Adult learning: what do we know for sure? *Training* 32:31–40, 1995, quote p. 33.

CHAPTER 17

Respectful Interaction: Working with the Older Adult

CHAPTER OBJECTIVES

The student will be able to

- Discuss in general terms Erikson's assessment of the developmental tasks in the later years of life

- Describe the roles of friendship and family ties among older people and how these ties can have an impact on an older patient

- Compare and contrast at least two psychological theories of aging

- List some basic challenges to well-being that present themselves in old age and the ways in which you, as a health professional, can help older people to meet such challenges successfully

- Describe how the health professional's attention to sensory impairment in older patients who require assistive devices can have a positive effect on the interaction

- Summarize the reasons an established time for treatment and a regular routine may be signs of respect toward older patients

- Discuss appropriate and inappropriate responses to a patient who has acute or permanent cognitive impairment

- List some values that may become highly prized among many older people, and suggest approaches that the health professional can use to optimize those values

I look at my mother. She's staring at the birds in the small cage across the room. Her rocker soothes her and her eyes close to slits. I take my thumb and trace her cheekbone. I rub the skin and watch it become young in my hands. The lines vanish, then reappear. Vanish, then reappear.

I remember being her young daughter, rubbing the rouge into her cheeks this way. She taught me how to find the bone and trace it. And then she placed the color on my finger and let me smooth it in. I could have stared at her forever. I still could.

My thumb moves softly from front to back, again and again. I watch the lines return and disappear. They will someday be the lines that already have begun to form across my own face.

J. Dyer[1]

One of the challenges confronting anyone who attempts to speak of old people is to earmark exactly when old age begins, even though it is a time of life everyone will enter if they are fortunate enough to live past middle age. According to many statements on social policy, eligibility for financial and other supportive benefits begins at age 65, but the usefulness of this age as a distinguishing line largely ends there. In fact, people's feelings that they are "old" usually are much determined by the presence of sickness, disability, or other factors rather than simply by their chronological age. For the purposes of this chapter, terms such as "elderly," "old," and "aged" will refer to individuals age 65 or older. The older population numbered 34.5 million in 1999. They represented 12.7% of the U.S. population, about one in every eight Americans.[2] Even though not all older Americans are sick, it is true that the average patient in a health care facility is older than 75 years of age. Thus, you will probably encounter older patients in your work as a health professional.

Almost every generality advanced about the older person is quickly countered by an individual's personal experience with a chronologically older man or woman. However, some processes that take place in a person as he or she advances in years differ little from one individual to another. In that perspective, the aged are those people in whom the process has taken place over a period of many years. This chapter provides an overview of physiological and psychosocial changes with a special emphasis on the psychosocial aspects of aging as they are relevant to respectful interaction. We urge you to study the burgeoning literature of aging further because the questions and clinical issues surrounding care of older patients are complex.

The days of "over the river and through the woods to grandmother's house" have disappeared in large segments of today's society. Indeed, a grandmother often discourages the visit because it will interfere with her scuba-diving lesson or her scheduled speech at a meeting concerning newly proposed city ordinances.

Where did grandmother go? Did the big bad wolf eat her? Did she at last find the Fountain of Youth? Neither grandmother nor grandfather has gone anywhere. Each is where the older person has always been—at the other side of time. It is society that has gone somewhere; the rapid societal changes taking place around older people give them greater opportunity for divergent roles than ever before. If they are unable to take advantage of these opportunities, as many are, then they are burdened with greater insecurity and more complex problems than were any of their predecessors. However, if they can make the best of these opportunities, their potential for an active and meaningful old age is excellent.

VIEWS OF AGING

"Aging is a highly individualized process that affects each person in unique ways. Aging is the result of the interaction among genetics, environmental influences, lifestyles, and the effects of disease processes."[3] This definition of aging is fairly straightforward, but there is much more to aging than mere physiological changes. Cultural and societal views of aging influence how you understand the aging process and how you work with older patients. The following are various views of aging, proposed by Gadow in 1980 and still relevant today, with some examples involving older patients.[4]

Antithesis of Health and Vigor

This is the negative extreme as far as views of aging go. Aging is the opposite of what we value most highly in our society—youth, vitality, strength, etc. This view is seen in health care when terms such as "degenerative" are used to describe physiological changes that accompany normal aging. Many elders view their health status as "fair to good" even with a number of degenerative conditions.

Unwelcome Reminder of Mortality

More than 70% of all persons who die in a given year are 65 years and older.[5] Death in old age is therefore more common and more "natural." "The effect of this view is that the more natural and acceptable mortality is thought to be for 'the elderly,' as they are sometimes called, the more unthinkable it is for the non-elderly, and the more the aged are avoided as symbols of the unthinkable."[6] Thus, one of the major problems of working with older people is that we have not come to terms with our own aging and mortality. The presence of the aged is an uncomfortable reminder of the future that is in store for all of us. Health professionals sometimes react to this discomfort by trying to avoid such patients whenever possible.

Underprivileged Citizens

Ageism as a type of discrimination and demeaning behavior were addressed in Chapter 3. In this view, old adults are treated as other oppressed groups in our society. They are the not readily accorded the respect they deserve but are forced often to rely on the benevolence of society in an attempt to make up for past and continuing discrimination. Programs such as Medicare and Medicaid, "senior discounts," and special services for "senior citizens" are examples of programs designed to redress shortcomings in society's treatment of older people as full citizens. Because we live in a youth-oriented society, older people often seem to have little importance. The young may have some guilt over this and therefore tend to be overly protective and patronizing. Such an attitude on your part toward an older patient will project a transparent insincerity that can be construed as disrespectful and annoying.

Aging as a Clinical Entity

This view of aging sets it apart from other life experiences shared by all human beings. Aging is seen as a clinical entity in its own right, something to be studied and analyzed through research. The subspecialties of "geriatrics" in health care and "gerontology" in the social sciences bear witness to the trend of separating out the unique features of aging. Although considerable positive developments have come from this view of aging, such as recognizing the special strengths of older patients as well as deficits, the risk remains that the aged will be treated differently from younger patients merely because they are old. An example of this can be found in a study of the recommendations medical students give to older (≥59 years) and younger (≤31 years) women regarding breast-conserving procedures. Although research has determined equivalent results between breast-conservation therapy and modified radical mastectomy, the medical students ($N = 116$) were biased by patients' ages when making recommendations. "They recommended breast-conservation therapy for a significantly higher percentage of younger patients than older patients (86% versus 66%)."[7] When age is inappropriately used to determine treatment options, it is a form of ageism. Fortunately, new theories of physical development show that some aspects of development can continue throughout the lifespan.

Older People as a Cultural Treasure

The most positive view of aging is to see people who have lived a long time as a source of wisdom and experience. Recent interest in obtaining oral histories from elders who have witnessed great and mundane historical events are evidence of this view. The past experience of the aged is of value to younger generations and fits well with Erikson's theory about the later stages of adult development.

NEEDS: RESPECT AND INTEGRITY

Several basic psychological and social processes are evident in the widely divergent lifestyles of today's older people. Erikson proposes that the success with which an older person can make psychological and social adjustments will depend on his or her ability to meet the most basic psychosocial developmental challenge of old age—that of integrity. In this last stage of human development, the person "understands, accepts, and loves the life he [or she] has led."[8] The

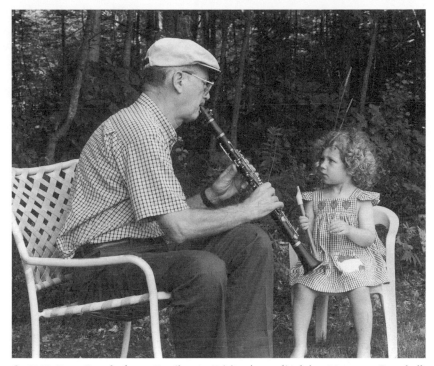

© 1995 Joan Beard, from *Family: A Celebration*, edited by Margaret Campbell, Peterson's (USA).

person "possesses wisdom" and is willing to share this wisdom with the younger generation.[9] The little girl and older man in the photograph perfectly illustrate this sharing of expertise across generations.

Health professionals are delighted, and sometimes awed, by an older person who expresses the breadth and depth of acceptance described by Erikson. These older people readily accept the psychological and social adjustments that confront them. However, some older persons despair of being old, the psychological and social adjustments of old age overwhelm them, and they find little from their past to support them in their present situation. Key psychological and social processes assist or deter older persons from achieving a sense of wholeness and integrity in old age. Some of these are discussed on the following pages.

The Psychology of Aging

One theory of aging, the disengagement theory, suggests that, even before their friends die, some people contribute to their own isolation. Cummings and

Henry, who first proposed this theory in the early 1960s, define disengagement as "an inevitable process in which many of the relationships between a person and other members of society are severed, and those remaining are altered in quality."[10] The central argument of the disengagement theory is that the severing of relationships is inevitable. They view disengagement as a normal process that occurs earlier for some than for others, depending on the person's physiology, temperament, personality, and life situation. Retirement, they propose, is society's permission for men to disengage, whereas widowhood serves the same purpose for women; the disengaged person eventually develops a high morale. Some of the postulates of the disengagement theory appear dated, such as the one regarding gender roles. Some critics questioned whether disengagement was a true indication of successful aging or desirable. Because Cummings and Henry's work was not based on longitudinally obtained data, there were questions regarding the developmental status of disengagement. However, even with all of its critics, the theory was one of the first attempts at a "grand theory" of aging and, as such, remains of interest to the field of gerontology.[11]

Subsequent studies and other theories present different views of the psychology of aging. Since the beginning of the 1980s, Baltes and colleagues have conducted a series of studies on psychological development from a life-span perspective. The central focus of this model of successful aging, called "selective optimization with compensation," is on the management of the dynamics between gains and losses.[12]

New theories of the psychology of aging, such as gerotranscendence (a shift in perspective from a materialistic and rational vision to a more cosmic and transcendent one) and gerodynamics/branching theory (based on general systems theory), have some of the components of past theories as well as novel ideas about the process of aging.[13, 14]

Recently, continuing active engagement with life has been identified as one of the manifestations of successful aging along with a low risk of disease and disease-related disability and a high level of physical and mental functioning.[15] This model of successful aging requires that older adults work to overcome the natural losses that occur with age. As you can see, there is still considerable disagreement about what counts as successful old age. Can you think of some problems that could occur clinically if you and a colleague differed in your definition of "good" old age?

Friendship and Family Ties

The amount of contact older people maintain with their families and friends varies greatly. Many persons lose a valuable source of natural physical contact and companionship with the diminution of friendship and family ties, whereas others remain actively integrated into family and community circles. If you take time to assess how much of a patient's need for physical contact is still being met by friends and family, you will understand a lot about their conduct during their time with you. It is not unusual for people to transfer their needs to health professionals once they have lost other contacts.

Friendships. Until the present ultramobile way of life in the United States, the acquisition of a single set of friends continued throughout early life and tapered off when one settled down in a community. One's job seldom changed during the entire period of employment, and, as a result, the community (and the friends therein) remained the same up through old age. In one sense, this is a secure mode of existence, but reliance on lifelong friendship carries with it the risk that, if these friends all die, the person will be left alone. Many people who have depended on lifelong friendships find it difficult to make new acquaintances at 70 or 80 years of age. Friendships have been demonstrated to influence a person's psychological well-being. An older person's attitudes toward friendships and the make-up of the physical environment play a role in the maintenance and development of friendships in old age.[16]

The older person's ability and desire to make new friends depend partly on the extent to which friendship has been considered an important individual value throughout life and therefore on the extent to which friendship skills have been cultivated. Another important determinant is the type of friendship the person established in younger years.

There are basically four types of friendship, which vary in number and importance over the years:

1. *Fusion* friendships, which are fused to other roles such as those involving family or occupation, increase or decrease in importance according to the person's present situation.

2. *Substitution* friendships are those into which the person channels energies that formerly were directed toward someone or something else.

3. *Complementary* friendships develop from situations in which another role (such as that related to occupation) and the friendship are mutually supportive.

4. *Competition* friendships are those that compete with another role.[17]

Therefore, an older person whose fusion or complementary friendship, made at an early age, centered on his or her occupation may find that after retirement the friend is very much alive but their friendship is dead. Conversely, a substitution or competition friendship may thrive after retirement because energy directed elsewhere can now be devoted to the friend. In this sense, the basis of a friendship is an important determinant of its longevity. In working with patients you can understand some important things by exploring who the person's friends are and how the friendships were generated and sustained.

Family. As we discussed in Chapter 14, the family structure is changing. Participation in that unit is one of the most lasting and significant roles a person assumes.

In married relationships or other long-term couple relationships the history is that the couple usually had an opportunity to spend much time alone together. When children become a part of the relationship, attention is transferred to them, and in many families much of the communication for many years takes place in the presence of at least one child. For persons with no children, jobs often become the center of attention. Only after the children have left home or the working years end is the couple alone again. Their attempts to reestablish direct communications are sometimes futile, causing them to withdraw, literally or symbolically, from the family. Other couples find this to be an opportunity to engage in activities together that they put off in their younger years.

In the present oldest population, those 85 years and older, there are many married or formerly married people. Older men are more likely to be married than older women are. You may work with elderly women who are not prepared to cope with financial and other business affairs because in their youth it was considered improper for women to be thus involved. You may work with elderly men who have never had to prepare a meal or wash clothes because it was considered improper for a man to do "woman's work." The death of a spouse can be extremely difficult for them. Sometimes they turn to children, nieces, or nephews for help. Elderly people often turn to siblings when they find themselves alone. A sibling has the added benefit of a shared history, as is evident in the following poem.

> Homecoming
> I
> after 45 years
> of writing letters
> & calling, Estelle sent word
> to find a contractor—
> she wants a home
> built next to her sister
> the house, brick & modern,
> is an oddity—
> sits prominently among shotgun houses,
> cows, chickens, fish ponds, bait shops
> & trailer homes
> Celeste walks the clay red road
> to her Oakland-California-sister—
> they have forty-five years to catch up on

II
Estelle & Celeste talk of the other two sisters
who died in their early 70s—
bring out boxes of black & white worn photos
Estelle rakes arthritic fingers
through Celeste's hair
conjuring memory
she parts the white/yellow-stained strands—
braids her sister's hair.[18]

A discussion of aging and family relationships must include a look at who is most likely to provide support for older people in times of illness. Social support systems for people who are ill include both informal systems (family and friends) and formal ones (community and social services). The informal support systems clearly are key for maximizing adjustment during old age and increasing overall well-being. As we discussed in Chapter 16, families provide the majority of care for older relatives. Many families struggle to provide this care as is evident in the following example.

> Dad may be desperately ill, demanding constant attention and unable to join the family and guests at dinner. Mom may be afflicted with Alzheimer's and can't follow a conversation. Grandma may be bedfast. And in as many cases as not, the woman of the house does the caretaking even though she is poor, busy with a job to stay above subsistence level, preoccupied with her own children, and untrained. In such circumstances—God forbid—there is no extra room for the ill or aged, and little patience or reason for hope.
>
> Caring in the home is still the great overlooked medical-social problem among all classes in the United States.[19]

It is no wonder then that this level of stress sometimes leads to elder abuse. Elder abuse can take several forms: (1) rights violations—such as denial of basic rights to adequate medical care or decent housing; (2) material abuse—defined as monetary or material theft; (3) physical abuse—which covers a variety of practices from omission (leaving a nonambulatory person in bed for long periods of time) to commission (beating or injuring the person); and (4) psychological abuse—a situation in which the person is debased and intimidated verbally.[20] Elder abuse is often not reported because the older person (or others) fear retaliation or believe that nothing will be done to change the situation. Just as with a child whom you suspect is being abused or neglected, you are legally responsible in all 50 states for reporting suspected elder abuse. It is important to add, unfortunately, that elder abuse is not isolated to the home setting. Elder abuse can occur in institutional settings as well such as domiciliary homes, nursing homes, day care, or even hospitals.

Where "Home" Is

A major challenge for older people is to decide where to make their home. Security, accessibility to services, transportation, and physical considerations due to bodily changes in aging are important variables. Reduced income and the desire to be near friends or relatives also often weigh heavily for people who have a choice of location. For about 4.3% of the older than 65 population in the United States, the nursing home becomes their last place of residence. This statistic can be somewhat deceiving if we look at a breakdown of nursing home residents in various cohorts of this population. Of people 65 to 74 years old, only 1.1% reside in nursing homes. About 4.5% of persons 75 to 84 years of age reside in nursing homes, but 19% of those 85 years of age and older do.[21] Primary reasons for admission to nursing homes include Alzheimer's disease and osteoporotic hip fractures.

Chapter 7 addresses how changes associated with illness are a challenge for any patient. You will benefit from bearing in mind that these same losses may have already occurred for the older person simply because he or she is old rather than because of illness or injury. The loss of a long-established place of residence, of consequence to anyone, is felt deeply by the older person because self-respect and the power to command the respect of others depend, in part, on independence. Although many patients experience the loss of independence as temporary, older people usually realize that each loss is a one-way street to more dependence. Moving out of one's home symbolizes dependence with a capital "D."

Each move of residence may have a greater significance for old people than for those of any other age group. For example, a woman who has been forced to move out of her long-established residence into her daughter's home and who then requires admission to the hospital for elective surgery that results in placement in a nursing home for rehabilitation certainly has grounds for feeling completely "undone" by the number of moves she has had to make in a short period of time. Thoughtful health professionals take these factors into consideration and are patient in helping the older person adapt accordingly. In fact, a key to respectful interaction with an older person is to promote as much stability in the place of residence as possible.

THE CHALLENGE OF CHANGES OF AGING

In the following section, some major losses described in Chapter 7 are discussed as they present themselves as challenges to many older people today.

Challenge to Former Self-Image

There is ample evidence to support that we have the potential to continue to develop throughout our lifespan, and our self-esteem can remain high or even grow stronger in older years. Some recognize talents they never knew they had or refocus their energies on other hobbies or projects. Consider the following poem and the primary values that guide each woman's daily activities.

Social Security

She knows a cashier who
blushes and lets her use
food stamps to buy tulip
bulbs and rose bushes.
We smile each morning as I
pass her—her hand always
married to some stick
or hoe, or rake.
One morning I shout,
"I'm not skinny like
you so I've gotta run
two miles each day."
She begs me closer, whispers
to my flesh, "All you need,
honey, is to be on welfare
and love roses."[22]

Some persons do not even notice the changes in how they look, seeing only what they want to see in the mirror. Unfortunately, other people cling not only to a former visual image, but begin to reject the changes brought about by aging. They see themselves as has-beens who are no longer valuable to society and cannot perform as they did in the past.

Retirement from a long-held job often poses a threat to self-image (and, subsequently, to self-esteem) in many older men and women. With almost all adults employed in the workforce at some time in their lives, more people than ever before will face the challenge of retirement. However, retirement is being postponed for many. In 1999, 12% of Americans aged 65 and older were in the labor force. (See the Bureau of Labor Statistics web site: www.dol.gov, Tables 3, 8, 15, and 31.) For most, retirement not only involves a substantial reduction in income but also signals a change in their daily activity. In a revealing study of 63-year-old workers from a variety of occupations in Sweden (where retirement is not a choice but required at 65 to 66 years of age), the soon-to-retire participants were more concerned about "doing" rather than identity after retirement.

As the person looks forward in time to retirement, a central issue becomes replacing time spent in work with other activity. Although work is only one part of the person's whole landscape of activities, it is a large part. The disappearance of work potentially leaves much of his or her landscape unfilled. At a minimum, retirement precipitates change in the person's whole activity pattern.[23]

To be sure, the amount of satisfaction a person has found in his or her work, the success or failure in achieving satisfying occupation in spheres outside of

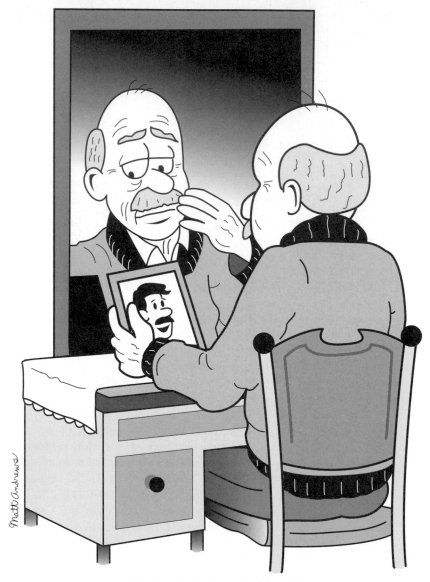

"... I haven't changed a bit ..."

work, along with a variety of other personal factors, will determine the significance of retirement.

To maintain their status as useful members of society, almost all old people need to be engaged in some kind of ongoing activity. This may be a job, a hobby, a volunteer service, or a club. Regardless of the activity chosen, they do need to have something to look forward to and to know that they are needed in a certain place at a certain time. However, there are some good reasons why many older people do not take advantage of activities that are available.

1. They may be shy about meeting new people, particularly if they have maintained one set of friends and acquaintances for many years.
2. They may be too physically ill to participate in ongoing activities.
3. They may have no way to get to them.
4. They may not be able to afford to go.
5. They may be afraid to go out at night or alone.

One or more of these reasons may also prevent them from seeking ongoing health care!

Fortunately, as the average age of our society grows, older people will become involved in continuous activities. For example, politics is one area in which the older-than-65 population has gained a powerful voice. Political involvement facilitates progress in legislation regarding their own interests and provides a broader perspective for legislation regarding society as a whole.

Physical Changes Characteristic of Aging

A high percentage of older people are remaining in good health longer than ever before. Perception is the process of making meaning out of experience, and largely depends on our sense organs. With aging the efficiency of both information gathering and making sense out of the information declines for most people. Visual changes include declines in acuity, speed of focusing, and accommodation in vision. With aging, adaptation to darkness usually declines too. Hearing losses are greatest in the high-frequency range. There is a steady loss in perception of body movement or kinesthesia. The older person may "adjust" to the losses gracefully. An example is an exchange that one of the authors had with her 92-year-old neighbor. As she walked into his living room, where the television announcer was blaring the Red Sox's latest play, she was surprised to see Tom planted in front of a blank screen. "Tom!" she shouted above the clamor, "There's no picture!"

"Picture tube went about a month ago!" he shouted back. "Can't see the screen anyway!" Tom, in spite of his good humor, would probably concede that the savings on the picture tube was not worth the price of failing eyesight. For people with sensory impairment, the start of each day must seem like, as Shakespeare put it, the "Last scene of all,/That ends this strange eventful history . . . /Sans teeth, sans eyes, sans taste, sans everything" (*As You Like It,* II, vii, 139). Your sensitivity to patients' feelings about this loss can have profound effects on the extent to which a patient feels respected by you.

Understandably, attention to a patient's sensitivity about such matters and attempts to help an older person with sensory deficits prepare for the day are critical components of showing respect.

We will not discuss musculoskeletal or neurological changes in the aging process because many health professionals learn these elsewhere. Posture, balance, strength, endurance, and other physical expressions of aging will vary, but overall wear and tear on the body will affect everyone in their later years. On the other hand, exercise has a positive impact on human beings of almost any age. Regular activity can reverse the decreased mobility that contributes to disease and disability in old age.[24] Furthermore, exercise has been shown to promote modest positive changes in cognitive functioning in the aged.[25] Given demonstrated improvements in so many areas, a prescription for activity seems indicated for most elderly patients.

One way of dealing with all of the physical changes that are a normal part of aging as well as those that accompany chronic and acute illness and injury is to share experiences with others who understand what the person is going through. A wonderful example of this can be found in the field study of older women in a neighborhood beauty shop by Furman. Because few of us get to interact with older people who are not related to us, this glimpse into the social life of elderly women is particularly enlightening.

> Customers exhibit a capacity for laughing at themselves, at their aches and pains, and at their intense engagement in such matters. For example, Blanche and Carmela, along with Claire, find themselves discussing various surgeries that they've had, stimulated by the fact that Blanche recently had cataract surgery. They first compare notes on that type of surgery; Blanche then talks about the hysterectomy she had years back, and so forth. Rather spontaneously, Blanche breaks into this discussion by saying, "Look at us, talking about cataracts, hysterectomies, hospitals!" They all laugh in this moment of self-recognition and amusement at themselves.[26]

Your sensitivity to changes, offering the person opportunities to talk about illness and loss and especially what changes mean for his or her feeling of well-being, is an avenue to respectful interaction, too.

Mental Changes Characteristic of Aging

In most respects, working with an older person is no different from working with a person of any other age. However, a few minor differences due to mental changes normative for all aging can enhance the health professional's success in working with older people.

All patients benefit from the security of a set schedule, and this may be especially true for many older persons. The security arises from the knowledge that, at least in this one small area, he or she is in control of the environment. Some older people continue to exercise complete control over the details of their existence, whereas others gradually lose this opportunity. Even if this control extends no further than the patient's telling the taxicab driver to hurry because he or she is scheduled to be in speech therapy in 13 minutes, that person's self-respect will have been bolstered by exercising this type of control.

More important, establishing a schedule may be a way of helping an older person maintain a proper orientation to the environment. Some institutional-ized older people become confused about the time of day and the date because they have few clues to orient them compared with the person who works 5 days a week or a peer who has more ongoing routine activity. But it is not that group alone. They will benefit from your thoughtfulness in this matter.

Besides setting a time, you can state the time limit of a certain treatment or test. For instance, if an apparently disoriented old man will be in the testing situation for ½ hour, he should be told this at the onset and at the end of the test. If he does not have a clock, one should be provided so that he can check the time in the interim.

An older person's sense of security, control, and orientation can be further enhanced if, in addition to being treated at the same time each day, the routine of the treatment or test is kept reasonably stable from one day to the next. If the treatment or testing situation varies significantly every day, the patient may feel that nothing about it is familiar; it may be an anxiety-producing experience every time the person reports to the health professional. Anxiety can greatly decrease the person's performance and have a detrimental effect on both the relationship with you and the patient's progress.

Establishing a routine does not imply that the treatment should be exactly the same each day. Monotony or boredom can be just as detrimental to the patient as anxiety. Rather, the ideal situation is a balance between the patient's need for stability and his or her continuing interest in life and need for stimulation.

INTERACTING WITH COGNITIVELY IMPAIRED OLDER PEOPLE

Cognitive impairment in the aged person can take many forms, and it is important that you study them in more depth than is appropriate to address in this book. We engage you in a general discussion about cognitive impairment and provide some general guidelines for respectful interaction with people suffering from brain syndromes that directly affect thought and speech processes.

Acute confusion or disorientation can be caused by a variety of factors, such as an infection, a fluid or electrolyte imbalance, or a cerebral vascular accident. It is important to determine the cause of confusion in an elderly patient and not just ascribe it to "being old." The following story illustrates how critical it is to understand the genesis of a change in mental status in an older patient.

> Family members brought an 81-year-old man, Abraham Steinman, who was in an acutely agitated and confused state, to the emergency depart-ment. The family stated that Mr. Steinman had gradually been getting more and more confused over the last few weeks and finally became

violently disturbed earlier in the evening. He was admitted to the adult psychiatric unit because he was physically violent to the staff in the emergency room. The distraught family said he had never had an emotional outburst in his life and could not understand his behavior. The next day a careful physical examination revealed that Mr. Steinman had bilateral pneumonia and some signs of kidney failure. His confusion and agitation had only been a symptom of his physical illness.

For such patients, acute confusion can be continual and may be increasingly profound, although you can help diminish the patient's suffering from disorientation at any given moment. Often, a useful approach is to not support the older person's constantly confused ideas, unless correcting them causes him or her to become violent, further disoriented, or deeply agitated. If an old man thinks he is in a hotel, you should try to correct him using a gentle reassuring voice and manner. If he confuses you with someone else, his mistake can be corrected by showing him your name badge and repeating your name. Chances are that he will be less frightened if the people around him are willing to help him clear up his mind, if only for a few minutes. It is a good general rule of respectful interaction to correct the person. However, you should also remember to listen with interest and politeness to the patient. Listening will help you to determine the depth of the confusion, ascertain the wisdom of trying to correct it, and, in some cases, discern that the patient is making sense within a context not immediately evident.

The seemingly confused person should be treated kindly. Such treatment should never be condescending, but it should reflect the gentle authority that gives the patient a sense of security. If the confusion is the result of a disease such as Alzheimer's disease or another form of dementia, many of the same principles apply. Some additional strategies for communicating with patients with dementia are as follows: use broad opening statements or questions, try to establish commonalties, speak to them as equals, and try to recognize themes in what the patient is trying to share with you.[27]

Sometimes medications can help the patient relax or in other ways be more comfortable, although with elderly patients it is best to be cautious with the use of drugs. Goals must be adapted according to what they can comprehend. Some patients may be unable to remember the simplest tasks from one testing or treatment period to the next and may never grasp the most elementary verbal instructions. Others, however, will be able to follow astonishingly complex procedures. It is your responsibility in such situations to approach each person as an individual and to not take for granted that all confused utterances are signs of organic brain changes. In some cases, the confusion will increase no matter what is done. However, none of these complications should deter you from first attempting, in a kind way, to correct the inaccuracies. With a great number of patients, this humane act is the key to respectful interaction.

ASSESSING A PATIENT'S VALUE SYSTEM

The mechanics of adjusting a hearing aid, setting a schedule, or correcting a confused-sounding statement must all be done in a way that supports the older person's value system. Otherwise, the person is reduced to nothing more than an object to be efficiently manipulated.

Chapter 1 listed some of the primary societal and personal values cherished by people in this society. Older people as a group can be expected to hold the same range and variety of values; no particular value can be ruled out automatically on the basis of age. However, the topics treated in this chapter can help you understand why so many older people adhere to some values more than others.

For instance, the primary good of self-respect will often be a more consciously prized value for older people because they perceive, correctly, that they are subject to loss of self-respect in an ageist society. Security, both financial and physical, may also be highly prized by older people because, again, for many of them the hold on it is more tenuous. Further, continued independent functioning is valued dearly when commitment to a nursing home is a threat or when activities that can be performed alone become increasingly limited. Listening for which values the older patient expresses as his or her most precious and then trying to set treatment goals accordingly will greatly enhance your success.

In working with older people, the most important challenge confronting you is resisting the tendency to stereotype them. Society's expectations of older people, many of which are inaccurate and outdated, are propagated through literature, television, and other popular media.

You can learn to appreciate individual differences among aged persons by increasing your contact with people who are older. Programs sponsored by churches, private organizations, and the government offer volunteer opportunities ranging from transportation to recreational activities to providing hot meals for home-bound persons. In some cities foster care facilities and other institutions where older persons live welcome young people who are interested in volunteering their services or visiting older people. Whether through volunteer services, organizations, or contact as a health professional, your challenge is to develop an acutely discriminating eye for individual differences.

SUMMARY

Care of older adults must be based on a sound understanding of the physiological and psychosocial aspects of aging. The major developmental tasks of old age are to find meaning and satisfaction with life as it becomes more and more difficult to keep up with everything that goes on in a busy world. The chief goal of care is to maintain and support the patient's self-esteem by affirming his or her strengths and discovering hidden resources. By keeping in mind a patient's emotional and social needs, you can help him or her retain dignity and self-respect. The secret to respectful interaction with older people is to keep their age-related problems in mind while concentrating on their individuality.

REFERENCES

1. Dyer, J.: *In a Tangled Wood: An Alzheimer's Journey.* Dallas, Southern Methodist University Press, 1996, p. 30.
2. Administration on Aging: *Profile of Older Americans: 2000.* Washington, DC, U.S. Department of Health and Human Services, 2000.
3. McConnell, E.S.: Conceptual bases for gerontological nursing practice: models, trends, and issues. In Matteson, E.S., McConnell, E.S., and Linton, A.D. (eds.): *Biological Theories of Aging in Gerontological Nursing: Concepts and Practice.* 2nd ed. Philadelphia, W.B. Saunders, 1996, pp. 3–73, quote p. 7.
4. Gadow, S.: Medicine, ethics and the elderly. *Gerontologist* 20(6):680–685, 1980.
5. Scitovsky, A.A.: The high cost of dying revisited. *Milbank Q.* 72(4):561–591, 1994.
6. Gadow, S: Medicine, ethics and the elderly. *Gerontologist* 20(6):680–685, 1980, quote p. 681.
7. Madan, A.K., Aliabadi-Wade, S., and Beech, D.J.: Ageism in medical students' treatment recommendations: the example of breast-conserving procedures. *Acad. Med.* 76(3):282–284, 2001, quote p. 283.
8. Erikson, E.H.: *Childhood and Society.* 2nd ed. New York, W.W. Norton, 1963.
9. Ibid.
10. Cummings, E., and Henry, W.E.: *Growing Old: The Process of Disengagement.* New York, Basic Books, 1961, p. 211.
11. Achenbaum, W.A., and Bengston, V.L.: Re-engaging the disengagement theory of aging: on the history and assessment of theory development in gerontology. *Gerontologist* 34(6):756–763, 1994.
12. Baltes, P.B., Reese, H.W., and Lipsitt, L.P.: Life-span developmental psychology. *Annu. Rev. Psychol.* 31:65–110, 1980.
13. Tornstam, L.: Gero-transcendence: a reformulation of the disengagement theory. *Aging (Milano)* 1:55–63, 1989.
14. Schroots, J.J.F.: Gerodynamics: toward a branching theory of aging. *Can. J. Aging* 14:74–81, 1995.
15. Rowe, J., and Kahn, R.: *Successful Aging.* New York, Pantheon, 1998.
16. McKee, K.J., Harrison, G., and Lee, K.: Activity, friendships and wellbeing in residential settings for older people. *Aging Ment. Health* 3(2):143–152, 1999.
17. Riley, M.W.: Friendship. In Riley, M.W. (ed.): *Aging and Society: A Sociology of Age Stratification.* Vol. 3. New York, Russell Sage Foundation, 1972, pp. 362–370.
18. Wren, A.M.: Homecoming (first appeared in *Afr. Am. Rev.* 27:1, 1993).
19. Marty, M.E.: The 'god-forbid' wing. *Park Ridge Center Bull.* 11(Sept/Oct):15, 1999.
20. Benton, D., and Marshall, C.: Elder abuse. *Clin. Geriatr. Med.* 7(4):831–845, 1991.
21. National Center for Health Statistics: An Overview of Nursing Home Facilities: Data from 1997 National Nursing Home Survey. Advance Data No. 311, March 1, 2000.

22. Bolz, B.: Social Security. In Martz, S. (ed.): *When I Am An Old Woman I Shall Wear Purple*, Watsonville, CA, Papier Mache Press, 1991, p. 127.
23. Jonsson, H., Kielhofner, G., and Borell, L.: Anticipating retirement: the formation of narrative concerning an occupational transition. *Am. J. Occup. Ther.* 51(1):49–56, 1997, quote p. 55.
24. Buckwalter, J.A., and DiNubile, N.A.: Decreased mobility in the elderly: the exercise antidote. *Physician Sportsmed.* 25(9):126–128, 130–133, 153–155, 1997.
25. Van Sickle, T.D., Hersen, M., Simco, E.R., Melton, M.A., and Van Hasselt, V.B.: Effects of physical exercise on cognitive functioning in the elderly. *Int. J. Rehabil. Health* 2(2):67–100, 1996.
26. Furman, F.K.: *Facing the Mirror: Older Women and Beauty Shop Culture.* New York, Routledge Press, 1997, p. 31.
27. Tappen, R.M., Williams-Burgess, C., Edelstein, J., Touhy, T., and Fishman, S.: Communicating with individuals with Alzheimer's disease: examination of recommended strategies. *Arch. Psychiatr. Nurs.* 11(5):249–256, 1997.

PART SIX

Questions for Thought and Discussion

1. An alert 92-year-old patient who has been in your care for several days arrives late for treatment one morning at your ambulatory care clinic. She explains that she missed her usual bus and had to wait in the rain and cold for the next bus to arrive. You begin to converse with her in your usual manner and very quickly realize that something is wrong; she does not answer your questions appropriately. Once or twice, she mentions her son (who, you know, was killed years ago in the service of his country), but her sentences are disconnected and incomplete.
   a. What possible reasons may there be for her apparent confusion?
   b. Where will you start in your attempt to diagnose her problem?

2. You are hurrying down the hospital corridor when you notice an acquaintance of the family, a bricklayer in his middle forties. You express surprise at seeing him there because he has always been the picture of good health. He tells you that he has had a heart attack. Suddenly he begins to pour out a blow-by-blow description of the incident. As he talks, he becomes increasingly agitated and finally bursts into tears, sobbing, "It's all over. I'll never be able to go back to my job or anything. What am I going to do?"
   a. What can you say or do right then to calm this man's immediate anxious state?
   b. Will you report this incident? To whom and why?

c. How can health professionals work together to treat the middle-aged person's anxiety about the long-term effects of illness on family, job, and self-esteem?

3. What do you dread most about growing old? What do you look forward to most? How do you think an older person's role will have changed by the time you grow old?

4. You are the supervisor of an adolescent unit in a hospital. The patient, a 16-year-old named Sam, is very mature for his age, and you have found him to be very thoughtful. Sam has cancer that you know has metastasized. His parents have decided with the surgeon that he should have an amputation, although all agree that the hope of saving him completely from the spread of the disease is negligible. One evening you notice that Sam is very withdrawn. He says, "My parents and the doctor are going to cut off my leg and they haven't even asked me what *I* think about it. I'd rather die than lose my leg."
a. What should you do?
b. To whom should you speak about this conversation? Why?

5. If you were asked to propose policies and plans for a family waiting area for a high-risk newborn unit in your institution, what would you suggest to the architects, decorators, and administrators? Why? What sorts of support services would you recommend for families in this situation?

PART SEVEN

Some Special Challenges

In this last section of the book we explore with you some special challenges you will face in your attempt to show respect for patients and their families during your interactions with them. We address two broad, diverse topics: patients who are dying and some other situations that we perceive as especially difficult for health professionals.

Human beings' understanding of dying and death is shrouded in mystery and, today, punctuated by our exposure to violence in the media and in our personal lives. Death rarely is portrayed as "natural." Persons whose lives are threatened by accident, injury, or illness may bring specific fears to the health professional and patient relationship—fears shaped by their personal experience and stereotypes. These responses and others by patients and their families are examined. We emphasize priorities that health professionals should set for such patients to show them the respect they deserve.

In the final chapter, Chapter 19, you have an opportunity to examine some situations that many health professionals identify as difficult. Now that you have read about and thought about different types of patients and situations, you have a better basis for thinking about disparities of power or status in the health professional and patient relationship and how role expectations may affect these interactions. You probably will be able to identify, too, why some patients are perceived as "difficult." In each of the examples our goal is for you to think expansively about your potential for respectful interaction in even the most challenging moments of your life as a health professional.

Chapter 18

Respectful Interaction When the Patient Is Dying

CHAPTER OBJECTIVES

The student will be able to

- Discuss the dying-death relationship and some sources of our understanding about dying and death
- Discuss denial in regard to its effects on respectful interaction
- Name four fears of dying that many persons experience
- List several factors that have a bearing on a patient's response upon learning that he or she has a terminal illness
- Describe six methods by which, according to historian Arnold Toynbee, humans have sought immortality, and discuss the importance of knowing these methods when trying to show respect for a patient
- Explain several areas of consideration in setting treatment priorities when a patient is dying
- Discuss ways to help maintain hope when a patient's condition is irreversible and will result in death
- Identify some important changes in focus that health professionals should seek when a patient is near death

---

The newspaper near his chair has a photo of a Boston baseball player who is smiling after pitching a shutout. Of all the diseases, I think to myself, Morrie gets one named after an athlete.

You remember Lou Gehrig, I ask?

"I remember him in the stadium, saying good-bye."

So you remember the famous line.

"Which one?"

Come on. Lou Gehrig. "Pride of the Yankees"? The speech that echoes over the loudspeakers?

"Remind me," Morrie says. "Do the speech."

Through the open window I hear the sound of a garbage truck. Although it is hot, Morrie is wearing long sleeves, with a blanket over his legs, his skin pale. The disease owns him.

I raise my voice and do the Gehrig imitation, where the words bounce off the stadium walls: "Too-dayyy . . . I feeel like . . . the luckiest maaaan . . . on the face of the earth . . . ."

Morrie closes his eyes and nods slowly.

"Yeah. Well. I didn't say that."

Tuesdays with Morrie[1]

This excerpt is from a book titled *Tuesdays with Morrie,* which chronicles the last months of a man's dying as it is recorded through the pen of his friend and former student. Here you catch them in one of their many exchanges, the young man trying to make conversation and the dying one bringing the narrative back to the heart of the matter—his own unique experience of dying. Of all the challenges you will face, your work with people who are dying will provide some of the greatest opportunities to use your skills as a professional.

"Terminally ill" is a term that is commonly used to describe people who are dying from a pathologic cause. Like all labels, it allows people in this group to be identified easily according to their special needs. At the same time, we refrain from using it in this chapter in large part because it is like a double-edged sword: it can further remove dying persons from others' caring by the fact that they belong to a group that carries many negative assumptions with it. One difficulty with the term is its generality. Persons such as Morrie, who suffered from amyotrophic lateral sclerosis (commonly known as "Lou Gehrig's disease"), may live for many months or years. Another person with a different condition may die within days or weeks. Still, both are labeled terminally ill. Many health professionals, as well as others, immediately place both people on the "critical list." One of the authors remembers a friend who had lived for more than 10 years with a malignant lymphoma. He went into the hospital for his periodic blood test. A health professional who had come back to work after a 5-year hiatus greeted him cheerfully, "Are *you* still around?" She was apparently astonished that this "terminally ill" patient had not died long ago! The patient recalled that although he knew her intentions were good, her greeting led to the most severe depression of his entire illness. As with all types of patients, the key is to look for the distinguishing factors that make this person's situation unique, and respond respectfully to the needs that arise out of that individual person's experience. And toward achieving that goal, a first step toward any health professional's understanding of a patient's situation is to gain some general idea of how death and dying are viewed within the larger society.

DYING AND DEATH IN MODERN SOCIETY

Children's experiences of dying and death have been studied in detail, highlighting some important differences in their understanding of and responses to dying and death compared with those of adults. We encourage you to acquaint yourself with these differences. However, we do not have the space to discuss them in detail here and therefore focus on patients who are past childhood.

Dying is first and foremost a personal event. Although individuals respond differently to it, one common thread shared by all is that they are going through a *process*. In addition, all persons share some awareness that the end of the dying process is the death event. What does this mean to a person? In the minds of many patients or their families you will meet, a known diagnosis and somewhat predictable range of symptoms make them feel robbed of the "natural" flow of life. The dying process feels unnatural, an imposition. A life-threatening condition generates new fears and concerns. Fortunately, for others it is also an opportunity to do some long-neglected business, put one's affairs in order, or pursue a postponed adventure, engendering new types of hope. Anticipation of the death event, too, creates its own concerns, fears, and hopes, many of which are rooted in religious and philosophical understandings of life and death. For most people death remains perhaps the ultimate mystery.

How *do* we gain an understanding of death?

In almost all cultures, death stories are an integral part of the stories passed down from childhood onward. They are the "great" stories, the material of the myths, in a culture. Notice the role death plays in snuffing out an enemy (but not the "good guys") in the following popular Western fairy tales:

> Down climbed Jack as fast as he could, and down climbed the giant after him, but he couldn't catch him. Jack reached the bottom first, and shouted out to his mother, who was at the cottage door. "Mother! Mother! Bring me an axe! Make haste, Mother!" For he knew there was not a moment to spare. However, he was just in time. Jack seized the hatchet and chopped through the beanstalk close to the root; the giant fell headlong into the garden, and was killed on the spot.
>
> So all ended well. . . .[2]

> Then Grethel gave her a push, so that she fell right in, and then shutting the iron door she bolted it. Oh how horribly she howled! But Grethel ran away, and left the ungodly witch to burn to ashes.
>
> Now she ran to Hansel, and opening his door, called out, "Hansel, we are saved; the old witch is dead!"[3]

Many Western childhood portrayals of the life-dying-death continuum show no connection between the two. (A notable exception is the childhood book *Wind in the Willows*, which some of you will have read or may now read to your own children.)

Both the health professional and patient may share beliefs about the "unnaturalness" of death rooted in many Western childhood stories. One of the most difficult misconceptions to correct is the belief that the patient's life-threatening condition is an enemy that always can be conquered if you, the health professional, try hard enough and if the patient is a good enough person (i.e., not the bad giant or witch).[4]

Of course, not all cultures have the same understanding of life and death. How might your relationship with a patient be different if, say, he or she grew up with the deep memory of this childhood story recounted by Mitch Albom, the author of *Tuesdays with Morrie* (whose conversations with his dying friend led him to read about how different cultures view death):

> There is a tribe in the North American Arctic, for example, who believe that all things on earth have a soul that exists in a miniature form of the body that holds it—so that a deer has a tiny deer inside it, and a man has a tiny man inside him. When the large being dies, that tiny form lives on. It can slide into something being born nearby, or it can go to a temporary resting place in the sky, in the belly of a great feminine spirit, where it waits until the moon can send it back to earth.
>
> Sometimes, they say, the moon is so busy with the new soul of the world that it disappears from the sky. That is why we have moonless nights. But in the end, the moon always returns. As do we all. . . .[5]

As you can begin to discern, in today's great mix of patients you will encounter, it is an important first step to try to gain some understanding of how death is viewed by what each of them learned from childhood stories and images. It will give you a starting place for your further deliberation about how to respect what they say, how they behave, and what their attitudes are toward various aspects of their interaction with you and others during their dying process. Having considered that, let us turn to additional insights that will help guide you in this situation.

Dying: Denial and Beyond Denial

It is often said that Western societies are death-denying. What can that possibly mean when all around us people are dying every day from illness, accidents, violence, old age, war, and other causes? Probably the best explanation is that although there is evidence everywhere of our mortality, we do our best to hold the inevitable at arm's length.

In many parts of Western culture, treatment of the dead body is one expression of a desire to deny death. The dead body is painted and dressed to make it appear alive, although a sign of life, such as a sigh or fluttering eyelash, would cause most people to rush screaming from the room. For the most part, however, denial has simply become more subtle. For example, a subtle denial of death is manifested in the incredible scenes of violence and killing viewed in films and on television as the line drawing on the next page illustrates. Even young children are exposed: they see the culprit killed but know that the same culprit will be on next week's show, having adventures in dangerous places.

To the viewer, death must seem a very exciting and not very permanent condition. Another demonstration of this denial is illustrated by the response of many people to the AIDS epidemic. Although it affects all population groups, AIDS is still often treated as a disease confined to small target groups in society: a "them but not us" perception of who could die from AIDS.

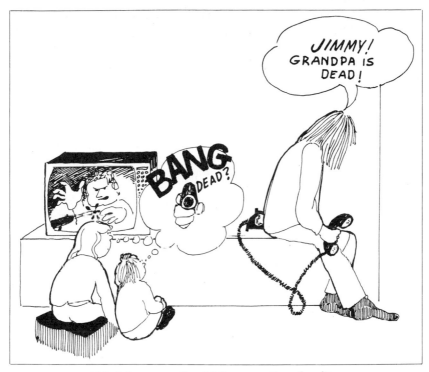

TV's influence on the child's perception of reality.

From the Swedish translation of *HPPI: Vård, Vårdare, Vårdad*, p. 242.

There are some positive dimensions of the denial of death for the person who is dying and for her or his family. The function of denial and its limitations are expressed well by a woman examining her own experience of having lung cancer:

> Our fear of death makes it essential to maintain a distance between ourselves and anyone who is threatened by death. Denying our connection to the precariousness of others' lives is a way of pretending that we are immortal. We need this deception—it is one of the ways we stay sane—but we also need to be prepared for the times when it doesn't work. For doctors, who confront death when they go to work in the morning as routinely as other people deal with balance sheets and computer printouts, and for me, to whom a chest x-ray or a blood test will never again be a simple, routine procedure, it is particularly important to face the fact of death squarely, to talk about it with one another.[6]

Cancer connects us to one another because having cancer is an embodiment of the existential paradox that we all experience; we feel that we are immortal, yet we know that we will die. To Tolstoy's Ivan Ilyich, the syllogism he had learned as a child, " 'Caius is a man, men are mortal therefore Caius is mortal,' had always seemed . . . correct as applied to Caius but certainly not as applied to himself." Like Ivan Ilyich, we all construct an elaborate set of defense mechanisms to separate ourselves from Caius. To anyone who has had cancer, these defense mechanisms become talismans that we invest with a kind of magic. These talismans are essential to our sanity, and yet they need to be examined.

Health professionals often are pivotal in determining how families will cope with a loved one's dying. Attentiveness to their need to deny the impending death or some aspects of it for a time can help them adjust to the momentous reality. At the same time, the following story of Beth Rice illustrates how we may unwittingly encourage a family's unhealthy, prolonged denial:

> When Beth Rice, a woman with AIDS, began to experience discomfort from her symptoms, the health professional advised her husband, "Better bring her to the hospital, where she can get better care!" Beth was admitted to the hospital, but, despite the best of care, the disease continued to run its debilitating course. The doctor then sent the patient to the intensive care unit, where she could get constant attention.
>
> In the intensive care unit, rehabilitation services were discontinued, and intensive care was implemented. Adult visitors were allowed to be with her for only a few minutes at a time. The nurses were kind, but firm, in restricting the family's visits. Eventually, the son and husband began to come less often, explaining to each other, "It's better for her, for there's really nothing more we can do for her, and she needs her rest." In addition, her two grandchildren were kept from her, as is the case in most intensive care settings. The adults rationalized this, too, saying, "It's better for them to be protected from this pathetic sight." When finally Beth lapsed into unconsciousness, the family realized that they had missed an opportunity to say good-bye to her as well as to fully admit how close to death she was.

All this was done by well-meaning, loving, grieving people who could not cope with the growing reality of death and who believed that they were doing what was most helpful for Beth. The institutional barriers they faced further encouraged—and at times required—them to seriously restrict their time with their loved one. What should have been done differently—by the families and by the institution? Often, families need assistance in figuring out what is going on and what they can do to support their loved one and each other.

Moving beyond denial toward a greater understanding is possible for many people, patients and family alike. One key is for them to become more familiar with their own feelings about and understanding of the death event itself. Three hundred years ago Jeremy Taylor suspected as much when he said, "In order to die well, look for death. Every day knock at the gates of the grave, then the grave cannot do you a mystery."[7] For many, however, knocking at those gates gives rise to fears and other responses associated with both dying and death.

RESPONSES ASSOCIATED WITH DYING AND DEATH

Because nearly all of us dread the thought of gradual and certain loss, the news of a life-threatening diagnosis is almost always disquieting. In the next section you have an opportunity to think about three of the most common fears, followed by some other responses patients and families may have.

Fears of Dying

What would be your biggest fears if you learned that you were dying? Most people can vaguely imagine what they would dread most; once the diagnosis is made, however, harsh reality intrudes and forces them to become acutely aware of their real fears. A patient's previous notions about the particular disease and the known experiences of others who have had the disease combine to create a vivid picture of what the patient believes to be ahead and gives rise to fears. The following are some of the most commonly expressed ones:

Fear of Isolation. The fear of separation from loved ones is often realized. The story of Beth Rice, who was first admitted to a hospital and then moved to the intensive care unit, is not uncommon.

Many persons are aware of the practice of being admitted to the hospital to die or of having to spend the final period of their lives in a care facility. It is not unusual for patients who have had several admissions to the hospital during a lengthy illness to announce during one of them that they will never leave the hospital again and often they are right. This awareness alters their response to those around them long before the final separation from life is imminent.

You will understand a patient better if you recognize that her or his anxiety about being abandoned by both family and health professional may be acute. The fear may be shown in complaints such as the following: "They are starting to ignore me"; "My family is busy with other things"; "The nurses skipped my medication this morning, so they probably are giving up on me"; "They spend more time with the woman in the next bed, but of course they know I'm dying." This worry about being abandoned when facing the greatest, or at least the final, event of physical life can be your cue to lend some extra support and encouragement. You can personally do little things to help the person gain greater self-understanding, even though the person cannot repay you with renewed functioning. If the person's friends and relatives are withdrawing, you can contact the institution's chaplain, social worker, or volunteer. These team members can help maintain a supportive atmosphere for a patient, and because they are institutional resources, they should be summoned without hesitation.

Fear of Pain. Fear of pain is also common in patients who are dying. Those who have known others who experienced a distressful end to life cannot be sure that their own dying will not be equally painful or worse. Fortunately, modern medicine has the potential to nearly obliterate the physical pain of dying, and hospice arrangements are explicitly designed to emphasize effective pain management. You should be mindful that, even in those patients who have persistent pain, the patient's suffering may be decreased by your compassion and caring. Also, it is well documented that the experience of physical pain is influenced negatively or positively by psychological states. For example, anxiety and depression have a heightened effect on pain, whereas distraction and feelings of security tend to diminish the suffering associated with pain.[8]

Fear of Dependence. In previous chapters fear of the loss of independence during illness, injury, and old age is examined. The attention given to these issues should signify the importance of continued independence when the person is in the process of dying. With rare exceptions, such people face certain and increasing dependence. Proof that they have thought about this is shown in their expressions of astonishment at having reached a point in their symptoms they had previously felt would be totally unbearable. Indeed, everyone has ideas of what he or she believes to be the "outer limits": loss of bowel and bladder control; sexual impotence; inability to feed oneself, to communicate verbally, or to think straight; unconsciousness; or other loss. Awareness of your own worries about dependence in some area of functioning will make you better able to understand your responses to what is happening to a patient.

Some health professionals also have to deal with their own feelings of pity toward a patient's plight. A student said to one of the authors about a patient he was treating, "I think I'm able to accept his blindness and the fact that he can't talk anymore, but what gets me is that no matter what I do for him he is going to get worse and worse and finally die. I feel so sorry for him that I can hardly stand to go into the room." Although feelings of pity are not uncommon for health professionals in this setting, they must be dealt with wisely.

What can you do when that happens? You were introduced to some alternatives in Chapter 12 when you were considering some detrimental consequences that can occur when pity takes over. For instance, some health professionals have to ask a colleague to assume responsibility for a patient because they find a patient's condition so horrendous that their effectiveness is hindered. Usually, such a radical measure is unnecessary, but it may be the best alternative in this difficult situation.

Patients' fears of isolation, pain, and dependence are basic, but there are other fears as well, such as the dread of suffocation and the fear that one's loved ones will not be adequately provided for. A person who dies suddenly in a car accident or plane crash or from a myocardial infarction may have long harbored these fears, but did not have a period of prolonged illness during which these fears surfaced. In the case of a long and progressively debilitating condition, sometimes the fears can be attended to. For instance, a man who has had trouble openly expressing affection to his wife may be able to do so by sharing his fear that she will not be adequately provided for. An indirect means of communication, such as writing a letter or telling a friend how wonderful she is, serves a similar purpose. You can be instrumental in making suggestions to help such a patient carry out her or his wishes if you get a hint that the patient desires to do so.

In summary, during their dying process, people must rely on their own best inner resources and the support of family, friends, and health professionals to sustain them as they face their fears. Any hesitance, embarrassment, or disdain you show when a person expresses a fear will exacerbate the suffering associated with it.

Fear of Death Itself

Why are we so afraid of the death event? Not everyone is, of course, and different cultures treat the moment of transition from alive to dead differently, but for many it is not something to relish. There are many possible reasons why a person might dread being "dead and gone": separation from loved ones, unfinished business, concern for the welfare of those left behind, the fear of being totally alone in some other world or other uncertainties about what comes after death, and the dread of annihilation, to name a few.

Probably for many people the greatest fear arises from the uncertainty of death. It is not what we know but what we do not know that scares us. The mystery of death baffles us all, and we are left groping for meaning beyond that provided by our own knowledge and experience.

Death and Immortality. The majority of people are taught that after this life there is something else. But that assumption is by no means held by everyone, including many who are religious. The varieties of religious beliefs are many, and there are wide variations in interpretation of the relationship of this life to the next, as well as of the meaning of illness and suffering when a person is faced with a condition that threatens to end physical life as he or she knows it.[9] In his now classic work, historian Arnold Toynbee traces, from a historical perspective, the ways in which people have tried to circumvent the finality of death and achieve immortality.[10] These ways include the following:

1. *Physical countermeasures.* Physical life is prolonged by providing the corpse with food and drink, and, in some cultures, even wives when a man died. This practice was common in ancient times and still exists in some parts of the world.

2. *Fame.* The dead person's image is preserved in poetry or inscription. War monuments, memorial rolls, and names inscribed in tree trunks are all examples. Plato encouraged his followers to achieve immortality through the fame of heroic deeds or scholarly pursuit as well as through procreation.

3. *Procreation.* Immortality is achieved through one's offspring. An example of this is illustrated in James Agee's novel *A Death in the Family*. When Jay Follet

is killed, one sees him emerging again in the person of his son Rufus. In a sense, Jay is reborn in his son. The possibility of procreation beyond one's own lifetime is now possible with the availability of sperm banks and banks for storing fertilized ova ("pre-embryos"). Cloning, although still experimental, produces genetically identical offspring to succeed the parent.

4. *Passing down one's treasures.* Family heirlooms including monetary trusts are constant reminders of their original owners, just as works of art such as paintings or books are reminders of their creators. Inanimate objects are the means of immortalizing a person.

5. *Submersion in ultimate reality.* Predominant beliefs in many religions, especially but by no means only those associated with Eastern religions such as Hinduism, propose that "death" is a process of birth and rebirth (e.g., reincarnation). The last step is not extinction but perfection, at which time one is absorbed into a "place" or into a "being" where complete unity of all beings is realized. Depending on the religion, the type of being one will become after humanhood and the opportunity for the final step into ultimate unity may or may not depend on the type of life one lived on earth during the human "phase." In Islam one may be transported through several levels of paradise depending on the type of life one lived.

6. *Resurrection of individuals.* Some people believe in the resurrection of souls only, whereas others believe that the actual human body will be restored. Most forms of Christianity believe in a literal, sudden bodily "resurrection" (sometimes referred to as the "rapture"), in which those—both dead and still living—who have lived holy lives will be immediately transported to heaven while others will be left behind forever to suffer the consequences of their sins. Other Christians have different versions of what it means to be "resurrected," although all share this basic belief.

Toynbee's six categories are useful for thinking about basic positions, but many groups (as well as individuals) combine aspects of these immortality-producing activities and beliefs. Recall the Arctic tribal belief (cited earlier in this chapter) that when a living being dies its miniature self finds another kind of being in which to reside, including a place to rest while awaiting where to go next. The Ho-Chunk peoples (now known as the Winnebago tribe—made up of the Iowa, Oto, Missouri, and central Algonquian Indians residing in the Midwestern states) believe that by living a clean life and enduring inevitable suffering, death will come but they will be reincarnated and eventually reach Heaven as a reward for their self-sacrifice on earth.[11]

You will meet individuals who talk with anticipation about "going to meet the Lord" while at the same time wanting to meet with their lawyer to be sure the bequest of their earthly belongings is in order. Knowing that any of these beliefs about immortality may influence the way an individual interprets the impact and meaning of his or her own impending death, you can be better prepared for comments from the patients or for rituals a patient and family engage in during the dying process. Go back over the six categories and try to think about conversations you have had with patients or families who held each of these positions.

Death as the End. A significant number of people in today's society do not view death as a precursor of immortality in any form. This view finds artistic expression in Tom Stoppard's play *Rosencrantz and Guildenstern Are Dead.* The two attendants, who believe through most of the play that they are accompanying Prince Hamlet to his death in Denmark, find out that, instead, they are going to be put to death. One of them reflects:

> Death isn't romantic, death is not anything.... Death is...not. It's the absence of presence, nothing more...the endless time of never coming back...a gap you can't see.[12]

From this standpoint, you could interpret a patient's fear of death as his or her dread of separation from things he or she values or wants to be around to experience: family, springtime, a growing bank account. There may be regret over not being able to reach a special anniversary or not knowing who will win the Super Bowl this year. To this person, death is viewed as an infringement on the deep wish for continued life, or "being." Try to construct a conversation you might have with a patient or family who does not believe in immortality. What themes are the most apparent?

All of these concepts about death can help you understand patients and their families when they share their feelings and ideas about death and how to prepare for it. When you can enter into such conversations with equanimity and express genuine interest in what the person wants or needs to say about death, you will be showing genuine respect for that person. Some specific methods are presented later in this chapter, but having now discussed basic sources of fear about dying that patients, families, and you and your colleagues may have, as well as common interpretations of the death event, let us turn to some other important responses besides fear.

Other Responses

What happens when a person learns that he or she has a condition from which death will result? As already noted, fears associated with dying and the death event may become more sharply focused. However, there are obviously other responses you can anticipate as well. For many, the first response is acute shock or grief, followed very quickly by denial. Some people die in denial, and others pretend to because they are afraid those around them would be too upset if the truth were known. For instance, a husband or wife might play out a game of deception to the end because each is convinced that the other would not be able to stand the shock of the information.

What happens to the person who finally cannot or does not want to deny it any longer? Such people may have some or all of the following other responses: depression, anger and hostility, bargaining behavior, or acceptance. In the 1960s, Elisabeth Kübler-Ross, a psychiatrist, introduced these responses as sequential "stages of dying"—a framework that has deeply influenced the approach taken by health professionals to dying patients in the subsequent years.[13] Today they are more generally viewed as a useful *range* of emotional-psychological responses a person may have rather than as sequential stages. Patients who go through a long process of dying are likely to feel all of these responses from time to time, and many times over. On one day, a woman denies her impending death; on another, she makes secret bargains with God about how long she can live; and on the following day, she feels the relief of acceptance, followed by a deep depression, and so on. Although the danger with any such framework is that you or your professional colleagues may tend to pigeonhole a patient according to the categories provided, we have found them to be a useful set of tools for thinking about what is happening to a person. The patient's basic personality structure before the present moment is an important factor in determining which kind of responses will predominate, too. How did the person deal with stress before learning that he or she had a life-threatening condition? Similar coping responses will probably surface in the present situation.

To further prepare yourself for working with such patients we suggest you pause here to engage in a reflection on your own life. Try to think about how you respond to stress. Can you imagine what you might be like as a patient or family member faced with the challenge of a dying loved one? If you have in fact had to face it, try to remember your overall types of responses. Another resource you can use was mentioned in Chapter 9, in which we highlighted how useful the writings of novelists, poets, essayists, and others can be. Many have recorded their experiences in this powerful situation, and it is to your advantage to avail yourself of these narrative accounts in preparation for your professional encounters with people who are dying.

Responses of the Patient's Family

The best and worst aspects of all family relationships are exposed when a family member is ill or dying. You will witness lifelong destructive patterns and the most intimate, loving characteristics of family relationships. The great majority of families are brought closer together by the experience, and their mutual support during this time is touching to observe. Despite this, for some health professionals, the members of the patient's family are viewed as intruders to be tolerated rather than as important people to be included. The experienced health professional knows that the family's presence may complicate the situation. At all hours of the day and night, they may ask questions, peek in on the patient, disrupt schedules, and aggressively offer suggestions. If the patient has not been told of the life-threatening nature of the condition, they whisper to you in doorways, trying to involve you in elaborate schemes to ensure continued deception. At the busiest time of day, they may stop you to tell you something, only to burst into tears.

Why is it important for them to be there? First, it is an absolutely critical means of coping with their own grief. Toynbee, at the age of 79, could reflect on the sadness he experienced when his wife died, and he gave this insight: "That is, as I see it, the capital fact about the relationship between living and dying. There are two parties to the suffering that death inflicts; and in the apportionment of that suffering, the survivor takes the brunt."[14] Regardless of whether Toynbee overstates the point, being in the presence of a loved one who is dying usually is comforting to the family. The astute health professional recognizes the agony the family experiences in anticipation of the loss of their loved one. The family sometimes goes through a series of reactions called "anticipatory grief" that parallels the symptoms usually seen in the acute grief that follows a death. You can watch for symptoms of acute grief such as the family member's tendency to sigh, complaints of chronic weakness or exhaustion, and loss of appetite or nausea. In addition, a family member may be preoccupied with what a person looks like, express guilt or hostility, and change his or her usual patterns of conduct.[15] As a result, the family's behavior in the presence of their loved one may appear altogether inappropriate for the welfare of the patient.

Except in extreme situations, family members should be an *integral* part of the treatment approach because the family is often a vital component of effective care. Family members not only need comfort but also provide it, they need to receive communications about the patient's status but often are also the best source of information, and they need to do their own grieving but can assist both the health professional and the patient in theirs as well. Sharing decision-making power with the patient and the family is one way of helping them to maintain their dignity.

SETTING TREATMENT PRIORITIES

There are several areas of consideration in setting treatment priorities when a patient is dying. First, what does the patient want and need to know?

Information Sharing

Traditionally it was considered unwise and uncompassionate to tell a person that he or she had a condition that appeared to be life threatening. The conviction was that a patient would give up hope. For the most part today in the United States, Canada, and many European countries, medical policies and practices take the position that a patient should be told of his or her diagnosis because the patient has a right to information about his or her health status. There is also a conviction that the duty not to harm is best realized by disclosure—the truth "sets free." The health professional's duty to protect the patient has been challenged by the idea that patients ought to assume more responsibility in the relationship, and to do so they must have all the necessary facts. In support of this, some states in the United States have passed laws that allow a patient to read the notations on his or her own medical record while other states permit the patient's lawyer to do so. Overall, the trend toward immediate access to formerly inaccessible information may eventually eliminate the question of whether or not a patient "ought to be told."

This trend toward openness is by no means shared universally or even by many of the cultures within the changing United States, Canadian, and Western European populations. At the very least, you must be attentive to clues you are receiving from the patient and family as to whether directly sharing this information with the patient is a culturally competent way to proceed. There may be an official spokesperson who should handle the situation, with or without your presence. Or other cultural norms may govern the way you will best be able to meet the intent of empowering and providing comfort to a patient through your honesty.

One consideration is the belief by many who advocate sharing the information that patients will find out anyway. For example, in *Endings and Beginnings,* a young woman's account of her husband's terminal diagnosis and eventual death, the author recalls that after exploratory surgery the doctor tried to be reassuring by saying they had found a "lymphatic tumor" but did not go on to tell them that it was an aggressive, life-threatening malignancy. In fact, that evening her husband reassures her that, since it was "lymphatic," it at least was not cancer. Their reassurance was short lived:

> That evening, as I left the hospital elevator . . . I was startled to have the head resident under Dr. C (the surgeon) turn to me and say, "Try not to worry; we'll do everything we can." It was clear there was much more going on than any of us was admitting.[16]

After that encounter the young couple spent many days trying to verify the simple truth, that in fact he had something that was very serious. In reflecting on the whole course of his dying, the author remembers that period as one of the most painful for both of them.

Do patients know? Probably some do and some do not. Whatever combination of considerations make up the physician's decision, many physicians are now telling patients with life-threatening conditions their diagnoses, usually in direct terms with emphasis on keeping communication channels open after the initial discussion.[17] In the end, there is no substitute for personalized, sensitive communication by all members of the health care team, initially and throughout the patient's course of interaction with them. Therefore, we explore that issue further now, to help you think about patients for whom it is culturally and individually appropriate for them to know their diagnosis.

The What and How of Telling

As you prepare to read this section, think about how you would like to be approached with the news that you have a life-threatening condition, and what you would like to have happen later so you would feel as if you had been treated with respect from the very start of your ordeal. If you are someone who for any reason absolutely would not want to know, try to think about how you will handle yourself with people for whom it is appropriate to know? If you would want to know, how can you become aware of when it is *not* appropriate for this information to be shared?

Responsivity and Responsibility. Sometimes health professionals think they have a responsibility to talk with the patient only if the patient asks. This is a "responsive" posture insofar as discussion takes place only in response to a patient's direct questions: "Am I dying?" or "Is it inoperable?" or "What can I expect?"

Although being responsive is important and this should always guide your conduct, sometimes it is helpful to the patient to be proactive as well. We have outlined some reasons for sharing information, and you will be treating the patient with respect if you are always ready to communicate those things he or she has a right to, and is ready to, know. Sometimes it is not within the boundaries of your professional role to communicate a diagnosis or prognosis directly, but you can always encourage this course of action with the physician or others whose legal/ethical responsibility it is.

Sharing Information: How Much and What Kind? The content of the information you or the appropriate team member reveals is important. When a diagnosis is known, naming it in words the patient really understands is imperative. Without this information, nothing else will make sense in the conversation. In most cases, however, stopping there is rarely helpful to the person.

Usually health professionals think it is helpful for the patient to have a prognosis. Patients often do ask; however, except in the rarest circumstances, the prognosis is not known with absolute certainty. Sounding the death knell on a given date in the future understandably would be disastrous for most patients anyway. Today physicians often talk about probability: "You have a 50 percent chance of a 5-year survival." This approach allows certain information to be transmitted to the patient and may permit the patient to learn what usually happens to people in similar situations.

At the same time, probabilistic information, given along with the diagnosis, has the power to leave a hollow feeling in the pit of a person's stomach, too. He or she must be able to understand the *meaning* of the diagnosis and prognosis. The patient who asks, "Am I going to die?" may be asking, "Do I have metastatic cancer of the breast?" *(diagnosis)* or "Where do I fall on the probability charts for a woman of my age?" *(prognosis)*. More likely, the person is really asking, "Am I going to be dying in a slow, painful way for the next few months?" "Will I turn yellow and wrinkled like my Aunt Susan did?" "Will I be slowly abandoned by my family and friends?" You will not be in a position to provide full assurance to counter every question a patient might have, but the following are several suggestions:

1. Disclosure of any information should come after careful consideration of the patient's need either to know or to not know at a given time. Someone must be attuned enough to the patient to perceive the person's mental and physical state at this given moment, and it is up to you to discern as fully as possible who that person is.

2. Different types of information are best provided by different significant people in the patient's life. We have already mentioned the need to ascertain cultural, ethnic, and other differences that may indicate the approach best taken by the team as a whole. It takes a combination of insight into the patient's needs, a measure of courage, and ready sympathy for the person's situation to talk effectively about difficult aspects of what is ahead for the patient. Depending on the circumstances, the best person may be a senior member of the patient's tribe or family, a member of the clergy, a family member, a physician, or another health professional. This can be worked out if the health care team is willing to make the effort to fully assess the situation.

3. All communication should be expressed in a vocabulary that the patient can understand. Ways of expressing the same information will differ dramatically from person to person. Deciding what type of vocabulary is appropriate means getting to know the patient beforehand, at least to the extent of reading the patient's clinical record.[18]

All of these suggestions leave communication channels open. They also all focus on how knowledge can best be shared once the team is convinced it should be.

Treating Losses and Fears

Previous sections of this book emphasize the importance of recognizing and understanding the patient's challenges, especially those in the form of losses. Those experienced by people with life-threatening conditions can span the whole range discussed in Chapter 7. However, this patient is facing the awesome prospect of losing everything associated with this worldly life, including physical identity. In *A Very Easy Death,* Simone de Beauvoir poignantly describes her mother, who has been dying from cancer over a period of several months:

> I looked at her. She was there, present, conscious and completely unaware of what she was living through. Not to know what is happening underneath one's skin is normal enough. But for her the outside of her body was unknown—her wounded

abdomen, her fistula, the filth that issued from it, the blueness of her skin, the liquid that oozed out of her pores. She had not asked for a mirror again; her dying face did not exist for her. . . .[19]

Many life-threatening conditions are accompanied by a gradual diminution of strength, endurance, control of movement, and sensory acuity. Helping the person and family adjust to each of the "little deaths" as they are experienced is a continuing challenge; your success depends on being attuned to the losses being suffered at any one time.

The fears outlined earlier in this chapter also call for your attention. For instance, you can "treat" (allay) the patient's fears of isolation by your continued presence. You cannot always assure patients that their loved ones will not "jump ship" when the going gets rough because sometimes families do. Observing this tapering off of supportive relationships is often very trying for you, let alone the patient. Relationships are bound to be altered during this time; some friends and relatives disappear because of indifference, despair, or exhaustion, and those who do not become more cherished. Health professionals often are eventually able to ascertain who, among the many at the onset, will endure. Often, it is wise to begin providing your own support to those who you judge to be the most enduring so that the patient will continue to have a community of support as the condition progresses.

In addition to your attentiveness occasioned by the necessary performance of technical skills, you may choose, as do many health professionals, to stop in and see a patient briefly or to talk with the patient's family from time to time after treatment has been discontinued. Sometimes a telephone call to the patient's home after discharge is a great source of comfort and encouragement to all there.

Of course, these means of maintaining human contact can present some difficulties. Tension arises over the establishment of priorities. Spending extra time with this person may subtract from time left for others. Judgment must be exercised in deciding how to proceed so that other patients receive their fair share of time and attention. Furthermore, sometimes spending extra time with the patient outside of the treatment or testing situation may encourage overdependence on you for things you cannot now or eventually be there to provide. The general rule is to be compassionately guided, aware that the patient and family are in a time of great turmoil and need.

Sometimes "treatment" takes curious forms when a person is dying. The authors have spoken many times of the following story, told by a physician friend.

> When she was an internal medicine resident, part of her day consisted of making rounds with the attending medical staff. Each day for several weeks, one of the patients they saw was a withered wisp of an old woman who was now semicomatose in this stage of a long bout with cancer. The old woman had no known relatives and was never visited by anyone, but

she lived on and on past the time the medical staff believed she would die. The group of physicians stood at the foot of the bed each day, studied her with bewilderment, read her medical record for signs of changes, said a few words to each other, and left. The resident believed that the old woman became tense during these discussions, and finally one day she mentioned it to her colleagues. They scoffed at the idea, saying the patient was too weak and too far gone to know what they were saying or that they were even there. The resident became increasingly troubled by the presence of this tiny patient, who was lying in what seemed to be a gigantic hospital bed. Finally, one time while on call, the resident was walking down the patient's corridor at 3 o'clock in the morning. For some inexplicable reason she was drawn into the patient's room. The woman looked no different than ever—very small, very alone, and very still. The resident shut the door, gathered the woman into her arms, and wept. Later that morning when the resident checked into the front desk, she was told that the woman had died at about 5 o'clock that morning.

It seems to us that the medical resident "treated" the patient with the human contact that the patient somehow needed to be released from her suffering. We know very little about the deep process of dying, but such acts of basic human caring may be the key to helping a patient face the unique challenges of the dying process.

Helping Patients Maintain Hope

The previous section briefly mentioned the importance of allowing the patient to claim fully the uniqueness of his or her dying to begin the search for meaning in the experience and maintain hope. The focus of hope will change over time, at least in part and not all at the same time, from a hope for cure to a hope for meaningful activities in the remaining period of life. The person's hope is therefore often directed toward events such as seeing a loved one another time, visiting a favorite place, or hearing a piece of music played.

Some hopes are less tangible: that one will be able to keep a positive spirit or sense of irony to the end; that one will be remembered and missed; or that a particular tradition will be carried on in one's absence. The previously sought long-term goals are put into perspective, and the patient focuses his or her hopes on the most important ones, knowing that some will no longer be attainable.

How can you help? Listen carefully to the patient express hopes and take seriously what the person says. Hope itself depends significantly on the attitudes of health professionals as well as on those of family and friends when the patient dares to disclose a hope. Your listening can help to maintain the person's feeling of worth and thereby provide a human context in which hopes may be expressed. Of course, health professionals can also often play a significant role in actually helping the patient realize some specific hope by making a few important telephone calls to the right people, by mentioning the patient's wishes to the family and others, or by other similar means.

In short, people faced with dying all hope that they will be treated kindly, that everything medically possible will be done for them, and that meaningful human exchange will not disappear. The health professional can assure the patient and family of these things by personally helping to effect them.

PROVIDING THE RIGHT TREATMENT AT THE RIGHT TIME IN THE RIGHT PLACE

Partially in response to the movement in several Western countries to reexamine the health professional's role in assisted suicide and euthanasia, much attention is being devoted to improving the methods of care at the end of life. Another factor leading to this focus (and partly resulting from it) is an improved understanding of physiological and other responses to agents designed to provide relief from pain or other disturbing symptoms associated with many life-threatening conditions. In other words, presently there is a much needed attempt to improve health care interventions for patients who are dying, both in terms of finding the right environment and in tailoring interventions to the appropriate time in the dying process.

Hospice and Home Care Alternatives

The hospice movement, which began in England and has spread to Canada, the United States, and many other countries today, has been a commendable attempt to provide treatment and care expressly designed to meet the needs of patients with life-threatening conditions and their families. Initially, hospice care was geared to the treatment of patients with cancer, but today hospice care is available for many other types of patients with irreversible conditions such as Alzheimer's disease, progressively deteriorating neurological conditions, and AIDS.

The hospice is often viewed as an alternative to the usual hospital and other institutional approaches to irreversible illness or the results of serious injury. Support is provided for the patient and family when cure or remission is no longer possible. The hospice setting is characterized by interdisciplinary health care approaches. Palliative (i.e., comfort-enhancing) measures that focus on symptom relief and psychosocial support rather than on life-extending interventions are utilized. When there is a family it, and not the patient alone, is the unit of care. In most hospice settings the primary caregivers are not physicians but family members, volunteers, nurses, social workers, and counselors.

In some locations, home care is supported sufficiently by government and/or insurance plans to make this a viable alternative for families. Some hospices are actually "without walls"; that is, they are designed to provide services within the home with devices such as hotlines, care networks, and respite programs for caregivers. Churches and other organizations sometimes become involved in these caregiving arrangements.

You and your patients will benefit from your acquainting yourself further with the functions and structure of the hospice and with the hospice and home care alternatives available in the communities where you work. This will prepare you to inform patients of these options when it becomes appropriate and to be active in the referral process. You may even find yourself drawn to these aspects of health care and be one of the growing number of professionals working in the hospice or home health care setting.

The Appropriate Treatment: Cure or Comfort?

From a clinical point of view, the treatment always must fit the situation. To do less is not acceptable. What constitutes "appropriate treatment" when the person is dying from a condition requiring the intervention of health professionals?

In the clinical practice focusing on people who have life-threatening conditions, the idea of palliation has played a central role. Palliative care (or, as it is commonly called, comfort care) traditionally was thought of as what health professionals can do when cure no longer is possible. In other words, it becomes appropriate when all else has failed. The problem is that from as early as the time of Hippocrates there was a suggestion that if cure was no longer possible, the disease had gone beyond the "art of medicine" and should not be interfered with by the doctor. So all too often palliation meant that dying patients received very little care. At the same time, you can understand that the idea of palliative care is important because applied appropriately it allows you to have better insight into how to respond well to patients' fears of abandonment, pain, and other distress associated with the dying process.

Today the growing focus on appropriate end-of-life care has shed new light on what palliative care entails. Comfort care goes well beyond the traditional hand holding at the bedside, as important as that continues to be. Comfort can be achieved for various patients through many varieties of intervention, such as painkillers, ventilators, dramatic surgical procedures, and psychological counseling, to name some. Moreover, there has been a rethinking of traditional medical, nursing, and other health care specialties into those that include palliative as well as curative aspects in their realm of expertise. Within medicine this may include anesthesiologists, physiatrists, internists, pediatricians, geriatric specialists, and surgeons, all of who often address chronic symptoms associated with dying. Anesthesiologists and oncologists regularly are involved as well. (You can draw parallels with other professional groups.)

Along with this heightened consciousness and technology there has also been a rethinking about the traditional assumption that the movement from "treatment" to "palliation" should be a linear progression as the patient's

Traditional Model for End-of-Life Care

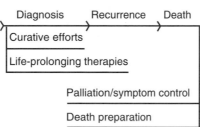

From Field, Marilyn J., and Cassel, Christine K. (eds.): *Approaching Death: Improving Care at the End of Life.* Committee on Care at the End of Life, Institute of Medicine. Washington, DC, National Academy Press, 1997, p. 85.

downhill course ensues. Using cancer as a model, the Institute of Medicine in the United States illustrates this progress, showing that traditionally palliation began well into the course of other treatments and would become the only form of intervention as the condition progressed.[20]

However, they conclude, a much richer and accurate approach that addresses the patient's many symptoms will not progress in such a tidy, linear way. Different combinations of education about how to prevent deterioration or the appearance of new symptoms, responsiveness to rehabilitative needs, acute care interventions and comfort measures all may remain appropriate from the beginning to the end of the patient's dying process.[21]

Other models that are fine-tuned to patients' and families' real needs also are being attempted. You are entering the health professions at a time when the attention being given to these issues will assist you in doing a better job than your forebearers in this important area of professional service have been able to do.

Revised Model for End-of-Life Care

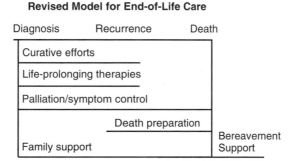

From Field, Marilyn J., and Cassel, Christine K. (eds.): *Approaching Death: Improving Care at the End of Life.* Committee on Care at the End of Life, Institute of Medicine. Washington, DC, National Academy Press, 1997, p. 85.

WHEN DEATH IS IMMINENT

The fears, challenges, and hopes associated with both the process of dying and death itself arise during the extended period of irreversible, life-threatening illness. However, at some point in the course of that illness it becomes apparent that the person will die soon. Persons who do not suffer from a prolonged illness as such also face the moment of imminent death: the accident victim, the attempted suicide or murder victim, and the young person going into battle.

Many people today do not have any customary rituals associated with the time of death, although you have a responsibility always to consider that a patient may have an urgent need to participate in a religious act appropriate to his or her faith and beliefs. These and additional factors make it necessary for health professionals to alter their treatment procedures and to judiciously attend to certain aspects of interaction. Three of the many ways that respect can be expressed are explained in the following discussion, and the reader will surely think of others.

Maximizing Comfort

The patient whose death is imminent should not be barraged with routine requests and procedures that no longer matter. As one woman sitting by her dying father's bedside asked dismayingly, "Does it *matter* if his bowels haven't moved on the last day he will probably be alive?"

Attempts to relieve pain by medication, massage, and other therapeutic means may have been started long before, and these should be continued unless the patient asks that they be withdrawn. Some people, if they know that they are experiencing the final days of their lives, find the torpor induced by heavy medication more troublesome than intense, unrelieved pain.

However, maximizing comfort goes beyond alleviating pain. It involves the relief of real or potential suffering. Suffering is a far more inclusive, personalized concept than pain, although pain may be one important factor. A friend relates that, on the last day before her 29-year-old husband died of cancer, she read to him, bathed him, nursed their 2-month-old daughter (who had to be sneaked up to the hospital room under a friend's poncho), sang songs he loved, and filled the room with apple blossoms. Friends came in to have "communion," which consisted of brownies and ginger ale, and her husband shared in it, although he had been nourished only intravenously for days.[22] The specific activities will vary from person to person, but it seems to us that she had the right idea of how to care for her husband in significant ways during their last day together. In addition, the health professionals who were involved helped the situation by allowing the family and friends their final day together. The woman says that one of the greatest gifts she received was being able to share this intimate time with her husband while still having the assurance that the health professionals were "on standby" if needed.

From this woman and others we can learn that probably the most meaningful act of caring the health professional can offer is to enable loved ones to be with the patient and each other. This may mean breaking hospital rules and readjusting one's schedule. It also means knowing who should be called if the patient's condition worsens and death appears near. Unfortunately, many patients die alone because health professionals, despite good intentions, sometimes do not take the necessary steps to ensure that the family is contacted at the appropriate time.

Saying Good-Bye

Many people find it difficult to say good-bye to a friend or other loved one who is going away. It is more difficult still when the person is dying—so much so that good-byes are seldom said, especially by the health professional to the patient and the patient's family. This is, however, something that you can do to show respect for the people and their situation when many other forms of interaction have been suspended. One psychiatrist offers this suggestion:

> What should be said is, I want you to know the relationship was meaningful, I'll miss this about you, or . . . it won't be the same, I'll miss the bluntness that you had in helping me sort out some things, or I'll just miss the old bull sessions, or something like that. Because those are things you value. Now what does that do for the other person? The other person learns that although it's painful to separate it's far more meaningful to have known the person and to have separated than never to have known him at all. He also learns what it is in himself that is valued and treasured by [you]. And some of those underlying, corrosive feelings of low self-esteem that plague people are shored up. . . .[23]

This encounter also allows the patient and his or her family to express similar feelings. There is often a real sense of closeness and gratitude felt toward the health professional and to be able to show it is a great relief.

In addition to what the exchange does for the patient and family, it is important to realize how much it can help in your own grieving.

Giving patients and families an opportunity to express gratitude to you may sound odd, but it is one way in which some patients and families can be assisted in their own grieving. When they observe that the health professional receives their thanks humbly, they will appreciate this show of human caring.

Other genuine expressions of your caring may be meaningful for the patient and family. A young mother told a physician friend:

> This may sound silly but one of the things that most sustained me the last few days was that night last week, when you believed Randy was going to die then, you had tears in your eyes.

Telling him that was a way of saying "thank you," and if he had not been able to receive it, she would have felt embarrassed or rejected.

Accepting Rejection

Having outlined some ways in which good-bye and thank you can be exchanged gracefully and meaningfully, you should also prepare yourself for the rare instances in which the patient and family reject your attempts to show respectful caring during this intense period of their lives.

Sometimes when a person is close to dying, he or she shuts out many people. Such a patient may not want to have anything more to do with you. There are many reasons for this. First, we have already discussed the great difficulty with saying good-bye or in showing affection under such trying circumstances. Second, there is the possibility that the person has accepted his or her death and no longer needs any people around. That such acceptance may occur has been well documented by those who have worked with a large number of terminally ill people. Although not necessarily so, it is more likely to occur when the approaching death has been preceded by a long illness. Third, you are not as important as loved ones, and the little energy the patient has is reserved for them. Fourth, the patient and his or her family may actually direct any anger they feel about the death toward you and other health professionals. The health professional who is the object of such anger may not even be the one who spent the longest or most significant time with the person, but rather the one who happened to be there at some crucial moment. Finally, you are inextricably linked to the whole setting in which suffering and dying have taken place. So much anguish may be associated with you and your professional environment that it is painful for the patient to be in your presence. The patient handles this difficulty by rejecting you along with other distressing aspects of the experience.

You should be prepared for the possibility that your final efforts and good intentions are neither wanted nor welcomed. On some occasions, you may feel hurt by these sudden or unexpected rebuffs and can do little more than forgive the person responsible for them. At times when hurt is present, support from your professional colleagues may become vital. Sharing feelings of failure, rejection, or bewilderment with an understanding colleague can be a balm for injured feelings and can give one the courage to try again in another such situation.

SUMMARY

This chapter scratches the surface of considerations that can be helpful to you in your attempts to show respect in the extreme life situation in which death is approaching for a patient in your care. The patient needs your professional skills, your compassion, and your wisdom in this situation. At the same time you are confronted with your own uncertainties and fears about dying and death along with the irony that, no matter what you do, the end result for this patient will be death. Your part in making the remainder of life for a dying patient as rich and worthwhile as possible may be the motivation you will need to sustain that person and his or her loved ones.

REFERENCES

1. Albom, M.: *Tuesdays with Morrie.* New York, Doubleday, 1997, pp. 88–89.
2. Jack and the Beanstalk (a traditional English fairy tale). In *The Arthur Rackham Fairy Book.* Philadelphia, Lippincott, 1950, p. 48.
3. Hansel and Grethel (a Grimm's fairy tale). In *The Arthur Rackham Fairy Book.* Philadelphia, Lippincott, 1950, p. 276.
4. Purtilo, R.: Ethical issues in end of life care. In *Ethical Dimensions in the Health Professions.* Philadelphia, W.B. Saunders Company, 1999, pp. 216–218.
5. Albom, M.: *Tuesdays with Morrie.* New York, Doubleday, 1997, p. 114.
6. Trillin, A.S.: Of dragons and garden peas: a cancer patient talks to doctors. *N. Engl. J. Med.* 304:669–701, 1981.
7. Taylor, J.: In Heber, R. (ed.): *The Whole Works.* Vol 2. rev. ed. New York, Adler's Foreign Books, 1971, p. 96 (first published in 1847).
8. Tolle, S., and Haley, K.: Pain management in the dying: successes and concerns. *BME Rep.* Fall 1998, pp. 1–2.
9. Hollinger, D.P.: The logical foundations for death and dying issues. *Ethics Med.* 12:3, 60–65, 1996.
10. Toynbee, A.: Changing attitudes toward death in the modern Western world. In Toynbee, A. (ed.): *Man's Concern with Death.* New York, McGraw-Hill, 1968, pp. 74–89.
11. Thomas, R.: The Ho Chunk (Winnebago) people. In Mondragón, D. (ed.): *Religious Values of the Terminally Ill: Handbook for Health Care Professionals.* Scranton, PA, University of Scranton Press, 1997, pp. 15–20.
12. Stoppard, T.: *Rosencrantz and Guildenstern Are Dead.* New York, Grove Press, 1967, p. 126.
13. Kübler-Ross, E.: *On Death and Dying.* New York, Macmillan, 1969, pp. 38–137.
14. Toynbee, A. (ed.): *Man's Concern with Death.* New York, McGraw-Hill, 1968, quote p. 271.
15. Vachon, M.L.S.: Emotional problems in palliative medicine: patient, family, and professional. In Doyle, D., Hanks, G.W., and MacDonald, M.: *Oxford Textbook of Palliative Medicine.* Oxford, Oxford University Press, 1993, pp. 735–738.
16. Albertson, S.H.: *Endings and Beginnings.* New York, Random House, 1980, p. 19.
17. Veatch, R.M., and Haddad, A.: Veracity: dealing honestly with patients. In *Case Studies in Pharmacy Ethics.* New York, Oxford University Press, 1999, p. 97–115.
18. Ramsden, E.L.: *The Person as Patient: Psycho-Social Perspectives for the Health Care Professional.* Philadelphia, W.B. Saunders, 1999, pp. 244–262.
19. de Beauvoir, S.: *A Very Easy Death* (O'Brien, P., trans.). New York, Warner Books, 1973, p. 89.
20. Field, M.J., and Cassel, C. eds.: *National Academy of Medicine Report Approaching Death: Improving Care at the End of Life.* Washington, DC, National Academy Press, 1997, p. 72.

21. Ibid, p. 76.
22. Albertson, S.H.: *Endings and Beginnings.* New York, Random House, 1980, pp. 19–22.
23. Cassem, N.H.: The caretakers. In Langone, J. (ed.): *Vital Signs: The Way We Die in America.* Boston, Little, Brown & Company, 1974, p. 255.

CHAPTER 19

Respectful Interaction in Other Difficult Situations

CHAPTER OBJECTIVES

The student will be able to

- Identify three potential sources of difficulties creating barriers to respectful health professional and patient interaction
- Discuss how disparities in power within the relationship can lead to anger and frustration on the part of the patient
- Identify attributes and behaviors of patients, such as manipulative, sexually provocative, or aggressive behaviors, that may challenge the health professional's ideal of compassionate care
- Reflect on personal expectations of what it means to be a "good" health professional and how this impacts interactions with patients
- Describe environmental factors that may contribute to difficulties in health professional and patient interaction
- List and evaluate guidelines for managing and, when possible, preventing difficult health professional and patient relationships
- List and evaluate techniques that can help to change a "difficult" working relationship and the surrounding environment

---

I can't stand the way Hal [another staff nurse] makes me get up and walk in the mornings. He knows I can't put weight on my leg, yet he insists that I do. He's the meanest nurse here, nothing like you. You really understand me. I bet I have an infection under my wound dressing, because Hal's so sloppy. I've tried to fire him as my nurse, but he just laughs. I have friends in high places in this hospital—I really could get him fired!

A "difficult" patient, as quoted by L. Nield-Anderson, et al.[1]

Many health professionals view working with dying patients and their families as one of the greatest challenges they face in health care. However, as you read in Chapter 18, working with patients who are dying can sometimes be full of joy as well as sorrow. Even though you might experience loss and grief when a patient you have cared for dies, there is often also an accompanying sense of satisfaction that you were able to make his or her death a little easier, a little less painful, or less lonely. There are other patient care situations in which you will not come away with a sense of satisfaction, but one of profound frustration. This chapter focuses on difficulties inherent in the health professional and patient interaction that have not specifically been addressed elsewhere in this book or that bear reemphasizing. We suggest that you refer to Chapters 11 through 13 to review the content on establishing relatedness, recognizing boundaries, and creating professional closeness. You will need to utilize all of these insights and skills in your work with patients who challenge your conceptions of what it means to be a "good" health professional. Moreover, you will have an opportunity to think about other factors that can create great frustration in the health professional and patient interaction, such as disparities in power and role expectations or an unsafe and negative working environment. We devote this last chapter to some summary statements about how to work more effectively with "difficult" patients and offer ways to effect change in "difficult" settings.

SOURCES OF DIFFICULTIES IN THE HEALTH PROFESSIONAL AND PATIENT INTERACTION

Generally, when you enter a relationship with a patient you have good reason to expect that things will go well, or if there are problems you expect that they can be resolved. However, there are situations in which even your best efforts cannot make things right. When this happens, a common response is to look for a place to lay the blame. For example, you might wonder what else you could have done for the patient, or you might reason that the patient was not ready for treatment, or you may become defensive and decide that the patient was disruptive, noncompliant, maladjusted, or any number of other negative labels. Difficulty relating to a patient may originate in the health professional, in the patient, or outside of the relationship in the setting in which the interaction takes place.

Sources within the Health Professional

As emphasized throughout this book, you bring a wealth of experiences, education, prejudices, and values to your interaction with patients and their families. All of these factors can affect how you react to a particular patient. For example, recall the discussion on transference and countertransference in Chapter 11: a patient may remind you of your third-grade teacher whom you particularly feared and disliked. This past experience can arouse intense emotional reactions in the present relationship. Additionally, your personality and how you deal with stress will play a large part in how you manage patient care situations that are interpersonally difficult.[2] In fact, your personality, more than your professional or demographic background, may explain why you react negatively to some patients and certain situations and have little difficulty with others.

For the health professional, the most reliable indicator of a negative emotional response is an unfavorable gut response or sense of discomfort in encounters with a particular patient.[3] If you are attuned to monitoring your feelings, then you can try to assess how much anger, fear, or guilt you bring to the interaction and try to manage those feelings before trying to manage the patient. Certain key words and phrases can help you identify the emotion that is being triggered (Table 19–1). After you identify the emotions, two questions often follow: "Why is this happening?" and "Where is this emotion coming from?"

Although it is a widely held belief, which has certainly been emphasized in this book, that health professionals should be nonjudgmental in their relationships with patients, it is a fact that some patients are more likable than others. More than 40 years ago, Highley and Norris asked their nursing students to identify major "dislikes" related to working with patients. The types of patients the students disliked can still be found in clinical practice today. The students reported the following dislikes:

1. Patients who feel bad and complain after everything has been done for them.

2. Patients who are not clean.

3. Patients who will not do what the health professional asks them to, will not cooperate, will not obey the rules.

TABLE 19–1. Key Words for Identifying Negative Emotions

Anger

Annoyance	Frustration
Bitterness	Hostility
Boredom	Irritation
Disappointment	Resentment

Fear

Apprehension	Hurt
Concern	Loneliness
Discouragement	Rejection
Emptiness	Sadness
Helplessness	Worry

Guilt

Anger at self	"I should have . . ."
"If only I had . . ."	"I wish I had . . ."

From Herbert, C.P., and Seifert, M.H.: When the patient is the problem. *Patient Care* 24(1):60, 1990.

4. Patients who are extremely demanding.

5. Patients who can help themselves but insist on the health professional doing everything.[4]

The common denominator in these dislikes is that either the patients made the students feel guilty because of their dislike for the patients, or, because they were never satisfied, the patients made the students feel inadequate as nurses.

Because this study was conducted in the 1950s, the students might not have mentioned some problems people are more self-consciously aware of today, such as patients who make sexually explicit remarks that cause embarrassment or aggressive patients who frighten or sometimes even physically harm health professionals.

These findings lead to another factor that is characteristic of health professionals and can cause difficulties in patient interactions: high expectations regarding the ability to help. As you progress through your program of study to become a health professional, the ideal is reinforced: you should be able to function effectively in all patient situations, and you are solely responsible for the success or failure of these interactions. This may not be what your teachers or we wish to convey, but it is often what health professionals feel at the beginning of their careers. Thus, long before you have a full complement of skills with which to deal with difficult situations, you may blame yourself for failing to meet the needs of a challenging patient. Before jumping to self-blame for not meeting these unrealistic expectations, you need to recognize that many errors occur before full competence is attained, and even then you should continue to work at establishing realistic expectations of yourself as a health professional.

Your perception of the patient's socioeconomic status also can influence your reactions to a patient. You are encouraged to review the content of Chapter 3 regarding appreciating differences and recognizing discrimination. A perceived difference in socioeconomic status can have a profound effect on the health professional and patient interaction. Papper noted:

> The very poor may be viewed as undesirable unrelated to their ability to pay. Even when the physician has genuine concern for the economically disadvantaged, he may because of his own background, unwittingly regard the extremely poor as *different*, with a flavor of *inferiority included in the difference*.[5]

Papper's personal observation of his medical colleagues was substantiated in a research study by Larson, who presented nurses with case studies in which the patient was identified as middle or lower class, with a more or less serious and more or less socially acceptable illness. The specific findings of Larson's study indicate that persons ranked as "lower class" were perceived as relatively passive, dependent, unintelligent, unmotivated, lazy, forgetful, noncomprehending, uninformed, inaccurate, unreliable, careless, and unsuccessful.[6] We return to

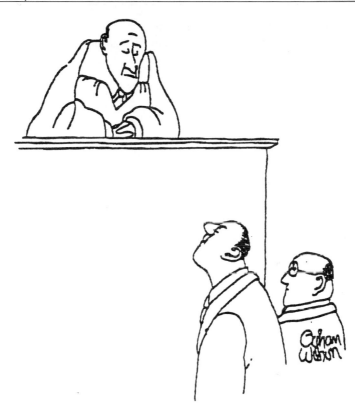

"You understand you're the sort of person I ordinarily wouldn't even speak to."
From Wilson, Gahan: *Is Nothing Sacred?* New York, St. Martin's Press, 1982.

the findings related to socially unacceptable illness later in this chapter because this also leads to the labeling of a patient as difficult or undesirable.

Socioeconomic differences between patient and health professional can surface in values about cleanliness. Most health professionals are from the middle or upper-middle class and hold certain values about cleanliness and other "correct" ways of being in the world. They not only are unfamiliar with the ways of poor people, but hold them in disdain. Persons in lower socioeconomic groups may be so concerned about basic human needs, such as food and shelter and so have little time or resources for luxuries such as bathing, that they appear not to care at all about cleanliness. Middle-class health professionals often, unconsciously, try to impose their values on patients concerning cleanliness. If neither the health professional nor the patient is aware of differences in socioeconomic status that generate values about bathing and hygiene, a struggle can ensue regarding cleanliness that is out of proportion to its importance in most patient care situations.

Sources within Patients

What makes a patient "undesirable?" Patients who do not comply with or sabotage treatment are generally labeled as problematic. Other types of behavior that commonly elicit a negative response from health professionals are violence, anger, or self-harm behaviors. In general, patients who do not affirm the health professional's identity, i.e., accept help and appreciate that help, are considered bad patients. The rejection of the health professional's help can easily be misread as rejection of the health professional. This rejection can take many forms, ranging from outright physical violence, to incessant demands, manipulative behavior, ingratitude, or sexually provocative behaviors.

As you can see from the list of dislikes that the students in Highley and Norris's study generated, the focus of the dislike easily moved from dislike for inappropriate or unacceptable behavior to dislike for the patient. For example, patients with illnesses that are socially unacceptable often are labeled as difficult even if their behavior is a model of compliance. People with communicable diseases such as sexually transmitted diseases or addictive disorders such as alcoholism or drug abuse are often viewed as unacceptable. Even if a health professional views alcoholism as a disease rather than a behavior a patient should be able to control, the patient who has a problem with alcohol is commonly rejected by most professional personnel.[7] Health professionals may project their own embarrassment about certain illnesses onto the patient.

Characteristics over which the patient has no power or ability to change, such as mental retardation, do not rate highly as factors in determining who is considered a difficult patient.[8] Thus, a large part of the label a patient receives depends on our role expectations of patients in general and of patients with specific characteristics. We return to a discussion of role expectations of patients and health professionals shortly.

Sources in the Environment

As we noted specifically in Chapter 10, the health professional and patient interaction takes place in a particular context. At times the context can be the source of difficulty in an interaction. For example, if the environment is strange and frightening, the patient or health professional may react in a fearful or angry manner. For many patients, a health care facility can be an extremely threatening place. Taken in this context, even a simple activity such as bathing can be viewed as menacing. Rader noted that for a person with apraxia (inability to execute purposeful learned motor acts despite the physical ability and willingness to do so), agnosia (inability to recognize a tactile or visible stimulus despite being able to recognize the elemental sensation), and aphasia (loss of language function either in comprehension or expression of words), symptoms often found in patients who have had a cerebrovascular accident, the standard nursing home bathing experience may be perceived as horrific. Consider these limitations, and place yourself in the patient's position.

A person the resident does not recognize comes into her room, wakens her, says something she does not understand, drags her out of bed, and takes off her clothes. Then the resident is moved down a public corridor on something that resembles a toilet seat, covered only with a thin sheet so that her private parts are exposed to the breeze. Calls for help are ignored or greeted with, "Good morning." Then she is taken to a strange, cold room that looks like a car wash, the sheet is ripped off, and she is sprayed in the face with cold and then scalding water. Continued calls for help go unheeded. Her most private parts are touched by a stranger. In another context this would be assault.[9]

An environment can be equally strange and intolerable to the health professional. For example, we have noted in other chapters that in community health practice health professionals may go into the unknown realm of the patient's living environment. One of us recalls a home visit to a small, run-down house literally butted up against the back fence of the holding pens for cattle at the stock market. The smell of manure was overwhelming both outside and inside the house. The elderly woman who lived there (and the subject of the home visit for management of diabetes) seemed oblivious to the odor. In fact, she had just finished hanging a load of clean sheets on the line to dry in her tiny backyard!

Similar stresses can arise in a hectic and crisis-ridden environment. Patients who are kept waiting in an overcrowded emergency room or office are more likely to be frustrated and hostile to health professionals when they are finally seen. Understaffing often leaves health professionals feeling frustrated and dissatisfied as they attempt to meet the needs of too many patients with too little time and resources. Overworked staffs worry about the effect of stretching themselves too thin and the impact this can have on patient care. The physical and psychological exhaustion resulting from excessive professional demands that can drain you have been aptly dubbed "compassion fatigue."[10]

Other environmental factors that make care difficult include the aesthetics of a space, crowding, and climate. One of us worked in a large acute care pediatric setting during the hottest months of the year with no air conditioning. As the temperature rose during the day, so did everyone's irritability; children cried more easily, and co-workers snapped at each other for the slightest offense. Only with the setting of the sun and the resultant drop in temperature did the atmosphere on the unit cool down as well.

Some settings in which the health professional and patient interaction takes place are tense and unpleasant because of the personal dynamics of the individuals who work in them.

Disparities of Power. We have noted several times in this book that patients are placed in a position of diminished power upon entering the health care environment. The content in Chapter 7 specifically discusses numerous losses that patients face because of illness or trauma: independence, social status and responsibility, and expressions of identity often are taken away from people upon entering a health care institution, and all of these factors contribute to feelings of powerlessness. A common reaction to powerlessness is anger, and a common target of anger is the most accessible and least-threatening health professional involved with the patient.[11] Thus, students are often the target for a torrent of rage from a patient that has little to do with the student or his or her abilities. Very few studies have explored patients' perceptions of this inequity in power, but in one study of mental health workers and patients, both groups reported an awareness of the struggle to gain or retain power and control. Patients noted that when health professionals demonstrated respect, took time with them, and were willing to give them some control and choice in their own care, feelings of anger were reduced.[12]

Role Expectations. Personality characteristics of "good" and "bad" patients initially described in the literature in the 1960s are familiar to health professionals today.

> A "good" patient has such attributes as emotional stability; he is cheerful, not overly anxious, and keeps his feelings under control. He communicates easily with the nursing staff, is cooperative, is appreciative, conforms readily to hospital routines and policies, and is thoughtful of the busy nurse's point of view. The "bad" patient is emotionally unstable; he may be highly anxious, depressed, and hostile. He may not communicate readily with nurses; he may challenge nursing actions or ask too many questions; he may be too independent. He is likely to be aggressive, impatient, unappreciative, unconforming to hospital routines and policies, and unsympathetic to the nurse's point of view.[13]

Because we are socialized not to use negative terms such as "bad," we substitute euphemisms to describe patients with the attributes listed above: they are described as disruptive, unmotivated, regressed, maladaptive, and manipulative. Patients who are perceived to be difficult to treat evoke intense negative-affective responses in the health professional that can work against establishing a positive, constructive relationship.[14] Furthermore, there is also a strong possibility that the professional's language exerts a powerful impact on thought and, consequently, action. Negative words lead to negative thoughts and actions regarding difficult patients. An example from rehabilitation medicine highlights the impact of language.

> Most rehabilitation staff have encountered patients who resist the best efforts to engage them in therapeutic activities. These patients seem not to want to be in rehabilitation. They may view therapies as trivial, irrelevant, uninteresting, or too demanding, and they must be constantly coaxed to attend; if they do attend, they do not participate. Staff members become quickly frustrated with patients who do not share the "rehabilitation perspective" that places a high premium on attaining maximal independent functioning. The patient's lack of involvement produces slow progress, proving the patient's point that therapy is valueless. This further

antagonizes staff members who, feeling professionally and personally offended, may diminish their efforts to engage the patient, thus producing a hostile standoff and virtually guaranteeing therapeutic failure. This is the fate of the "unmotivated" patient.[15]

Any patient behavior that is inconsistent with expected patient role behavior (read "good patient behavior") could negatively influence the care of patients. Not only might you be tempted to diminish your efforts in the care of a difficult patient, but you might also resort to distancing yourself from the patient. Unfortunately, avoidance and distancing may result in the reinforcement of deviant behavior as a patient response to nonsupportive care. In extreme cases, health professionals have been known to respond to difficult patients with their own version of negative behavior. In a study of nurses by Podrasky and Sexton, vignettes describing a variety of negative patient behaviors were used to elicit the following responses describing actions these professionals would take or like to take, including, "I have to keep myself from hauling off and whacking her once," "I would restrain her just a little bit too tight," and "I'd make her stay in the wet bed for a long while."[16] More profound and perhaps life-threatening consequences can result from a health professional's negative reactions to a patient. In a national study of transplant coordinators, a full 62% revealed a belief that a hostile or antagonistic patient should *not* receive an organ transplantation.[17] The irony and tragedy in such findings is that expressions of anger and frustration (behavior that can be labeled as hostile) may be a natural response by patients to chronic illness.

Most health professionals are able to control these kinds of strong emotional reactions and continue, at least marginally, to meet their obligations to the patient. The result is a sort of "grudging attention," i.e., the patient gets the minimal care that he or she needs and nothing more. Grudging attention occurs because of a combination of factors. Once a negative label is attached to a patient, it is difficult for health professionals to look past it and process other data about the patient. Negative labels often get "passed on" until a patient develops a bad reputation.[18]

It is as if we see only one aspect of the patient. Couple these stereotypes about the difficult patient with idealistic role expectations of ourselves as caring, nonjudgmental, and capable of reaching every patient, and the result is an interaction devoid of everything but going through the motions.

Although it is important to work toward the goals of acceptance and constructive problem-solving, sometimes the only solution is to do what you must for the patient and then leave. This is exactly what happened in the case of a sexually aggressive patient who made lewd propositions and repeatedly exposed himself to his caregivers. The health professionals in this case responded with grudging attention as follows:

> By now Mr. Leland was getting only the absolute necessities—no extras. After all, who wants to sit down and chat with someone who talks about nothing but his sex

life—or yours? Once our professional responsibilities were met, we avoided Mr. Leland. He couldn't fail to notice this, and as a result his demands for attention become angrier and more disruptive.[19]

Going through the minimal motions of care is a temporary, and not very effective, solution to a much larger problem. Often it results in guilt on the part of the health professional and can result, as in the case of Mr. Leland, in an escalation of the very behavior that led to avoidance in the first place. Although the following quote refers to nurses, the same can be applied to all health professions: "If patients interpret a nurse's manner as uninterested, or if they overhear pejorative comments, they fear that they won't be cared for adequately. It's as valuable to examine staff's behaviors as it is to understand a patient's motivations."[20]

DIFFICULT HEALTH PROFESSIONAL AND PATIENT RELATIONSHIPS

In this section, we introduce you to two patients who share some of the attributes that have been identified as undesirable or difficult by most health professionals. As you examine some of the character traits and behaviors of the two and the nature of the relationship between the patient and health professional, perhaps you will gain insight into your own values and attitudes and begin to prepare yourself for how you will respond.

The Aggressive Patient

Consider the story of Alex Peterson and Claire Chui:

> Alex Peterson was admitted for treatment of a *Pseudomonas* infection of his sinus and respiratory tract. In addition, he had developed some bleeding from his nose after being seen by the ear, nose, and throat specialists at the outpatient clinic. Alex looked considerably older than his 24 years due to a history of intravenous drug addiction, several attempts at drug rehabilitation, and finally a diagnosis of AIDS. He had a history of petty theft, prostitution, and imprisonment. Alex seemed to enter the unit with the intent to harass the staff. Despite a slow, but steady, recovery from the infection that led to his admission, he endlessly asked for pain medication. The physicians on Alex's case could find no reason for the constant demands for pain medication. A psychiatric consultation determined that Alex was competent, but had a diagnosis of antisocial personality disorder. The health care team decided to decrease the amount of analgesics Alex could receive. Even though Alex was informed of this plan, he still asked any staff member he could find for pain medication. Other members of the team had warned Claire Chui, a medical technologist, that Alex would probably ask her for pain medica-

tion when she went to draw blood. She felt she was prepared for her interaction with Alex. She kept telling herself, "Just stick to business. Draw the blood. Be firm, but gentle." She stated when she entered the room, "I am here to draw a blood sample." When Alex asked Claire for something for pain, she responded, "I will not discuss your pain medication with you." As Claire bent over to lower the side rail on Alex's bed, Alex seized Claire's head, kissed her full on the mouth, and thrust his tongue in her mouth as well. Claire immediately reported Alex's actions to the unit supervisor and her colleagues. When the unit manager confronted Alex with his inappropriate behavior, Alex reacted with a shrug and said, "I didn't hurt her, did I? Why did she get so rattled?"[21]

How would you describe Alex's behavior? In other words, how would you view Alex after this incident? Can you identify several reasons why the rest of the staff might not want to spend time with Alex? Put yourself in Claire's place for a minute and ask yourself how you would feel. Would you be able to work with a patient after an incident like this?

Alex would be characterized as a difficult patient for several reasons. His background sets him apart from the health professionals who are trying to care for him. He has led a life on the margins of society. He has engaged in unacceptable social behaviors such as intravenous drug use and prostitution, which carry with them increased risk for AIDS. His diagnosis places him at risk for stereotyping and stigmatizing. Alex is anything but a model of cooperation in the health care system. Alex also falls into the diagnostic category of "antisocial," which includes the inability to regulate impulses, delay gratification, and relate to others except by intimidation and manipulation. (This explains why Alex cannot tolerate pain of any kind nor comply with the plan to decrease his pain medication. He tries the only method he knows: constant verbal harassment, and, when that does not work, physical intimidation.) Alex is not respectful of the usual boundaries established between patient and professional. The final section of this chapter explores some specific techniques to show respect for Alex as a person while managing his antisocial behaviors.

The Self-Destructive Patient

Sometimes the most difficult patient is not the one who commits actions that are outrageous or inappropriate, but one who shrinks from constructive action and resorts to self-harm behavior such as that encountered in the story of Violet Mercer and Tina Kramolisch.

Tina Kramolisch worked evenings and weekends in a busy, urban emergency room as a technician while she finished her last year of professional preparation. Tina often commented to classmates that you really do not have a taste for what it is like in practice without the experiences you find in an emergency room. In fact, Tina felt as if she had seen it all and was quite proud of her ability to work with different types of patients in various levels of distress. However, after taking care of Violet Mercer, Tina wondered if she was ready to care for all types of patients.

Tina entered the holding area where Violet Mercer lay absolutely still on the examination cart under a sheet. When Tina said Violet's name, there was no response, so Tina gently touched the woman's arm. Violet flinched so violently at the touch that it startled Tina as well and she jumped back from the cart. Tina was even more shocked at how Violet looked. Violet murmured, "You scared me." The words were somewhat difficult to understand as Violet's lips were swollen and split in one corner. Violet had lacerations, contusions, and swelling all over her face. Tina had never seen anyone so badly beaten. Tina noticed old bruises and injuries all over Violet's body as she conducted her intake assessment. Tina knew the physician would have to confirm it, but she was also certain that several of Violet's ribs were fractured. Because Tina had been trained to work with women who had been abused, she knew the right questions to ask and did so. Violet admitted, very cautiously, that her husband, Donnie, had lost his temper and done this to her. Tina reported her findings to the nurse and physician, and they set into motion the services and protection the health care system can offer battered women. In fact, Donnie was being treated down the hall for a scalp laceration that Violet had inflicted as she tried to defend herself. The police who brought both of the Mercers into the emergency room were waiting outside Donnie's room to see if Violet would press charges. Tina was holding Violet's hand as the rib binder was put into place when the nurse entered the room and said, "The social worker can take you to the women's shelter after you talk to the police." Violet did not look up as she said in a flat voice, "I've changed my mind. I don't want to press no charges. I'll just go home with Donnie." Tina was speechless as she watched every effort to change Violet's mind fail. Tina felt hot tears of frustration and anger run down her cheeks as she watched Violet and Donnie walk out of the emergency room arm-in-arm.

Why do you think Tina felt a combination of frustration and anger with Violet? What would your reaction be? In this case, the perception of Violet Mercer as a difficult patient is of a whole different nature than that of Alex Petersen. Whereas Alex committed actions that were disruptive and inappropriate, Violet is compliant and willing to accept professional intervention—to a point. In Violet's case, the perception of difficulty rests to some extent on the invalidating effects of Violet's behavior on Tina and the other health professionals caring for her. In the eyes of the professionals, intervention in Violet's case should include more than merely suturing her cuts and bandaging her broken ribs; it should also include offering her a way out of an abusive, potentially life-threatening situation. When Violet fails to accept the help that is offered to her, the primary treatment goal is thwarted, and the health professional's role as a therapeutic agent is invalidated. Both Alex Petersen and Violet Mercer challenge the very notion of what it means to be a "good" health professional. They make us realize that, although we are generally able to effectively help patients, sometimes it is not possible to do so even with our best efforts. There are some techniques that may help you in working with difficult patients of all types, and we also share some ideas about changing a difficult working environment.

SHOWING RESPECT IN DIFFICULT SITUATIONS

When patients are uncooperative, manipulative, angry, or help-rejecting, this is not a license to show disrespect toward them as persons. You will have to be responsive to your own feelings of disgust, fear, anger, and so forth, as well as manage their unacceptable behavior. An appropriate place to start is to show respect by initially refusing to believe that you are dealing with a person whose character is flawed. The behaviors and attitudes may be the result of a treatable or modifiable factor. For example, one of your first determinations is to make certain that the patient has received a thorough, understandable explanation of the treatment or therapy in question. The patient may also be unmotivated or uncooperative if he or she has not been shown the respect of participation in establishing personally meaningful goals. After these more obvious problem areas are explored and resolved and problems still persist, you can turn to the following types of behavior that have been found to be effective in working with difficult patients.

As a general rule for all types of difficult situations, a deliberate, consistent approach is often helpful. Sometimes this is referred to as "setting limits." Setting firm limits is a part of setting boundaries with all patients but with additional safeguards given the extremity of the situation. By setting forth clear, consistent expectations in a nondefensive manner, you can help strengthen the patient's inner control. However, when you are involved in setting limits, respect for the patient must govern. You should ask yourself whether the limits you are setting are arbitrary—that is, do they stem from your need to be in control or to punish the patient—or whether the patient's welfare would indeed be best served by establishing external limits. Any plan to set limits should be agreed upon by all members of the health care team to avoid the potential for a patient to "split" the staff, i.e., divide staff into all good or all bad. To avoid division of the staff, good communication lines between all members of the team is essential. For example, the patient may use charm and flattery to manipulate some staff members but make disparaging and critical comments about their co-workers.[22] Refer to the scenario that opened this chapter. How would you react to this patient's comments? What if you thought that your colleague Hal was incompetent? How would this affect your response to the patient?

It is also helpful to focus on a patient's unacceptable behaviors rather than on the patient himself or herself. This allows for open communication and avoids negative labeling that tends to stick to patients and obscure the real problem. One way to avoid negative labeling of patients is to be honest with them and tell them exactly how you feel. Again, your honest comments should be directed at the patient's behavior and not at the patient. This way you can share your reactions and still not humiliate the patient.

On a broader basis, you can encourage the development of an environment that is respectful of everyone. Such a setting encourages patients' rights to ask questions and challenge the system's rules and practices. If just a single member of the health care team prompts the patient legitimately to question his or her care, the rest of the team could come to see the patient as "difficult." Having patients ask about the care they receive and make decisions about their care must be considered the normal, desired state.[23] The safety of health professionals should also be encouraged in a respectful environment. There must be practices and policies in place to give people like Claire Chui some protection from harassment, abuse, and so forth. You may find yourself in an environment that is amenable to change through education and support for staff. In fact, the support of supervisory staff in the form of validation and insight is an essential component of an environment that fosters positive health professional and patient interactions.

As you gain experience working with difficult patients in challenging settings, you can use this experience to effect change. However, if you find yourself in a work environment that routinely fosters negative stereotypes, lack of respect for workers and patients alike, and there is little hope for improvement, the only resolution might be to seek another position rather than endure the stress that is inherent in that type of situation.

In summary, here are general guidelines for showing respect toward difficult patients, keeping in touch with your own values, and making the system more responsive to both:

1. Avoid the use of derogatory labels as a means of reducing your frustration or anger.

2. Remember that the caring function is as important as other interventions.

3. Do not have unrealistic expectations of your own power as a health professional to force compliance.

4. Do not expect to change aspects of the patient's situation beyond your control.

5. Take care of your emotional well-being.

6. Try to help change the underlying social and institutional conditions or attitudes that lead to devaluing behavior by health professionals.[24]

7. When interacting with an aggressive patient, "Assure that exit is possible for both you and the patient; Monitor your body language and tone of voice;

Avoid pointing your index finger or putting your hands on your hips in a threatening stance; Avoid sarcasm or loudness."[25]

8. Work to affirm policies and practices that encourage respect of everyone while assuring their physical and emotional safety.

9. Recognize your limitations.

Although all of your efforts as a health professional should be directed to acknowledging negative biases and keeping them in check, you may find that you cannot operate in the best interest of a given patient, no matter how much you try. If it comes to letting a patient go, be certain that you are referring him or her to a capable professional and not abandoning the person. Respect includes everybody, but as humans we come in all shapes and forms, so the wise health professional recognizes that difficult patients and situations will arise.

SUMMARY

This final chapter makes suggestions about respectful interaction with types of patients whom many health professionals find difficult to treat without negative feelings or behaviors intruding on the relationship. Sources may be the patient's personality and behavior, societal stereotypes, your own countertransference and learned behaviors or the opinions of your peers. The environment in which the relationship takes place can also add to frustration, anger, and other negative responses by both parties. Despite such challenges, your responsibility to show respect for the patient as a person remains and can be expressed through attempts to use behaviors that provide an opportunity to minimize the negative aspects of the relationship.

REFERENCES

1. Nield-Anderson, L., et al.: Responding to the 'difficult' patient: manipulation, sexual provocation, aggression—how can you manage such behaviors? *Am. J. Nurs.* 99(12):26–34, 1999. quote p. 28.
2. Santamaria, N.: The relationship between nurses' personality and stress levels reported when caring for interpersonally difficult patients. *Aust. J. Adv. Nurs.* 18(2):20–26, 2000.
3. Herbert, C.P. and Seifert, M.H.: When the patient is the problem. *Patient Care* 24(1):59, 1990.
4. Highley, B.L., and Norris, C.M.: When a student dislikes a patient. *Am. J. Nurs.* 57(9):1163, 1957.
5. Papper, S.: The undesirable patient. *J. Chron. Dis.* 22:777, 1970.
6. Larson, P.A.: Nurse perceptions of patient characteristics. *Nurs. Res.* 26(6):416–420, 1977.
7. Harlow, P.E., and Goby, M.J.: Changing nursing students' attitudes toward alcoholic patients: examining effects of a clinical practicum. *Nurs. Res.* 29(1):59–60, 1980.
8. Podrasky, D.L., and Sexton, D.L.: Nurses' reactions to difficult patients. *Image* 20(1):16–21, 1988.

9. Rader, J.: To bathe or not to bathe: that is the question. *J. Gerontol. Nurs.* 20(9):53, 1994.
10. Leon, A.M., Altholz, J.A.S., and Dziegielewski, S.F.: Compassion fatigue: considerations for working with the elderly. *J. Gerontol. Soc. Work* 32(1):43–62, 1999.
11. Staples, P., Baruth, P., Jeffries, M., and Warder, L.: Empowering the angry patient. *Can. Nurse* 90(4):28–30, 1994.
12. Breeze, J.A. and Repper, J.: Struggling for control: the care experiences of "difficult" patients in mental health services. *J. Adv. Nurs.* 28(6):1301–1311, 1998.
13. Sarosi, G.M.: A critical theory: the nurse as a fully human person. *Nurs. Forum* 7(4):352, 1968.
14. Gallop, R., Lancee, W., and Shugar, G.: Residents' and nurses' perceptions of difficult-to-treat short-stay patients. *Hosp. Comm. Psychiatry* 44(4):352, 1993.
15. Caplan, B. and Shechter, J.: Reflections on the "depressed," "unrealistic," "inappropriate," "manipulative," "unmotivated," "noncompliant," "denying," "maladjusted," "regressed," etc. patient. *Arch. Phys. Med. Rehabil.* 74(October):1123, 1993.
16. Podrasky, D.L. and Sexton, D.L.: Nurses' reactions to difficult patients. *Image* 20(1):19, 1988.
17. Neil, J.A. and Corley, M.C.: Hostility toward caregivers as a selection criterion for transplantation. *Prog. Transplant.* 10(3):177–181, 2000.
18. Juliana, C.A., et al.: Interventions by staff nurses to manage "difficult" patients. *Holistic Nurs. Pract.* 11(4):1–26, 1997.
19. Stockard, S.: Caring for the sexually aggressive patient: you don't have to blush and bear it. *Nursing* 21(11):72, 1991.
20. Nield-Anderson, L., et al.: Responding to the 'difficult' patient: manipulation, sexual provocation, aggression—how can you manage such behaviors? *Am. J. Nurs.* 99(12):26–34, 1999, quote p. 31.
21. Daum, A.L.: The disruptive antisocial patient: management strategies. *Nurs. Manage.* 25(8):49, 1994.
22. Ibid.
23. Staples, P., Baruth, P., Jeffries, M., and Warder, L.: Empowering the angry patient. *Can. Nurse* 90(4):28–30, 1994, quote p. 30.
24. Purtilo, R.: *Ethical Dimensions of the Health Professions.* 3rd ed. Philadelphia, W.B. Saunders, 1999, p. 240.
25. Nield-Anderson, L., et al.: Responding to the 'difficult' patient: manipulation, sexual provocation, aggression—how can you manage such behaviors? *Am. J. Nurs.* 99(12):26–34, 1999, quote p. 30.

PART SEVEN

Questions for Thought and Discussion

1. You are in a patient's room performing a procedure. The patient, who has a type of cancer that is always fatal, has been told of his condition. While you are there, a man visiting a patient in the next bed begins to

describe the horror of his wife's last days before she died of cancer. The patient becomes increasingly tense and finally begins to sob.

   a. What can you do to console or reassure this patient?

   b. How could you have helped to prevent this situation?

   c. Should you report this incident? To whom and why?

2. Under what conditions would your life seem no longer worth living? What course would you take to show respect for a patient whose life is very similar to these conditions?

3. If you were truly able to plan your own death (age, setting, cause, persons present, etc.), what would be your most preferable way to meet your death? Least preferable?

4. You are working in an outpatient clinic in an economically depressed area of the city. A disheveled woman comes in dragging three young children behind her. One of the children begins to whine that she is hot. You are in the receiving area and see the woman hit the child so hard the child falls to the floor and begins to scream. The woman looks at you in panic. You are already late for your next appointment. Your next patient is anxiously waiting to be seen and looks with scorn at the woman and you.

   a. What feelings does this scene trigger?

   b. You probably think there are some things you should do in this situation, but what would you really like to do?

   c. What does this teach you about the possible difference between your emotional and "professional" reaction to this extreme situation?

5. In a small group, brainstorm major "likes" related to working with patients. After compiling the list, look for the common denominator or theme. What does this tell you about your expectations of patients?

6. What types of difficult patient care situations make you (or, if you are still a student, do you *think* will make you) the most uncomfortable? Identify two or three concrete interventions you would take to effectively deal with the situations you identified.

7. What type of policies or guidelines can be developed to foster better relationships with difficult patients? How would they help? What sort of supervisory support would you find most helpful?

Index

Note: Page numbers in italics indicate figures; those followed by t indicate tables.

Physical comfort. *See* Comfort
Physical space, 175–177, 210
Physician competencies, 223
Piaget, Jean, 247, 248
Pinch, W. J. E., 250
Pity, 214–216
Play
    in children, 259
    need for, 101–102
    in toddlers, 253
Plot, 150
Poetry, 150–151
Point of view, 150
Policies. *See* Laws/policies
Political activities, 276
Power disparities, 343–344
Prejudice
    origins of, 37
    toward elderly individuals, 43
    toward gays and lesbians, 50
Primary goods, 12
Primary relationships, 274–275, 281
Privacy, 117
Private-sector relationships, 23
Procrustes, 115
Professional boundaries
    explanation of, 208–210
    illustration of, 207–208
    keys to maintaining, 219–220
    making determination of, 210
    physical boundaries and, 211–214
    psychological-emotional boundaries and,
        214–219
Professional closeness
    attention to details to establish,
        225–229
    finding comfortable intimacy level for,
        231–233
    illustration of, 223, 224
    integrity and, 224–225
    paying attention to establish,
        225–227
    reality testing and, 229–230
Professional values. *See also* Values
    examples of, 10
    explanation of, 6, 9
    health care professionals and, 9–11
Professionalism
    conceptions of, 209, 210
    explanation of, 9
Professions
    explanation of, 9
    values held by, 9–11
Proxemics, 175–177
Proximodistal, 247
Psychological comforts, 115

Psychological-emotional boundaries
    caring too much and, 217–219
    overidentification and, 216–217, 220
    pity and, 214–216
Psychosocial development
    in adults, 272–274
    in elderly individuals, 292–293
    in toddlers, 248–249, 252, 258
Public-sector relationships, 23

Q
Qualitative research, 67
Quantitative research, 67

R
Race, 40, 41. *See also* Diversity
Rader, J., 342
"A Rare and Still Scandalous Subject"
    (Solly), 151
Rawls, J., 12
Reality, 148–149
Reality testing, 229–230
Reassurance, 192, 194–195
Recreational activities, 300–301
Referrals, 85–86
Rehabilitation Act of 1973, 27
Reich, W., 198
Reincarnation, 320
Rejection, 334
Relationships
    building trust in, 190–195
    communicating to forge, 66–67
    dual, 213–214
    fragility of, 127–131
    frameworks of interaction in helping, 193
    primary, 274–275
    stigma and, 133–135
    uncertainty and, 132–133
Religious beliefs
    about death and dying, 319, 320
    patient-provider interaction and, 49
    respect for, 135–137
Research skills, 67–68
Residence, impact of place of, 47–48
Respect. *See also* Values
    for children, 260–262
    for difficult patients, 349–351
    in difficult situations, 349–351
    as empowerment, 203–204
    explanation of, 4–5
    for infants, 250–251
    for malingering patients, 124–125
    for need for solitude, 96–98
    for others, 98–99
    in patient-provider communication,
        158–159 (*See also* Communication)